Case Studies in Neuropsychological Rehabilitation

Case Studies in Neuropsychological Rehabilitation

BARBARA A. WILSON

MRC Applied Psychology Unit, Cambridge, and
Oliver Zangwill Centre for Neuropsychological Rehabilitation, Ely

New York   Oxford
OXFORD UNIVERSITY PRESS
1999

Oxford University Press

Oxford   New York
Athens   Auckland   Bangkok   Bogotá   Buenos Aires   Calcutta
Cape Town   Chennai   Dar es Salaam   Delhi   Florence   Hong Kong   Istanbul
Karachi   Kuala Lumpur   Madrid   Melbourne   Mexico City   Mumbai
Nairobi   Paris   São Paulo   Singapore   Taipei   Tokyo   Toronto   Warsaw

and associated companies in
Berlin   Ibadan

Published by Oxford University Press, Inc.,
198 Madison Avenue, New York, New York, 10016
http://www.oup-usa.org

Library of Congress Cataloging-in-Publication Data
Wilson, Barbara A.
Case studies in neuropsychological rehabilitation / by Barbara A. Wilson.
p.   cm.   Includes bibliographical references and index.
ISBN 0-19-506598-0
1. Brain damage—Patients—Rehabilitation—Case studies.
2. Clinical neuropsychology—Case studies.   1. Title.
[DNLM: 1. Brain Injuries—rehabilitation case studies.
2. Brain Injuries—psychology case studies.   WL 354 W746c   1999]
RC387.5.W545   1999   616.8′043—dc21   DNLM/DLC   for Library of Congress   98-23697

1005204175

9 8 7 6 5 4 3 2 1

Printed in the United States of America
on acid-free paper

*This book is dedicated to
my granddaughters
Rosie and Francesca.*

Preface

Since 1979 I have assessed over 600 people with acquired, nonprogressive brain injury. The largest subgroup consisted of people with traumatic head injury, followed by those with stroke, encephalitis, hypoxic brain damage, and cerebral tumor. Many of these patients were also seen for rehabilitation of their problems. This book describes the progress of 20 of these patients in some detail. I have selected for inclusion those who taught me most. Some had particularly severe cognitive problems, some showed ingenuity in overcoming their problems, some helped me to see neuropsychological problems in a different way, and all reinforced the view that people with brain damage are first and foremost people rather than amnesics, aphasics, agnosics, or whatever.

I hope this book will persuade psychologists, neuropsychologists, neurosurgeons, and therapists that rehabilitation for brain injured people is not only worthwhile but also essential. For each of the 20 cases I shall try to present a clear clinical description, which will not simply be a neuropsychological report but an account of what their problems mean to the patients and their families. I shall provide details about assessment, treatment, and long-term outcome. Where possible I will note how I would do things differently if I were to begin again. Although theoretical models from cognitive and behavioral psychology have influenced both the assessment and treatment of these people, theoretical model building is not the main purpose of my work. Rather, I have been motivated by the desire to improve the quality of life of those referred to me by enabling them to reach greater levels of independence, to return to work, to reduce stress on their families and carers, and to solve their particular neuropsychological problems resulting from brain injury.

Cambridge, England   B. A. W.
January 1998

Acknowledgments

My greatest debt is to the 20 brain injured people and their families described in this book. I have learned a great deal from all of them and hope this book will go some way to improving the chances of rehabilitation for others with acquired brain injury.

Some of the work presented here has been referred to in other publications: Jay (Ch. 4) was described in Wilson, J. C. and Hughes (1997a), also in Wilson, J. C. and Hughes (1997b); Clive (Ch. 6) has been reported in Wilson and Wearing (1995) and in Wilson, Baddeley, and Kapur (1995); a paper on Lorna (Ch. 8) has been submitted to Cortex (Wilson, Balleny, Patterson, & Hodges, submitted); Jason (Ch. 9) was one of the people described in Wilson (1994); Ted (Ch. 13) was the patient reported in Patterson and Wilson (1990); Derek (Ch. 14) was referred to in Wilson (1987), Wilson (1994) and in Wilson and Patterson (1990); Jenny (Ch. 15) was also described in Wilson (1994) and was also the subject of two papers (Davidoff & Wilson, 1985; Wilson & Davidoff, 1993); Kirsty (Ch. 17) was one of the four patients reported in Wilson (1997) and Sarah (Ch. 20) was briefly described by Wilson (1988). I am grateful to Psychology Press for permission to reproduce (in part) the papers on JC (Ch. 4) and Ted (Ch. 13); to Blackwells for permission to reproduce (in part) the chapter on Clive (Ch. 5); and to Cortex for permission to reproduce Jenny's illustrations (Ch. 15).

I also thank the following colleagues for help with the assessment, investigations, and rehabilitation of the people described here: Alan Baddeley, Heather Balleny, Sally Carr, Linda Clare, Janet Cockburn, Jules Davidoff, Hazel Emslie, Jonathan Evans, Caroline Ferber, Philippa Garety, Anne Hankey, Jill Hazan, Dot Henry, John Hodges, Sandra Horn, Malar Hunt, Narinder Kapur, Jackie Knibbs, Anne Lodge, Peter McGill, Lindsay McLellan, Sue Maynard, Nicky Moss, Karalyn Patterson, Gary Patton, Graham Ratcliff, Louise Russell, Agnes Shiel, Caroline Trimnell, Anne Watson, Deborah Wearing, Klaus Willmes, and Andy Young.

Thanks are also due to Psychological Corporation for permission to reproduce the "American Liner" story in the chapter about Clive; Michael Oddy and the staff at Clive's home for permission to visit; to all the staff at Rivermead Rehabilitation Centre, Oxford during the period 1979–1985 when and where many of the brain injured people were first seen, and to the staff at Angela's day center for permission to visit. Finally I thank the three people who enabled this book to come to fruition: Jeffrey House for persuading me to embark on the book, Julia Darling for her patience, hard work, support, and help with the typing and references, and to my husband Mick for help with the redrafting. If I have left anyone out, please forgive me. My memory is not what it was a few years ago.

References

Davidoff, J. & Wilson, B. A. (1985). A case of associative visual agnosia showing a disorder of pre-semantic visual classification. *Cortex, 21,* 121–134.

Patterson, K. E., & Wilson, B. A. (1990). A ROSE is a ROSE or a NOSE: A deficit in initial letter identification. *Cognitive Neuropsychology, 7,* 447–477.

Wilson, B. A. (1987c). Single case experimental designs in neuropsychological rehabilitation. *Journal of Clinical and Experimental Neuropsychology, 9,* 527–544.

Wilson, B. A. (1988). Remediation of apraxia following an anaesthetic accident. In J. West & P. Spinks (Eds.), *Clinical psychology in action* (pp. 178–183). John Wright & Sons.

Wilson, B. A. (1994). Remediation of acquired dyslexia: A 6–10 year follow-up study of seven brain injured people. *Journal of Clinical and Experimental Neuropsychology, 16,* 354–371.

Wilson, B. A. (1977d). Semantic memory impairments following non-progressive brain damage: A study of four cases. *Brain Injury, 11,* 259–269.

Wilson, B. A., Baddeley, A. D. & Kapur, N. (1995). Dense amnesia in a professional musician following herpes simplex virus encephalitis. *Journal of Clinical and Experimental Psychology, 17,* 668–681.

Wilson, B. A., Balleny H., Patterson, K., & Hodges, J. (1998). Myotonic dystrophy and progressive cognitive decline: A common condition or two separate problems? (Manuscript submitted).

Wilson, B. A., J. C., & Hughes, E. (1997a). Coping with amnesia: The natural history of a compensatory memory system. *Neuropsychological Rehabilitation, 7,* 43–56.

Wilson, B. A., J. C., & Hughes, E. (1997b). Coping with amnesia: The natural history of a compensatory memory system. In A. J. Parkin (Ed.), *Case studies in the neuropsychology of memory* (pp. 179–190). Hove: Psychology Press.

Wilson, B. A., & Davidoff, J. (1993). Partial recovery from visual object agnosia: A 10 year follow-up study. *Cortex, 29,* 529–542.

Wilson, B. A., & Patterson, K. E. (1990). Rehabilitation and cognitive neuropsychology: Does cognitive psychology apply? *Journal of Applied Cognitive Psychology, 4,* 247–260.

Wilson, B. A., & Wearing, D. (1995). Prisoner of consciousness: A state of just awakening following Herpes Simplex Encephalitis. In R. Campbell & M. Conway (Eds)., *Broken Memories* (pp. 14–30). Oxford: Blackwell.

Contents

IV LANGUAGE IMPAIRMENT

V REMEDIATION OF ACQUIRED DISORDERS OF READING

VI PERCEPTUAL AND VISUOSPATIAL PROBLEMS

VII BEHAVIOR AND SELF-CARE SKILLS

Some of the people described in this book were happy for me to use their real names and true autobiographical details. Others wanted their names changed and agreed to the names selected. Some wanted both the name and identifying details changed. I was unable to contact a few patients and in these cases I have changed their names and certain details to avoid identification.

SETTING THE SCENE

1

PATIENTS AND THEIR PROBLEMS

Many neurological conditions give rise to brain damage. Most patients referred to neuropsychologists are likely to have experienced one of the following:

1. Traumatic head injury following a road traffic accident, fall, industrial or sporting accident, or assault.
2. Cerebral vascular accident (stroke).
3. Viral infection of the brain, particularly encephalitis.
4. Hypoxic brain damage following, for example, such insults as myocardial infarction, respiratory arrest, carbon monoxide poisoning, or anesthetic accident.
5. Wernicke-Korsakoff syndrome following chronic alcohol abuse and poor nutrition.
6. Brain tumor.
7. A degenerative disease such as Alzheimer's disease, Huntington's disease, Parkinson's disease, multiple sclerosis, or dementia associated with acquired immunodeficiency syndrome (AIDS).

Although common as causes of neuropsychological deficit, degenerative disorders are not a common reason for admission to a rehabilitation unit and will not be discussed further here. For an up-to-date account of dementia, the most frequently encountered degenerative disorder, the reader is referred to Cummings and Benson (1992); and Huppert et al. (1994). Because they are most likely to be seen in rehabilitation centers, the remaining diagnostic groups are described briefly later.

TRAUMATIC HEAD INJURY

The sequelae of head injury may result from both direct physical damage to the brain, and from secondary factors, such as vascular disturbance, anoxia, and cerebral edema. Teasdale (1991) and Mendelow (1991) provide detail on etiology.

Severity of head injury is usually judged by the depth and duration of coma, and post-traumatic amnesia (PTA). *Coma* has been characterized as ". . . not obeying commands, not uttering words, and not opening the eyes" (Jennett and Teasdale, 1981). *Post-traumatic amnesia* (PTA) has been defined as ". . . a period of variable length following closed head trauma during which the patient is confused, disoriented, suffers from retrograde amnesia, and seems to lack the capacity to store and retrieve new information" (Schacter and Crovitz, 1977).

The Glasgow Coma Score (GCS) (Teasdale and Jennett, 1974) is used frequently to measure the depth and duration of coma. The GCS is composed of three sections involving eye opening, verbal responses, and motor responses. The original 14-point scale of the GCS, later extended to 15 points, provides an uncomplicated, easily scorable, objective measure of coma. Within each section, the worst possible response is scored 1 and the best possible response is scored 4, 5, or 6, depending on which component is being measured and which version of the test is being employed. The operational definition most often used is that a combined score of 8 or less means the patient is in coma and 9 or more means the patient is out of coma. Wilson et al. (1994) discuss some of the difficulties that may occur with the GCS.

Turning to PTA, one of the main problems is the lack of agreed upon criteria for assessing its presence or absence. Russell (1932), for instance, asked the patient, "When did you wake up?" That is, "When did you stop being confused and start to remember coherently?" In 1946, Russell and Nathan were of the opinion that the patient is usually able to date the time from which continuous memory is present. Schacter and Crovitz (1977) believe the idea of continuous memory to be important because recovery from PTA may be sporadic, with "islands" of normal memory functioning interspersed with confusion. Other authors have used "PTA" synonymously with "coma" (e.g., Kløve and Cleeland, 1972). Still others have differentiated between disorientation and amnesia in the posttraumatic period (Moore and Ruesch, 1944). Sisler and Penner (1975) have argued that there are three distinct components of PTA: namely, disorientation, anterograde amnesia (AA), and retrograde amnesia (RA). It would appear that PTA does not necessarily begin at the moment of injury. In a study of American footballers, Lynch and Yarnell (1973) questioned four players who were concussed during play. When questioned immediately following the blow, all realized what had happened to them, and three of them could describe the situation of the game immediately preceding the blow. When questioned again between 3 and 20 min later, all had forgotten this information. This suggests that information was registered but was not consolidated or retrieved appropriately.

As recovery from PTA includes the ability to restore and retrieve information, what are we to make of those patients whose memory problems do not resolve? Are we to regard amnesic patients as still in PTA? Wilson et al. (1992) compared memory and attention functioning in three groups of patients: (1) those in PTA, (2) those with the amnesic syndrome, and (3) those with chronic memory impairment following severe head injury, but who were no longer in PTA. A control group of people with orthopedic injuries was also tested. Patients in PTA differed from all other groups on semantic processing, verbal fluency, and simple reaction time. The results suggested that PTA is not solely a disorder of memory and orientation as indicated by tests of PTA, but includes slowness and impaired retrieval from semantic memory. For a further discussion of PTA see Snow and Ponsford (1995).

Survivors of traumatic head injury (THI) usually but not always show reasonable recovery of motor functioning, may have behavior problems, and almost always have cognitive problems, particularly with attention, speed of information processing, memory and executive functioning (Wilson, 1987b). These will be addressed later. Ponsford et al. (1995) provide a comprehensive account of THI and rehabilitation strategies for these patients.

CEREBRAL VASCULAR DISORDERS

There are two main kinds of cerebral vascular disorder: those resulting from hemorrhage and those resulting from infarction or blocking of the blood vessels in the brain. The term "stroke" is used to describe both of these processes and is "the outward manifestation of a localized sudden interruption of the blood supply to some part of the brain" (Wade et al., 1985, p. 6). Hemorrhages may be intracerebral or may occur in the subarachnoid space following a ruptured aneurysm. Infarction may be due to thrombosis of the cerebral blood vessels or to an embolus which lodges in these vessels.

About 10% of cerebral vascular disorders are due to subarachnoid hemorrhage (Teddy, 1991). Despite their small numbers, they are important because they tend to affect a younger age group who are less likely to suffer from more widespread cerebral vascular disease. The usual cause is rupture of an intracranial aneurysm that bleeds into the subarachnoid space surrounding the brain. Sometimes a sub-arachnoid hemorrhage results from a ruptured angioma, but in some 20% of cases no structural cause can be found (Teddy, 1991). Aneurysms are usually found at the forks of cerebral arteries, and certain sites are more commonly in-volved than others. The anterior communicating artery is one site frequently as-sociated with ruptured aneurysm. This lies between the frontal lobes and is close to the anterior hypothalamus. Other commonly involved sites are the middle cerebral artery and the posterior communicating artery. in addition to the hemor-rrhage, ischemia (restricted blood flow) may result from spasm or occlusion of as-sociated vessels (Lishman, 1987).

Memory problems and executive deficits are not uncommon following anterior communicating artery aneurysms. Intracerebral infarction or hemorrhage may give rise to language deficits if the lesions are in the left hemisphere. Visuospatial deficits are common following right hemisphere strokes and bilateral infarction of the posterior cerebral arteries may result in a classic amnesic syndrome. (For a more detailed description of the neuropsychological sequelae of stroke see Bogousslavsky and Caplan, 1995).

ENCEPHALITIS

Encephalitis is an inflammation of the brain caused by a virus. If meningeal irri-tation is also present, then the disease is sometimes called meningoencephalitis. Oxbury and Swash (1991) say that viruses can affect the brain in at least two major ways. They may invade the brain and destroy the host cells or they may lead to an allergic reaction within the brain and/or the spinal cord. Herpes simplex virus encephalitis (HSVE) is probably the most common form of en-cephalitis seen in patients referred to British rehabilitation centers. Several are described later in this book. Herpes zoster, related to the chicken pox virus, is sometimes seen and occasionally brain stem encephalitis, as described by Bicker-staff (1957). Angela discussed in Chapter 21 suffered from this form of en-cephalitis. Postinfection encephalitis, for example, following influenza or vacci-nation may also give rise to cognitive deficits. In some cases the etiology remains unknown.

The typical picture of most forms of encephalitis is of a rapidly developing ill-ness, with headache, prostration, vomiting, and irritability. Impaired conscious-ness is usually encountered, although this may range from mild sleepiness to deep coma. Delirium and epilepsy are common in some varieties. Focal neuro-logical signs vary greatly, depending on the major site of inflammation. For ex-ample, if the brain stem is the most affected area, then quadriplegia and dysarthria may result; however, when the main site of infection is the temporal lobes, then a classic amnesic syndrome may be observed. In some cases, no residual effects may be seen. In others, permanent sequelae range from mild neurological signs to severe global intellectual impairment.

HYPOXIC BRAIN DAMAGE

Disruption or cessation of the brain's supply of oxygen can have disastrous results on cognitive functioning. Common causes of cerebral hypoxia include cardiac failure, respiratory arrest, and carbon monoxide poisoning. Less frequently cerebral hypoxia may occur following anesthetic accident, attempted hanging, or near drowning.

Neuropsychological deficits in patients with hypoxic brain damage include memory deficits (Kapur, 1988, Hopkins et al., 1995), executive problems (Lezak, 1995), apperceptive agnosia (Farah, 1990), and severe widespread cognitive deficits (Parkin et al., 1987). Some patients remain in a persistent vegetative state with no observable cognitive functioning at all. For a review of neuropsychological deficits in 18 patients with hypoxic brain damage, see Wilson (1996).

ALCOHOLIC WERNICKE-KORSAKOFF SYNDROME

Chronic alcohol abuse may give rise to the Wernicke-Korsakoff syndrome. Wernicke encephalopathy is an acute reaction to severe thiamine deficiency. The symptoms include ocular–motor abnormalities, ataxic gait, confusion, and disorientation. Although commonly associated with alcohol abuse, it can also result from severe malnutrition or carcinoma of the stomach. It was Malamud and Skillicorn (1956) who first demonstrated the connection between Wernicke encephalopathy and Korsakoff syndrome. The two groups of patients differ only in the acuteness or chronicity of the disorder with Korsakoff syndrome being the residual and often permanent effect. Victor et al. (1971) say 54% of Wernicke encephalopathy patients show little or no improvement in memory functions. Wernicke encephalopathy is therefore now seen as a precursor of the Korsakoff syndrome.

Korsakoff first described the syndrome in 1887, with severe amnesia as the central feature. The disorder is one of the most frequent causes of amnesia and one of the most widely studied. It differs from confusional states in that there is clarity of consciousness and intact perception (Hecaen and Albert, 1978). Many patients show lack of insight into their memory difficulties (Zangwill, 1977). Kapur (1988) suggests this is due partly to the forgetting of instances of memory loss and partly to apathy secondary to frontal lobe disorder. Unlike demented patients, Korsakoff patients show relatively intact intellectual functioning although, as Kapur (1988) points out, those with a pure amnesic syndrome represent only a subset of Korsakoff's patients as a whole, with others showing additional cognitive deficits. The severity of impairment also differs considerably among patients (Wilson, 1987a).

BRAIN TUMOR

Tumor is a general term referring to any abnormal swelling, but *brain tumor* usually refers to a neoplasm (new growth). Intellectual deficits are common and may be progressive or fluctuate from one occasion to another (Lishman, 1987). In addition to the destructive effects of the tumor itself, there may be displacement of neighboring structures, generalized swelling, disturbance of cerebral blood flow, and disturbance in the flow of cerebrospinal fluid (Kapur, 1988). The three main types of brain tumor are *gliomas* (arising from glial cells in the brain), *metastases* (which are secondary to a primary tumor elsewhere in the body), and *meningiomas* which arise in the meninges, i.e., the linings of the brain.

The type of deficit shown by tumor patients depends on (1) the intracranial pressure, (2) the nature of the tumor, (3) the location of the tumor, and (4) the individual's response to the tumor. Raised intracranial pressure is responsible for many of the symptoms and for fluctuating levels of consciousness. Malignant tumors such as gliomas typically lead to greater cognitive impairment than benign tumors such as meningiomas. Tumors in the third ventricle are particularly likely to result in an amnesic syndrome (Thomas et al., 1991). Frontal lobe tumors are likely to be mistaken for dementia particularly when both lobes are affected and the tumor develops in the midline (ibid.). Lack of insight is typical (Lishman, 1987) and thus there are similarities with Korsakoff patients. Patients with corpus callosum deficits may show severe memory impairments and other cognitive difficulties. General impairment may be seen after temporal lobe tumors although Wilson (1987d) describes a temporal lobe tumor patient with a severe but specific verbal memory deficit. Parietal tumors may result in unilateral neglect if in the right hemisphere and dysphasia if in the left. Occipital tumors can lead to visual recognition difficulties.

Tumors of the posterior fossa (e.g., the cerebellum, cerebellopontine angle, and brain stem) are less likely to result in cognitive deficits than those tumors described above unless the raised intracranial pressure is such that hydrocephalus occurs (Lishman, 1987).

Although the seven diagnostic groups reported here encompass most of the patients referred for rehabilitation, this list is not exhaustive. We have not discussed, for example, those with epilepsy. Rather than a specific cerebral pathology, epilepsy refers to clinical phenomena. Nevertheless, many brain injured people will have epilepsy. It is common for example, after penetrating brain injury, and is also commonly associated with tumor. Thus most patients with epilepsy seen in neurological rehabilitation centers will typically have one of the conditions described above. Occasionally I have been asked to see people with idiopathic epilepsy (Wilson, 1991b), that is where the epilepsy is not associated with another condition. In these cases the cognitive deficits appear to be secondary to hypoxia sustained during the seizures. Kapur (1988) gives a good account of memory impairment and epilepsy.

Other patients not included are those whose problems result from electroconvulsive therapy (ECT), psychiatric disorders such as schizophrenia (Frith, 1992), or functional amnesia where there may be some organic damage as well (Kopelman, 1995). Nevertheless the main groups have been described and all but one of the patients reported in this book fall into one of these categories. The one exception, Lorna (Chapter 8), has an autosomal dominant disorder, myotonic dystrophy, together with a slowly progressive cognitive deterioration.

The Nature of Problems Seen After Brain Injury

Brain injured people present with a variety of problems, the nature of which depends in part on the site, extent and severity of the damage, and the age at which it occurred. Inappropriate early treatment, particularly for those with traumatic head injury (THI), may also add to resulting problems (Wilson et al., 1994). Motor, sensory, emotional, social, behavioral, and cognitive problems are common after many kinds of brain injury. A few people may face all these problems while others may experience just one or two. Neuropsychologists may be involved in the treatment of any and all of these problems.

Although motor problems are most likely to be treated by physiotherapists who are trained to prevent deformities and contractures and to understand how to reteach motor skills, neuropsychologists can assist physiotherapists in enhancing the likelihood of rehabilitation success. They can do this in several ways. For example, knowledge of learning theory can be harnessed to improve motor learning. Robertson and Cashman (1991) improved the walking ability of a stroke patient through providing auditory feedback which increased the number of times the patient placed her heel properly. Behavioral assessment and task analysis can be used to measure and understand motor disorders. Wilson and Powell (1994), for example, describe behavioral assessment leading to a young head injured woman tolerating physiotherapy exercises. In addition Carr and Wilson (1983) describe cooperation with a skin-care regime in a man with spinal cord injury and pressure sores.

Many head injured people show good motor recovery if this is measured by functional mobility (McKinlay et al., 1981) although they may have more subtle motor deficits. Brain stem damage, for example, can lead to difficulty controlling fine movements. Damage to the cerebellum may lead to gross tremor and a staggering gait. Frontal lobe damage may cause difficulty in initiating movements or may result in the poor sequencing of motor movements involved in such tasks as making a cup of coffee or changing bed linen. Focal lesions following, for example, stroke or tumor can lead to permanent and intractable motor impairments.

Sensory impairments are also common after central nervous system damage. Hemiplegic stroke patients frequently lose sensation in their paralyzed limbs and may, as a consequence, damage themselves by trapping a leg in the spokes of a wheelchair or by burning an arm as a result of leaving it too close to a radiator. Visual sensory deficits are common following stroke, head injury, tumor, and other kinds of brain damage. Some studies have suggested it is possible to reduce hemianopia in stroke patients (Zihl, 1995) although others have disputed this (Pommerenke and Markowitsch, 1989). Even if reduction of hemianopia is unachievable, hemianopic patients can be taught to compensate for their visual field loss through, for example, improved scanning (Kerkoff et al., 1992). It is even possible to reduce other visual deficits such as myopia through treatment procedures. Collins et al. (1981) improved the short-sightedness of nonbrain damaged people and Thomas (reported in Wilson, 1991a) achieved the same effect with a young head injured woman whose poor visual acuity resulted from a motor cycle accident.

Auditory sensory problems are less frequently encountered, although occasionally head injured people become deaf as a result of the accident. It is sometimes possible to teach these people sign language or another alternative communication system. Typically these programs are implemented by speech and language therapists but neuropsychologists may also take on such treatment either alone or working together with the speech and language therapists. Once again, principles from learning theory and other branches of psychology should enhance learning.

Emotional and social difficulties including fear, anxiety, depression, and social isolation, are faced by perhaps the majority of brain injured people. Prigatano (1995) believes that dealing with the emotional effects of brain injury is crucial to rehabilitation success. Depression and anxiety may be expected in about two-thirds of patients with THI (McKinlay et al., 1981). Traumatic head injury patients are also likely to face social isolation (Talbott, 1989; Wilson, 1991b). Emotional changes are also seen frequently in stroke patients. Those with right hemisphere lesions are likely to show denial or indifference to their problems (Weinstein, 1991) whereas those with left hemisphere lesions are more likely to show "a catastrophic reaction." Patients with brain stem strokes may show extreme emotional lability (Ross, 1983). Of course, emotional and social problems may also occur for nonorganic reasons such as problems with mobility, financial restrictions, or fear of what might happen in the future.

In an excellent review of emotional and psychosocial problems after brain injury, Gainotti (1993) distinguishes three main factors that cause these problems. First are neurological factors that provoke disturbances by the disruption of the specific neural mechanisms subserving the regulation and control of emotional and social behavior. Second are psychological or psychodynamic factors involving attitudes toward the disability arising from awareness of the disability and its implications for the patient's quality of life. Third are the consequences of the functional impairment on the patient's social network and social activities.

Most clinical psychologists and some neuropsychologists are well placed to deal with the emotional and social consequences of brain injury. Anxiety management procedures, cognitive therapy, and other methods for dealing with depression, family therapy, and social skills training can all be applied to brain injured people as well as to those whose mental health problems arise from psychiatric causes.

Behavior problems, frequently seen at some stage in people with severe head injury may worsen over time if not treated properly (BPS Report, 1989). They certainly cause great stress for families and caregivers (Brooks, 1984). Livingston et al. (1985) say that families of head injured people show twice the level of psychiatric dysfunction than can be expected in the general population.

The growing awareness of the importance of behavioral management programs is reflected in a number of publications in recent years (Wood, 1988; Alderman and Ward, 1991; Wilson, 1991a; Hanlon et al., 1993; Alderman and Burgess, 1994). Common problems associated with severe head injury include yelling and swearing. Less common but more difficult to manage are physical violence and sexually offensive behaviors. Such problems may result in patients being admitted to long-term psychiatric care. Even very severe behavioral disturbance, however, may respond to behavior modification regimes (Wood, 1984; Eames, 1989; Alderman and Ward, 1991; Alderman and Burgess, 1994). Shiel et al. (submitted) provide some tentative evidence that violent behavior is more likely to occur in THI patients who do not receive rehabilitation.

Finally, we address cognitive problems. These are probably of most interest to the majority of clinical neuropsychologists. Cognitive problems almost always occur after severe THI and frequently follow other causes of brain damage. Disorders of learning and memory, information processing, planning and organizational problems, slowness of intellectual activity, and communication are all common after THI (Ponsford et al., 1995). Less common are the agnosias, apraxias, and aphasias although these are often found after stroke, hypoxic brain damage, and some tumors.

The late 1970s to the early 1980s have seen an increasing interest in the management and remediation of cognitive deficits (Diller and Gordon, 1981; Trexler, 1982; Uzzell and Gross, 1986; Wilson, 1987d, 1997a, b; Seron and Deloche, 1989; Riddoch and Humphreys, 1994). Cognitive rehabilitation programes are now found in many rehabilitation centers. These may be part of the "holistic programs" of Ben-Yishay (New York) Prigatano (Phoenix), and Christensen (Copenhagen) (Wilson et al., in press) or specifically tailored to particular cognitive problems such as memory (Wilson, 1995a,c), attention (Sohlberg and Mateer, 1989), executive deficits (Alderman et al., 1995; von Cramon and Matthes von Cramon, 1992), and language (Byng and Coltheart, 1986). Whatever the approach, the aim of cognitive rehabilitation is to enable brain injured people and their families to live with, manage, by-pass, reduce, or come to terms with cognitive deficits resulting from an insult to the brain (Wilson, 1989f). This is achieved through a process whereby brain injured people work together with health service professionals to remediate or alleviate cognitive deficits. Cognitive, emotional, and behavior problems are far more likely to impede return to work or independent living than the more obvious physical problems. Although physical restrictions can indeed be traumatic for the individual concerned, physically handicapped people can and do achieve independence, hold down jobs, and make rational decisions about their lives. However, people with cognitive handicaps, may have impaired judgement and be slow to learn new things; they may be unable to remember what they were doing a few minutes ago, and be very slow to process information. As a consequence, they may remain permanently dependent on their families. Furthermore, many are unaware of the extent of their problems and may think they can do things just as well and just as quickly as they were able to do before the brain injury. Such lack of insight is likely to impede rehabilitation efforts. Behavior problems can exacerbate the situation. People with tantrums and poor self control are not readily tolerated in society. Apathy and indifference reduce the chances of obtaining and holding down a job. Personality changes, mood swings, inappropriate social behavior, concrete thinking, and loss of sense of humor all reduce the chances of successful reintegration into society. This book tells the story of 20 brain injured patients faced with one or more of the problems outlined above. None of these people were restored to their former levels of functioning and all had to contend with the permanent effects of brain injury. Nevertheless, all overcame their difficulties to some extent. They achieved this through a mixture of determination, help from their families, and the efforts of the rehabilitation staff with whom they came into contact.

Before considering the cases of these individuals, it is necessary to discuss more generally the principles and practices involved in rehabilitation so that the reader can more easily relate specific treatments, which are described later in this book to broader issues in rehabilitation as it is currently understood.

2

PRINCIPLES AND PRACTICES
OF REHABILITATION

Rehabilitation is a two way process. Unlike treatment, which is given *to* a patient, rehabilitation is a process in which the patient, client, or disabled person takes an active part. Professional staff work together with the disabled person to achieve the optimum level of physical, social, psychological, and vocational functioning. The ultimate goal of rehabilitation is to enable the person with a disability to function as adequately as possible in his or her most appropriate environment.

RESTORATION AND RECOVERY

In the early days and weeks following brain injury, attempts are usually made to restore lost functioning. Thus therapists working with stroke patients who have lost the ability to walk and talk will try to teach the patients to walk and talk again. After a while, however, if restoration of function has not occurred, therapists are likely to adjust their objectives and perhaps concentrate on the goal of wheelchair independence or teach an alternative communication system. Both of these are acceptable approaches to rehabilitation.

It is not always easy to decide when attempts toward restoration of function should be abandoned. In the early days, weeks, and even months after brain injury recovery or partial recovery may be rapid. Even though rate of recovery slows down, it may nevertheless continue for several years (Robertson and Wilson, in press). It is probable that natural recovery can be enhanced or facilitated through rehabilitation. For example, lesioned animals placed in stimulating, enriched environments show greater recovery than animals left in unstimulating, barren environments (Gentile et al., 1978; Kolb, 1992). Enriched environments also appear to lead to greater cortical recovery (Black et al., 1987; Mayer et al., 1992) Furthermore Mayer et al. (1992) showed that rats given striatal neural transplants benefited from transplants only when they were also given opportunities for learning. It is likely that enriched environments for humans also lead to greater recovery. Brain injured patients placed in unstimulating rooms are likely to do less well than those receiving rehabilitation.

Stimulation has been shown to change cortical activity in brain injured humans (Lindgren et al., 1997). In their study, 14 patients with organic solvent–induced toxic encephalopathy participated in a 10 week visual imagery training, following which a change in right hemisphere regional blood flow was observed during activation. Hemiplegic stroke patients also show greater recovery when forced to use their weak limb through immobilization of the nonaffected limb (Taub et al., 1993).

COMPENSATION

Attempts to restore lost functioning fall into one category of rehabilitation. There are several others including teaching or enabling people to compensate for their deficits, and psychotherapy to address emotional problems and enhance self-esteem. Counselling, education, and support are other methods that are frequently tried. Prigatano (1995), Jackson and Gouvier (1992), and Wilson (1995c) address some of these issues. Our concern in this section is compensation. This widely used strategy in rehabilitation is particularly likely to be employed when the rate of natural recovery has slowed down or stopped altogether. Compensation can be achieved in several ways. For example, one can avoid or by-pass certain problems through restructuring the environment. Compensation is thus achieved by removing the patient's need to function in a particular way. The function is provided in or by the environment. As an example, consider people who are totally paralyzed from the neck down. With appropriate equipment they can control their physical environments through a voice-activated control mechanism or by using their mouths to control a stick. By using these mechanisms they can open and close doors and windows, turn the pages of a book, answer the telephone, and so forth. The disabled person controls the structured environment through his or her mouth and no longer needs the use of limbs to do this. Similarly a person with severe intellectual impairments can be enabled to function in a suitably structured environment with signposts, labeling of doors, reminders from staff, and alarms that alert carers if the person wanders off. "Smart houses" for people with cognitive deficits are already being designed for people with dementia (Slaven, 1996, personal communication) in an attempt to "disable the disabling environment." These environments, controlled by computers, video links, and telephones can, for example, remind people about toilets, baths, and medication, ensure showers are the right temperature, and turn electrical appliances on and off.

It might be possible to achieve compensation through anatomical reorganization whereby the undamaged areas of the brain take over the function of the damaged area. Although we know this can happen in babies and infants (Kohn and Dennis, 1978), it is often at the expense of other functions (Dennis and Kohn, 1975) and it is less clear to what extent this happens in adults. Robertson and Wilson (in press) consider this in further detail.

Perhaps the two most important methods of compensation in neuropsychological rehabilitation are (1) teaching people to use their residual skills more efficiently and (2) finding an alternative way to achieve a desired outcome. In the former approach one assumes that some residual functioning remains. Thus people with amnesia do not lose all memory functioning and can possibly be helped to use the little that remains more effectively. This might include allowing extra time to learn new information and making associations between the new information they are trying to remember and old information they already know. Mnemonics, for example, probably work because they allow previously isolated items to become integrated with one another (Bower, 1972). Many of the memory therapy techniques described by Wilson (1987d) follow this approach. Rehearsal techniques such as Landauer and Bjork's (1978) method of expanding rehearsal have been employed by Moffat (1989) to teach new words to a woman with nominal aphasia, and by Camp and Schaller (1989) in their work with Alzheimer's patients. In both of these studies people were helped to use their residual skills more efficiently.

Finding an alternative solution to a problem or relying upon an intact cognitive skill to compensate for one that is damaged is one of the most long-standing procedures in rehabilitation. Zangwill (1947) believed it to be an important approach in rehabilitation and gave as an example teaching people with a right hemiplegia to use their left hands. Later Luria et al. (1969) described the principle of "functional adaptation" i.e, if you cannot do something one way, find another way to do it. Many of the aids provided by occupational therapists for activities of daily living can be described as functional adaptations. Equipment for disabled people provides an alternative solution to tasks such as dressing, eating, and cooking. This practice also works well in cognitive rehabilitation. Teaching dysphasic people to communicate with sign language (Skelly, 1979) or visual symbols (Gardner et al., 1976), "talking books" for people who are blind, and the use of memory aids for people with amnesia are all examples of compensation through finding an alternative solution. Wilson (1995d) and Wilson and Watson (1996) discuss the development of compensatory behavior in people with severe memory problems. They also consider which characteristics predict good use of compensations.

These different approaches to rehabilitation are not mutually exclusive and can be used in combination. For example a memory impaired person may be helped by (1) reorganizing the environment to reduce the load on memory, (2) being taught to use external memory aids i.e., use a functional adaptation approach, and (3) by being encouraged to use residual skills more efficiently when learning new information through employing mnemonics and rehearsal strategies. It should be noted, however, that severely memory impaired people rarely use mnemonics spontaneously. Therapists or relatives typically supply the mnemonics whose main value is that their use leads to faster learning. Wilson (1992) offers more detailed discussion of the use of mnemonics with memory impaired people and Clare and Wilson (1997) provide suggestions for families and carers of memory impaired people to get round some of the everyday difficulties.

ASSESSING INDIVIDUALS AND PLANNING APPROPRIATE REHABILITATION PROGRAMS

The successful programs described by Prigatano (1986) and Christensen and Teasdale (1995), and the many treatment studies in the journal *Neuropsychological Rehabilitation* suggest that there is more than one way to plan an effective rehabilitation program. What I intend to do here is describe my own approach. Until very recently, I did not work in a holistic program although I have employed some of the principles from such programs. I frequently collaborate with occupational therapists and to a lesser extent speech and language pathologists and physiotherapists when trying to work out a rehabilitation plan for an individual patient. Other neuropsychologists working in similar situations might find this cooperative approach helpful. Those working in different environments might be able to adopt and adapt some of the ideas that follow in this chapter.

Referrals might come from one of a number of sources including the patient's general practitioner, neurologist, or neurosurgeon or an occupational therapist, a speech and language pathologist, the National Head Injuries Association, or a family member. If a family member approaches me, I ask for a medical referral, saying something like, "Ask your G.P. or consultant to write to me requesting an assessment of your difficulties and advice on management and rehabilitation."

The next step is to arrange an initial interview with the patient and one or more family members. I begin by asking for a brief account of what happened to the patient and what the patient and the relatives hope to achieve through this referral. If the reply is something like, "I want my memory back," or "I want you to teach me to read again," I explain that it is not always possible to restore lost functioning but we can certainly try to find ways to help with everyday problems.

The next step is to arrange a neuropsychological assessment to build a picture of the cognitive strengths and weaknesses and, at the same time, to start gathering information about the everyday problems faced by the patient and the family (Wilson, 1991c). I consider this two-pronged approach to assessment to be important because (1) we need to know the cognitive abilities and deficits in order to build a map of what is and is not cognitively possible for the patient, (2) we need to know how the problems are manifested in real life and what the people involved consider to be important, and (3) we need to individualize treatment and not follow a "packaged" approach. Such individualization involves the identification of problems from the patient's point of view (Wilson, 1989a).

Individualized treatment programs are needed because they can be directed at the manifestations of the patients' problems as they affect general well-being. Such programs can be designed to overcome specific problems that patients experience in their day-to-day lives. This does not mean that each rehabilitation program is unrelated to any other program: the factor linking individual programs together is a general framework and recourse to theory to provide principles and models to form a starting point for the assessment and planning of a management or remediation strategy (Wilson, 1989b).

How might a clinical neuropsychologist refer to theory to improve assessment and therefore treatment programs for brain injured patients? Assessment for rehabilitation, like any other assessment, is conducted in order to answer questions. The nature of these questions determines the assessment procedure used. In the case of a brain injured patient it is important to know a patient's cognitive strengths and weaknesses. Is there intellectual impairment? Is speed of processing information slower than one would expect for the patient's age? Is memory functioning affected and if so, which aspects of memory are intact and which are impaired? What kind of language (or perceptual or reading) disorder is present?

Before treatment is planned, answers to such questions must be considered. Formal psychological and neuropsychological tests can usually answer these sorts of questions reasonably well. Formal, standardized tests used by neuropsychologists have been influenced by a number of theoretical approaches. The psychometric approach, for example, is based on statistical analysis and includes measures of reliability, validity, and performance of a selected sample of a given population. (See Anastasi, 1982, for a succinct account of the characteristics of psychological tests.) The Wechsler Adult Intelligence Scale and the Wechsler Adult Intelligence Scale-Revised (Wechsler, 1955, 1987) are two examples of tests influenced by psychometry. Obviously, when a trained rehabilitation clinician uses a test of this kind, more than a mechanistic documentation of results should be produced. The use of such a test should be contextualized by the clinician's understanding of the test's place in theory; the clinician should understand the principles on which the test has been created and the relevance of data collected in support of the instrument's standardization, validity, and reliability. Without such an understanding, it is unlikely that good diagnosis will follow testing.

The identification of such neuropsychological syndromes as agnosia and apraxia requires a different form of assessment, in which the examiner must eliminate or exclude explanations for a particular problem. For example, to diagnose the recognition disorder known as visual object agnosia, the examiner must eliminate poor visual acuity and naming disorders as explanations of the failure to recognize objects. Lezak (1995) discusses both theoretical and practical considerations in her comprehensive account of the characteristics of neuropsychological assessment.

The development of theoretical models in the field of cognitive psychology has provided a rich source of theoretical support for the assessment of brain injured people. For example, the working-memory model (Baddeley and Hitch, 1974) has influenced the assessment of neurologically impaired people, particularly those with Alzheimer's disease and other memory disorders. This model has enabled clinicians to assess separately the individual components of working memory, visual and verbal memory, and semantic and episodic memory. Furthermore, the model helps explain or predict such differences as those seen between people with short- and long-term memory deficits. Similarly, the dual-route model of reading (Coltheart, 1985) has led to a more careful and systematic analysis of acquired disorders of reading. (See Wilson, 1987d and Wilson and Patterson, 1990, for a more detailed discussion of these issues.)

Localization studies from neuropsychology provide another approach to assessment, in which the examiner attempts to assess deficits in, for example, the functioning of the right and left hemispheres, the frontal lobes, the temporal lobes, and so forth. The Halstead-Reitan battery (Halstead, 1947; Reitan and Davison, 1974) is an example of this approach. The battery was originally used to discriminate among patients with frontal lobe lesions or between frontal patients and normal controls.

Although these theoretical approaches to assessment offer relatively sophisticated diagnoses of individual patients, they do not and indeed cannot address other important issues arising from cognitive and neuropsychological deficits. Here I am thinking of the effects on patients, how their daily lives will be altered, and how changes after neurological insult will also affect the lives of relatives.

The enormous personal and social problems confronted by patients and their relatives in their home environments is a major concern for those working in rehabilitation. Because these problems are not a primary concern for theorists working in such areas as localization, neuropsychological syndromes, or cognitive psychology, there is the danger of a split developing between theorists and practitioners. Indeed, I believe these different perspectives have led to division between theorists and practitioners in the past. But this division has very little substance and simply requires greater understanding of differences in role and purpose on the part of the protagonists to ensure that theory and practice are mutually supportive whenever this is possible and appropriate.

For those working in rehabilitation, there is an approach to assessment that is both theoretical and practically applicable to problems encountered in the everyday lives of patients. Behavioral assessment can bridge the gap between diagnosis and treatment in ways that other forms of assessment cannot. It is a major force in rehabilitation precisely because it can address a problem as it affects a patient's well-being. In behavioral assessment one can ask questions such as the following: What problems cause the most distress to a patient's family? How many times does this person ask the same question in the course of a day? Does this person bring a notebook to therapy sessions? Does this person remember to put on wheelchair brakes before transferring to the toilet? When questions like these are answered a relevant treatment can be implemented.

Behavioral interviewing scales, checklists, and direct observation can all be used to identify and monitor the everyday implications of neuropsychological impairment (see Wilson, 1987d, 1989d, 1991a, for further discussion). One of the ways in which behavioural assessment differs from standardized testing is that it is usually part of the treatment process itself. Behavioral assessment identifies problems for treatment and can evaluate the effectiveness of that treatment. Consequently, the therapist or psychologist continues to assess the patient while treatment is progressing. Treatment can thus be modified or altered in response to information obtained. It is this inherent dynamism that is so useful to the rehabilitator: doors are always kept open, and alternative routes can be tried in the pursuit of making life more bearable for the patient, and the behavior of the patient more conducive to tolerable living. Behavioral assessments have emerged from learning theory and from models of behavior modification.

Finally in this section I want to emphasize that there is no one right way to assess a brain injured patient, and no one discipline can answer all the questions that arise during rehabilitation. When assessing a particular patient, the neuropsychologist should draw from all the disciplines I have mentioned and should keep in mind that theoretical principles and models are not necessarily static, but are there to be modified in the light of experience. Above all, good theory is dynamic and can grow as knowledge is extended. The neuropsychologist who continually relates practice to theory, who keeps up with current academic discussion, is likely to find that rehabilitative work is indeed supported by a sturdy theoretical framework. There would appear to be four main approaches to cognitive rehabilitation in operation today. These are discussed briefly here. For a more detailed discussion see Wilson, (1991d, 1995e, 1997a).

COGNITIVE RETRAINING

This approach assumes that it is possible to remediate underlying cognitive deficits (or teach patients to deal with these deficits) by exercise, practice, and stimulation. Thus it is similar to the "mental muscle" approach (Harris and Sunderland, 1981.i.Harris & Sunderland, 1981) in that it assumes appropriate exercises can improve well-being or strength. Such programs typically involve the presentation of exercises for patients to work through. These exercises are often computerized. Sohlberg and Mateer (1989), Parenté et al. (1989), and Gianutsos (1992) are among the proponents of this approach.

The main drawback of the cognitive retraining method is the lack of evidence for its success (Wilson, 1982; Miller, 1984; Glisky, 1995). In a review of computerized cognitive rehabilitation Robertson (1990) found no evidence of significant changes in memory, visuoperceptual, or visuospatial functioning of computerized training and minimal or conflicting findings with regard to language and attention functions. Further studies including Sturm and Willmes (1991), Gray et al. (1992), and Ponsford (1995) have supported Robertson's earlier conclusion.

In addition this exercising approach fails to address (1) the functional or everyday problems arising from cognitive deficits, i.e., it tackles impairments rather than disabilities, (2) the emotional, social, or behavioral consequences of brain injury, and (3) the question of generalization. Cognitive retraining would be justified if improvements on training tasks generalized to real life problems but there is, as yet, no good evidence of this.

COGNITIVE NEUROPSYCHOLOGICAL THEORY

Approaches to cognitive rehabilitation derived from theoretical models of cognitive neuropsychological functioning argue that before a cognitive deficit can be treated one needs to have in mind a model of how that function is normally achieved (Coltheart, 1991). These models identify, often very precisely, the deficits experienced by brain injured clients and rehabilitation strategies influenced by these models are often held in high esteem (see, for example, Coltheart et al., 1994; Mitchum and Berndt, 1995). Once the deficit has been carefully analyzed, treatment is selected to fit in with the theoretical interpretation of the impairment. The treatment itself, however, typically involves practice at the damaged component of the model.

Even among cognitive neuropsychologists there are critics of this approach (Caramazza, 1989; Wilson and Patterson, 1990; Baddeley, 1993). The main drawback is that although such theoretical models are useful in identifying the nature of the impairment and for explaining observed phenomena, they provide little information on the treatment itself. In other words they tell us *what* to treat not *how* to treat. Furthermore, this approach is typically used with patients having pure or single cognitive deficits whereas, in clinical practice, most patients have mixed deficits. I am not critical of the models themselves as they have been valuable in furthering our understanding of cognitive impairments and in the development of assessment procedures. My point is they are limited as tools for cognitive rehabilitation and, once again, fail to take into account the social and emotional sequelae of brain injury.

COMBINED APPROACHES

These approaches typically combine theories and methodologies from several fields particularly neuropsychology, cognitive psychology, and behavioral psychology. Neuropsychology provides an understanding of the organization of the brain; cognitive psychology provides a way to conceptualize cognitive functioning and behavioral psychology provides a number of treatment approaches that can be modified for brain injured people together with a structure for analyzing problems and evaluating treatment effectiveness (Wilson, 1987d, 1989c, g, 1992).

The main drawback of these approaches is that they, too, fail to address the emotional and social or noncognitive aspects. In practice this failure may be more apparent than real as anxiety management strategies and cognitive behavior therapy are usually well understood by practitioners of the combined approaches. Nevertheless it is true to say that patients' beliefs about brain injury, emotions, and self-esteem are not always seen formally as part of the cognitive rehabilitation. Furthermore, it is common practice to focus on one aspect of cognitive dysfunction such as language, attention, or memory rather than addressing a broader spectrum.

THE HOLISTIC APPROACH

This approach was pioneered by Diller (1976), Ben-Yishay (1978), and Prigatano (1986) who believe one should not separate the cognitive, psychiatric, and functional aspects of brain injury from emotions, feelings, and self-esteem. Holistic programs include individual and group therapy in which patients are taught to be more aware of their strengths and weaknesses, helped to accept and understand these given cognitive exercises, helped to develop compensatory skills, and provided with vocational counseling. Such programs appear to result in less emotional distress, increased self-esteem, and greater productivity (Prigatano, 1986, 1994).

There are two main drawbacks connected with the holistic approach. First, their programs are expensive to run although some studies (e.g., Cope, 1994 and

Mehlbye and Larsen, 1994) suggest that costs can be recouped in a few years through greater productivity. Second, they have not been rigorously evaluated. Although they have probably been subjected to more research than other approaches (Cope, 1994; Diller, 1994), this activity has not as yet encouraged evaluations at a sufficiently penetrating level.

II

LIVING WITH MEMORY DISORDERS

Amnesia and organic memory impairment are commonly seen after many types of brain injury and can be extremely handicapping. People with the classic amnesic syndrome have great difficulty learning and remembering most kinds of new information. Immediate memory as assessed by a forward digit span task is normal. There is usually a period of retrograde amnesia, that is, a loss of information acquired before the onset of the amnesia. This period of retrograde amnesia or gap in memory is variable in length and may range from a few minutes to decades. Previously acquired semantic knowledge about the world and implicit memory (i.e., remembering without awareness or conscious recollection) are typically intact in amnesic patients. Other cognitive skills such as language, attention, perception, planning, and organization are unimpaired.

People with a pure amnesic syndrome are relatively rare as most memory impaired people do have additional cognitive deficits and people with these additional problems are described in the next section, Part III. In this section three young men are described with pure or classic amnesic syndromes: Jack who attempted suicide with carbon monoxide, Jay who became amnesic following a brain hemorrhage at the age of 20 when he was a law student, and Alex who sustained hypoxic brain damage during a diving accident while he was on holiday in Australia.

It is certainly easier for people with a pure amnesic syndrome to compensate for their memory problems. If there are no difficulties in other areas of cognitive functioning, and particularly if executive skills, such as planning, organizational, and attentional skills are intact, then it is possible to bypass or overcome everyday memory problems (Wilson and Watson, 1996). The three young men described here were all able to compensate for their difficulties to a lesser or greater degree. Jack adjusted well to his problems, Jay showed impressive use of external memory aids, and Alex was able to return to paid employment, get married, and have a daughter.

Despite these impressive achievements life is not easy for any of them. Jack is not able to work, Jay puts enormous effort and energy into remaining independent, and Alex is both easily fatigued and constantly struggling to keep his life on an even course.

Although some improvement occurred in each of these three people in the early stages, restoration of memory functioning was not the goal of rehabilitation and was not achieved. The goal of any brain injury rehabilitation is rarely to restore lost functioning, instead it is to reduce the everyday problems and to enhance quality of life. Together with the health service staff and their families, all three young men have been successful in achieving these goals.

3

JACK: COMING TO TERMS WITH AMNESIA

BACKGROUND

Although apparently happy and healthy, Jack attempted suicide with carbon monoxide poisoning when he was 19 yr old. Following resuscitation he sustained a generalized epileptic convulsion and remained unconscious for 20 min. For several months after this he suffered from subclinical seizures. Nine months later all seizure activity had ceased and his electroencephalogram (EEG) was normal. He was left however with a major problem of severe memory impairment, and was referred to me for help 8 mo after his suicide attempt.

I made an appointment to see Jack and his parents and they traveled by car from their home approximately 20 miles away. It was clear that the suicide attempt had been a complete surprise to Jack's parents although it had been a predetermined and planned event. Jack had taken equipment with him in the morning before leaving ostensibly for work. He was found in a parking lot some hours later by the police who thought he had been unconscious for about 2 h. He was taken to the hospital, treated with hyperbaric oxygen therapy, and was considered lucky to be alive.

Jack's parents said their son had always been shy, lacked confidence in dealing with others, and preferred to "stay in the background." He had a particular talent for writing, he was a good artist, and was imaginative and sensitive. He had hoped to have a career in the media and this was on course until halfway through his "A" levels when (as his parents found out later) he became involved with a girl whom they claimed was a "bad influence." Jack's work deteriorated, he failed to attend his classes while continuing his friendship with the girl. After performing poorly in his examinations, he took an unskilled job where he worked for a short time before the suicide attempt.

The family appeared to be close. Their interaction was warm and caring. Jack's parents were, however, still hurt by the words of the psychiatrist who saw them soon after Jack's resuscitation. They remembered the psychiatrist saying words to the effect of, "What you see is what you get. He won't change much from how he is now." They felt their hopes were dashed and the future looked very gloomy.

When asked to give some examples of how Jack's memory problems affected his everyday life, his mother said,

> He never remembers where the car is parked and gets embarrassed if he has to look in his book. He gets confused about arrangements with his friends. He double books: for example, he records one appointment at home and then meets someone in the street and arranges another meeting with that person. He loses everything: pencils, his wallet—everything. It would be worse except I move things to obvious places. He never remembers what he has spent his money on and he forgets to carry out any plans he has made for himself, like sorting out his video tapes.

Jack, himself, was rather quiet during the initial interview although he appeared to be pleasantly mannered and his behavior was appropriate. He obviously could not remember much about what had happened to him since the suicide attempt nor the few weeks before it. He was probably embarrassed although he appeared to be dignified and sensible.

During this initial interview I explained that although we probably would not be able to restore Jack's memory functioning, we would, nevertheless, be able to help him overcome some of the everyday problems resulting from his impaired memory. I proposed the following plan of action. First, I would assess Jack's memory, thinking, concentration, and so forth to build up a picture of his strengths and weaknesses. We would require two or three sessions, each of 2–3 h, to do this. Meanwhile, I wanted Jack's parents to keep records of his everyday failures at home so we could identify the frequency and severity of particular memory difficulties. Following this I said I would offer Jack some individual and group memory therapy.

Jack and his parents agreed to this. We set a time for the next appointment, I said I would prepare some record sheets for the parents for next time, and I gave them an information booklet to read. The booklet, written for the National Head Injuries Association, was entitled *Memory Problems after Head Injury* (Wilson, 1989e) although, as I explained to the family, the information contained in the booklet applied to memory problems following other conditions, including anoxic brain damage. Today I would have given them a copy of *Coping with Memory Problems* (Clare and Wilson, 1997) as this covers a wider range of problems and provides suggestions for families on how to get around some of the difficulties.

THE ASSESSMENT

As noted in Chapter 2, Jack had both a neuropsychological and a behavioral assessment. The neuropsychological assessment was briefer than I usually give, partly because Jack's problems were more straightforward than some patients and partly because it seemed expedient to begin treatment fairly quickly, given the family's anxiety and the gloomy picture they had been given earlier. Jack was assessed on the Wechsler Adult Intelligence Scale-Revised (Wechsler, 1981b), the Wechsler Memory Scale-Revised (WMS-R; Wechsler, 1987), The Rivermead Behavioural Memory Test (RBMT; Wilson et al., 1985), the Autobiographical Memory Interview (AMI; Kopelman et al., 1990), the Rey-Osterreith Complex Figure (Osterreith, 1944), the Graded Naming Test (McKenna and Warrington, 1983), and the Modified Wisconsin Card Sorting Test (Nelson, 1976). The results can be seen in Table 3.1.

Table 3.1 shows that Jack's verbal IQ was in the high average range of ability with his performance IQ in the superior range. Although not assessed in great depth, there was no evidence of language, perceptual, or executive deficits. His memory, however, was severely compromised. On the WMS-R he was in the very impaired range for both general memory functioning and delayed recall. His visual memory was not good but was significantly better than his verbal memory. His recognition memory on the Recognition Memory Test was poor and his performance on a test of everyday memory, the RBMT, was in the severely impaired range. Furthermore his results on the AMI were typical of someone with organic amnesia in that he had a particularly poor recall of facts and events from the past year with a better recall of events earlier in his life.

A behavioral assessment was carried out in order to identify (1) the particular problems Jack faced in his everyday life, (2) those problems for which Jack and his parents considered they needed help, and (3) the coping methods they presently used.

This information was obtained through self-report measures in the following manner. First, Jack and his parents were interviewed and asked a series of questions about Jack's current memory problems. These questions, which can be seen in Table 3.2, were based on a rating scale devised by Kapur and Pearson (1983).

In each case Jack and his parents were asked to compare Jack's current memory for certain activities with his memory before the suicide attempt. The main purpose of this rating scale was to determine whether Jack had insight into

Table 3.1. Jack's Main Neuropsychological Test Results

Wechsler Adult Intelligence Scale-Revised

VERBAL SUBTESTS	AGE SCALED SCORES	PERFORMANCE SUBTESTS	AGE SCALED SCORES
Information	11	Picture completion	11
Digit span	14	Picture arrangement	17
Vocabulary	14	Block design	15
Arithmetic	9	Object assembly	14
Comprehension	11	Digit symbol	10
Similarities	14		
Verbal IQ	113	(High average)	
Performance IQ	126	(Superior)	
Full scale IQ	121	(Superior)	

Wechsler Memory Scale-Revised

General memory index	< 50	(Very impaired)
Visual memory index	78	(Below average)
Verbal memory index	51	(Impaired)
Attention/concentration	97	(Average)
Delayed recall	< 50	(Very impaired)

Rivermead Behavioural Memory Test

Screening score = 1 (Maximum 12)⎱
Standardized profile score = 3 (Maximum 24)⎰ (Severely impaired)

Recognition Memory Test

Words	Age scaled score	< 3	(Very impaired)
Faces	Age scaled score	4	(Impaired)

The Autobiographical Memory Interview

	PERSONAL SEMANTIC		AUTOBIOGRAPHICAL INCIDENTS	
Childhood	18/21	(Normal)	4/9	(Probably abnormal)
Early adult life	15/21	(Probably abnormal)	5/9	(Borderline)
Recent (past year)	12/21	(Definitely abnormal)	3/9	(Definitely abnormal)
Total	45/63	(Definitely abnormal)	12/27	(Definitely abnormal)

Immediate Memory Span

Corsi blocks	5	(Average)
Forward digits	7	(Average)
Backward digits	4	(Low average)

(continued)

Table 3.1. Jack's Main Neuropsychological Test Results (*continued*)

Rey-Osterreith Complex Figure

Copy	36/36	(Above average)
Delayed recall	3/36	(Severely impaired)
Percentage retained	8.33	(Severely impaired)

Wisconsin Card Sorting Test (Nelson's 1976 modified version)

Categories	6	
Total errors	6	Normal
Perseverative errors	1	

Graded Naming Test

16/30   (Average)

Table 3.2. Memory Rating Scale

	Rating		
HOW IS YOUR MEMORY FOR:	ABOUT THE SAME	SLIGHTLY WORSE	VERY MUCH WORSE
1. The date	0	1	2
2. The month	0	1	2
3. The names of people you have known for a long time	0	1	2
4. The names of people you have met only once or twice before	0	1	2
5. The faces of people you have known for a long time	0	1	2
6. The faces of people you have met only once or twice before	0	1	2
7. How to get somewhere you knew well	0	1	2
8. How to get somewhere you have been to only once or twice before	0	1	2
9. Where you have put something	0	1	2
10. What you have been told	0	1	2
11. What you have read	0	1	2
12. Any other memory problems not yet covered (please specify)	0	1	2

his problems. The measure here was the degree of consistency between Jack's report and his parents' report. In fact, they were in very close agreement suggesting Jack was well aware of his problems.

The main areas of difficulty, rated as very much worse by both Jack and his parents were:

Item 4: Remembering names of people met only once or twice before.

Item 9: Where you have put something.

Item 10: What you have been told.

Item 11: What you have read.

Under item 10, Jack's mother and father expanded saying Jack frequently lost track of a conversation. Jack also added that he forgot details of telephone conversations arranging meetings and so double booked.

Jack and his mother and father were also asked to keep a weekly memory diary for 2 wk, to identify with some degree of precision how often particular problems occurred in everyday life. The diaries were prepared from work carried out by Alan Sunderland (personal communication) and can be seen in Table 3.3.

Table 3.3. Memory Diary

Every evening over the next 7 days, go through the diary and indicate against each question, how many times that problem happened to you during that day.

If it occurred once put 1 in that square.

If it occurred twice put 2 in that square.

If it occurred three times put 3 in that square, and so on.

	Please enter day of week
If you should forget one evening, don't guess.	
Try to complete it regularly for a week.	Day 1 *Wednesday*
We want YOUR opinion. Don't ask anyone to help you fill it in.	Day 2
	Day 3
If it did not apply to you during the day put 0.	Day 4
Carry on until you have completed 7 days.	Day 5
	Day 6
	Day 7

Date and time of next visit: _____

(continued)

Table 3.3. Memory Diary (*continued*)

	Day 1	Day 2	Day 3	Day 4	Day 5	Day 6	Day 7
1. Forgetting where you have put something. Losing things around the house.							
2. Failing to recognize a place that you are told you have often been before.							
3. Finding a television story difficult to follow.							
4. Not remembering a change in your daily routine, such as a change in the place where something is kept, or a change in the time something happens. Following your old routine by mistake.							
5. Having to go back to check whether you have done something that you meant to do.							
6. When thinking of the past, forgetting when something happened. For example, whether it was yesterday or last week.							
7. Completely forgetting to take things with you, or leaving things behind and having to go back and fetch them.							
8. Forgetting that you were told something yesterday or a few days ago, and having to be reminded of it.							
9. Starting to read something (a book or an article in a newspaper or magazine) without realizing you have already read it.							
10. Letting yourself ramble on to speak about unimportant or irrelevant things.							
11. Failing to recognize, by sight, close relatives or friends that you meet frequently.							
12. Having difficulty in picking up a new skill. For example, having difficulty in learning a new game or in working some new gadget after you have practiced once or twice.							

(*continued*)

Table 3.3. Memory Diary (*continued*)

	Day 1	Day 2	Day 3	Day 4	Day 5	Day 6	Day 7
13. Finding that a word is "on the tip of your tongue." You know what it is but you can't find it.							
14. Completely forgetting to do things you said you would do, and things you planned to do.							
15. Forgetting important details of what you did or what happened to you the day before.							
16. When talking to someone, forgetting what you have just said. Maybe saying, "What was I talking about?"							
17. When reading a newspaper or magazine being unable to follow the thread of a story, losing track of what it is about.							
18. Forgetting to tell somebody something important. Perhaps forgetting to pass on a message or remind someone of something.							
19. Forgetting important details about yourself, e.g., your birthdate or where you live.							
20. Getting the details of what someone has told you mixed up or confused.							
21. Telling someone a story or joke that you have told them once already.							
22. Forgetting details of things you do regularly, details of what to do, or at what time to do it.							
23. Finding that the faces of famous people seen on television or in photographs, look unfamiliar.							
24. Forgetting where things are normally kept or looking for them in the wrong place.							

(*continued*)

Table 3.3. Memory Diary (*continued*)

	Day 1	Day 2	Day 3	Day 4	Day 5	Day 6	Day 7
25. **a.** Getting lost or turning in the wrong direction on a journey, a walk, or in a building, where you have OFTEN been before.							
b. Getting lost or turning in the wrong direction on a journey, a walk, or in a building, where you have been only ONCE or TWICE before.							
26. Doing some routine thing twice by mistake. For example, putting two lots of tea in the teapot, or going to brush/comb your hair when you have just done so.							
27. Repeating to someone what you have just told them or asking them the same question twice.							
28. Any other memory or concentration difficulties? If so, please describe.							

Problems mentioned most frequently were:

- Forgetting where the car had been parked
- Double booking appointments
- Losing belongings
- Not being able to account for money spent
- Forgetting to do something planned.

The third self-report measure was a questionnaire about the compensatory strategies used by Jack. This can be seen in Table 3.4.

Jack completed the questionnaire and his parents were asked to confirm the accuracy of his responses. The main compensatory aid used by Jack was a small diary he usually carried with him. Sometimes he wrote things on pieces of paper that he frequently forgot to transfer to a more permanent system. He also had a large diary by the telephone at home. This, too, led to problems because information recorded in the large diary during a telephone conversation was not always transferred to the small diary. Jack's mother often retrieved his belongings and put them in obvious places so Jack could find them easily. Thus although Jack was using compensatory memory strategies, the system was not well organized or foolproof.

Table 3.4. Memory Aids		
DO YOU USE:	BEFORE ACCIDENT/ ILLNESS	NOW
1. An alarm clock to wake you up?		
2. A clock or watch to tell you the date?		
3. A watch with a timer?		
4. A diary (appointments)?		
5. A journal (log book)?		
6. A notebook and/or notes to yourself?		
7. A personal organizer?		
8. Lists of things to do or buy, e.g., shopping list?		
9. Writing on your hand (or elsewhere)?		
10. Calendars/wallcharts, etc.?		
11. A dictaphone or tape recorder (or special calculator)?		
12. Asking other people to remind you?		
13. Leaving objects in an unusual place as a reminder?		
14. Visual imagery (i.e., turning words or names into pictures)?		
15. Alphabetic searching?		
16. Mental retracing or events?		
17. PQRST?*		
18. Any other method to help you remember?		
*PQRST, *Preview, Question, Read, State, Test.*		

TREATMENT

By now Jack was ready to begin his memory rehabilitation. We arranged for him to come once a week for a 1 h individual session followed by lunch at the hospital and then a 2 h group session with four other memory impaired people. Jack and his parents were keen to begin. On a more practical note, it was agreed that one of his parents would bring him each week and collect him after the group meeting.

Individual Therapy

Using the findings from the neuropsychological and behavioral assessments, together with further discussion with the family members, the following plan was proposed.

Jack was intelligent and apart from severe memory impairment he had no additional cognitive problems. He should, therefore, be able to learn to compensate for his memory difficulties and to learn some mnemonic strategies. We would select a few problems identified from the memory diary and see if we could teach Jack to overcome these problems. We would first try this in the hospital and on the hospital grounds. If successful we would try to ensure generalization to Jack's house. I have written elsewhere about generalization (e.g. Wilson, 1987d, 1995c) which is often a major problem in rehabilitation effectiveness. Learning in one situation does not mean the skill or information learned will automatically be seen in another situation. It is often necessary to teach generalization (Wilson, 1995).

The problems selected for Jack's treatment were:

1. Forgetting where he had put his belongings.
2. Leaving belongings behind.
3. Double booking appointments.
4. Forgetting where the car was parked.
5. Not completing planned activities.

The strategy adopted for the first problem was to always place his belongings in a particular location. At the beginning of each session, three coins of different denominations were placed in three locations. The locations remained constant at each visit. As the coins were placed in the three locations Jack was asked to make an association between the coin and the place, e.g., penny = *Penny Dreadful* book on the bookshelf. At the end of the session Jack was asked to find the coins. During individual sessions at the hospital, Jack improved dramatically at this task. Meanwhile, he and his mother cleared and organized his shelves and storage spaces at home, labeling them to encourage Jack to put things in the proper place. His parents also prompted him to always put his keys, wallet, and other possessions in the same place.

The second problem, forgetting to take belongings with him when he moved from one place to another, was tackled in the following way. The main strategy was to pause and look around whenever he left one place to go to another. This was practiced by having Jack put two objects on the table at each session. One was always his diary and one was a different object (changed each week), such as his wallet or keys. He was then invited to go to another location in the hospital. Before leaving he was required to stop and look around, systematically check his pockets, and ask himself if he had left anything. This was practiced every week. Although the diary was never left behind, Jack needed reminding to retrieve the novel object. During the last 6 wk of the 12 wk individual therapy, however, Jack reliably remembered both items. Once again, his parents were asked to repeat this exercise at home to ensure generalization.

The third problem, double booking, was tackled more directly. The problem arose because of having two diaries and using odd scraps of paper to record arrangements. Jack needed the two diaries, one small enough to carry around with him and one larger family diary for everyone to use. The solution was to ensure that all relevant information was recorded in both places. During his individual sessions Jack practiced transferring information from written notes on loose paper to his small diary. The main benefit came from persuading Jack's parents to remind him to go through his diary every evening to ensure information was recorded in both places. The double booking ceased to be a major problem almost immediately.

Problem number four was forgetting where the car was parked. This was annoying and embarrassing for Jack. Six parking lots at the hospital were used to help Jack overcome this problem. Each week a car was chosen at random in one of the six parking lots and Jack was asked to remember its location using three cues. The first was to check for any landmarks such as a nearby gate or air vent and record this, the second was to record the parking lot number from 1 to 6, and the third was to envisage the location of the parking lot on an imaginary question mark (the six parking lots could be conceived as being in the shape of a question mark). It will be remembered that Jack's visual memory was less impaired than his verbal memory. Furthermore, Jack was an artistic young man who reported thinking in images. Using visual imagery therefore seemed suited to his personal style. He adopted the cue system for the parking lot readily and soon became very good at remembering the location of the car selected for that particular week. Unfortunately, locating was harder to generalize to his own home environment as his parents usually parked in a multistory parking lot. In these circumstances, Jack had to rely more on recording sufficient information in a notebook.

The fifth problem, remembering to carry out planned activities was tackled with a memo board. During his individual sessions at the hospital, Jack was requested to carry out three activities that were noted on the memo board. Each had to be carried out at a certain time. As each was completed, Jack was supposed to cross it out. At first, this was the least successful of the five strategies as Jack forgot to look at the board. When we decided to use an alarm on a kitchen timer to remind Jack to check the board his performance improved. Meanwhile he was using a similar system at home and the problem there eased. The weekly appointments calendar at home can be seen in Table 3.5.

At the end of the individual session and just before lunch, one or both of Jack's parents joined the session to spend about 10 min summing up the results of the

Table 3.5. Appointment Calendar

TIME	WEEK OF OCTOBER 9–15						
	MONDAY OCT. 9	TUESDAY OCT. 10	WEDNESDAY OCT. 11	THURSDAY OCT. 12	FRIDAY OCT. 13	SATURDAY OCT. 14	SUNDAY OCT. 15
8–9 A.M.							
9–10 A.M.							
10–11 A.M.							
11–12 A.M.							
12–1 P.M.							
1–2 P.M.							
2–3 P.M.							
3–4 P.M.							
4–5 P.M.							
5–6 P.M.							
6–7 P.M.							
7–8 P.M.							
8–9 P.M.							
9–10 P.M.							
10–11 P.M.							
11–12 P.M.							
12–1 A.M.							

day. This was also an opportunity for Jack's mother and father to discuss any particular problems or anxieties encountered that week.

At the end of the 12 wk period, Jack seemed ready to move on. It was possible to set up a 6 wk work trial with the medical illustrations department in the hospital. Jack came once a week to help catalogue the video tape library. I explained Jack's memory problems to the staff members and kept in touch during the 6 wk trial. Jack fitted in very well and the staff appeared to enjoy having him.

Jack had enjoyed his individual sessions and his work trial. He and his parents were pleased with his progress.

The Memory Group

The group Jack attended was similar to that described in Evans and Wilson (1992) which, in turn, was loosely based on the Rivermead Memory Group described by Wilson and Moffat (1984). Apart from Jack, there were four other brain injured people in the group: three men and one woman. The woman and two of the men had sustained a severe head injury, the other man had sustained a subarachnoid hemorrhage as a result of a ruptured aneurysm on the anterior communicating artery. Jack was the most severely memory impaired but was also the most intelligent member of the group and he was the only group member without additional cognitive deficits. I ran the group with the help of a clinical psychology student, although on other occasions my co-worker had been an occupational therapist, a speech and language therapist, a physiotherapist, or a nurse.

During the first group session we talked about the aims of the group, explaining that we did not expect to restore or repair damaged memory systems, but we would help group members to understand how memory worked, and we would introduce them to certain memory aids and compensatory strategies in order to deal with everyday problems. We also explained that we hoped to reduce some of the anxiety and other emotional consequences of memory impairment.

Following the first introductory meeting, a typical memory group session would start with some orientation questions such as the year, month, date, and names of group members. The more impaired members were given easier questions to try to ensure success. We usually spent some time discussing a particular problem such as, "How do you tell people you have a memory disorder?" We might role play various ways of achieving this. Most weeks we practiced using a particular compensatory strategy or technique. For example, an electronic organizer or day book might be demonstrated and practiced. Considerable discussion took place about the use of notebooks, diaries, and other compensations. Jack was good, both at using such external aids and at entering into the discussions about their value. However, he refused to practice or even consider using a pocket tape recorder, although some of the other group members found this to be useful. Jack's reluctance seemed to be due to the fact that he feared the information would become public and that he would lose control of confidentiality. Whatever the reason, this reluctance illustrated the importance of allowing individual choice over memory strategies to be employed and for therapists to take personal style and preference into account when recommending compensatory techniques. Homework was set and reviewed each week. Homework tasks usually required group members to remember to do something, such as listen to a particular radio program, make a birthday card, or find an item of news from the local newspaper to discuss. The rationale for the homework was to help members generalize strategies learned in the group to the home environments. Sessions usually ended with a memory game such as "Concentration" ("pairs"), which proved to be a great favorite of all participants. Memory games were played not only because of face validity but also because they enabled members to practice using strategies for novel tasks. The refreshment break was an important group activity when the staff members made the tea or coffee, giving the group members a chance to talk informally about their difficulties and to share experiences on coping with specific problems.

Jack was a thoughtful and respected member of the group and I can remember being especially pleased when I saw him exchange telephone numbers with another young man during the break. Although a normal everyday occurrence for nonbrain injured people, this exchange brought home the isolation frequently experienced by many people with memory impairments.

Family members were asked to keep weekly records of the use of memory aids and strategies for the several months the group ran. Jack showed an increase in the number of occasions he used an aid or strategy from a total of 204 per week at the beginning of the group to 385 per week at the end. He used his notebook or diary most often and here the increase was from 100 times per week at the beginning of the group to 200 at the end. He also increased the number of times he wrote lists. This ranged from 14 per week at the beginning to 100 per week at the end. His use of a wall chart or a notice board at home increased from 0 at the beginning to 15 at the end. The use of the alarm on his watch remained constant at 20 throughout, whereas asking to be reminded of something decreased from 50 per week at the beginning to 35 per week at the end. This, no doubt, reflected Jack's increase in self-sufficiency through use of external aids.

Anxiety and depression were measured with the Hospital Anxiety and Depression (HAD) Scale (Zigmond and Snaith, 1983). Jack's scores on the Depression Scale were consistently low during the whole period of group therapy, indicating that he did not feel depressed. In contrast his scores on the Anxiety section of the HAD was very high at the beginning. However, this rapidly declined over the first few weeks of the group sessions. Jack also commented that he had enjoyed meeting people with similar problems. In short, although Jack's general memory functioning had not improved (when reassessed with the RBMT) he had shown a marked increase in the overall use of memory aids and strategies and a reduction in clinical levels of anxiety.

Later Rehabilitation

Soon after Jack's successful work experience with the help of the sympathetic medical illustrations department, he was accepted at a local college for a course in media studies. I wrote an explanatory letter to the college authorities explaining the nature of Jack's problems and how these were likely to affect his studies. I also kept in touch with Jack's tutor for the 1st yr of the course. At about the same time Jack and his parents began the process of trying to get his driver's license back. This had been revoked because of the nature of his original illness.

Once again I wrote to the authorities explaining that although Jack had severe memory problems he had no perceptual, visuospatial, or concentration problems that might affect his driving ability. He had plenty of common sense so that if he did get lost because of his amnesia, he would be able to telephone home or extricate himself in some other way. Jack's driving license was soon returned.

JACK TODAY

At the time of writing it is now 6 yr since Jack's suicide attempt. Although he finished his college course, he did so with difficulty. He still lives with his parents and is not employed, although he has a close circle of friends and is busy with his own film studies. He has come to terms with the limitations imposed upon him and offers valuable insights into memory impairments. He uses his less impaired visual memory as far as possible. He says,

> Without any effort, I can remember details of my favorite films and I use this to aid me. The visual nature of the films themselves can trigger a sequence of memories; I remember seeing Scorcese's remake of *Cape Fear* in March 1992. I saw it by myself and didn't discuss it with anyone afterwards, but the effect this finely crafted piece of cinema had upon me has helped me to remember that experience with crystal clarity. I remember where I sat in the cinema, the pub I went to after the screening, and even details of the drive there.

However, Jack also admits that life is often more difficult than this. He says,

> But often, especially when I have to venture out of this private realm, it doesn't come so comfortably. Being continually made aware of mistakes, especially mistakes that I can't help but make, and being forced to challenge my own inability can result in personal humiliation. I may be asked to do things that I have taught myself not to do as part of my own memory disciplines.
> Whilst studying, one lecturer asked me to quickly relay a message to another elsewhere in the building. Thrown by the audacity of this educated man, who was fully aware of my limitations, I left the room and promptly forgot the message, where to go, the name of the lecturer who'd sent me, and how to return to the room I had originally been sent from. I was lost. And I can't recall what came of that incident. But the feeling of indignation, frustration, and fear from that incident has stayed with me. Many of my recent memories are like this. They start off relatively clear and then fade off as I relate the story to myself. And I often find that as faithful to the truth as many of my recollections may be, some are tinged with pure fiction, as if without even realizing it, I am filling in the gaps, the empty times with fabricated notions of the past. And like a game of Japanese whispers, sometimes the more I think about these memories, the less truthful they probably become. But then I am in no position to say whether this is in fact the case. I cannot gauge how accurate any of my memories are.
> I use triggers to aid me, no, I *rely* upon triggers and visual cues to help myself as best I can to organize my mind and construct a kind of database from which I can access material. I also use a diary for appointments and I carry a notebook with me al-

ways, using it with a religious devotion to make written notes on where I am going, where I leave my car, who I am going to see, and afterwards, notes on the consequences of such events so that I can transfer important material that I may wish to look back upon or refer to at any point in the future. That is my material memory.

I lead a basic lifestyle. I strenuously avoid what I would call "high-risk" situations. That is, situations in which my memory difficulties would leave me lost and disoriented. I don't *ever* travel to unfamiliar places unless I am accompanied or have a detailed written guide (and even then I find concentrating difficult in stressful situations or if I am late for an appointment, for example). If I visit the cinema or theater, I must make sure that I won't have to leave my seat during the screening as I would not be able to find my way back. I can't perform basic sociable tasks such as taking orders to buy a round of drinks or noting the names and faces of new acquaintances. In fact, I am sure that on many occasions I have met people who are not aware of my condition, and then upon not recognizing them on a second meeting, will have appeared rude and impolite.

I don't read novels. I will never be able to take a job. Familiarizing myself with the location of the workplace, the nature of the job, the names of my employers and colleagues, the plan of the building, the extent of my responsibilities, etc. would take many many weeks. In fact it would not be possible. As I hope you can imagine, even a job involving nothing but menial tasks would pose serious problems.

The condition of my memory also affects me on many social and personal levels. Conducting relationships can be difficult whereby notions of trust can seem so fragile and arguments can turn a genuine poor memory incident on my part into a 'deliberate' act of spite in the eyes of another. And on the other hand, gestures of kindness by others may go without thanks and may appear to have been unnoticed or not appreciated. To those unfamiliar with the many quirks of the condition, I must appear sometimes extremely dismissive and rude.

I'm finding it very hard to write this. Not only is it becoming clearer to me that it is impossible to accurately describe the experiences, the feelings, but without checking, re-checking, and re-reading the text above several times over, I have no way of recollecting what I've already written. Frustration is constantly waiting at the wings.

Frustration can come as a result of many symptoms, but not anymore from the disruptions in my routine which rarely occur unexpectedly. And having a complete memory is not a possible goal, so I cannot feel frustrated for not reaching it. Frustration comes from much smaller, subtler things. Being accused of not using my memory aids is infuriating, particularly when such comments come from those who know I depend upon them. Sometimes of course, I don't forget certain things but may make a mistake just as anyone else might. And to then have someone casually and dismissively assume that I've forgotten, whereby I have, for once, managed to *remember* is a very cruel blow indeed.

I have lost many cherished personal items to people who borrowed them and never returned them. Of course there is no malice involved and I do willingly let people borrow such things as any friend would, and I do make a note of who has taken what. But then it is so easy to lose these notes too.

My memory limitations are not so much a problem anymore. I don't mourn the loss of my memory as I can't remember what it used to be like. The condition has helped me evolve, I think, into a different type of person. Although I may have become more sensitive, I have also, ironically, become more cerebral, my thinking more esoteric, and I am very comfortable with this. I think it suits my character.

4

JAY: COMPENSATING FOR AMNESIA

BACKGROUND

Jay was born in 1965. After leaving school he went to a university to study law. During his 2nd yr there, at the age of 20 yr, he sustained an epileptic seizure and collapsed during a tutorial. He was admitted to the accident and emergency department of the local hospital where he had two further seizures. A computed tomography (CT) scan carried out soon afterwards, showed a large subarachnoid hemorrhage arising from the left occipital region. A subsequent arteriogram showed a left posterior cerebral artery aneurysm. The aneurysm was clipped 3 wk later.

About 5 wk after the hemorrhage Jay was admitted to a rehabilitation unit for a further 5 wk treatment. On admission to rehabilitation he was reported to have a marked loss of memory and to be unable to remember anything from one minute to the next. His other cognitive abilities appeared to be largely intact and there was no dysphasia. Neurological examination revealed a dense right hemianopia with macular sparing and diplopia plus some meningeal irritation.

Although Jay's diplopia had resolved when he was discharged from rehabilitation he still had the hemianopia. He was referred to me for advice on the management of his memory difficulties about 4 mo after the hemorrhage. He was seen as an outpatient approximately once every 2 wk for a period of 6 mo. Three yr later he was seen again for follow-up and since then he has been seen approximately once every 6 mo.

Much of Jay's rehabilitation was conducted independently by Jay himself and his family. Initially however he was seen for a neuropsychological assessment and an investigation was carried out to see which strategies might be viable for managing his problems in everyday life.

Jay's sister accompanied him for the first few appointments and she and her father were the primary caregivers at that time. Other members of the family, notably Jay's aunt, were also closely involved in his care. I learned that Jay was the youngest of four children and the only son. He had been a clever student and obtained a scholarship to a prestigious university.

Following his hemorrhage Jay did not realize he had memory problems and considered problems with his eyesight to be of more concern. After a few months, however, awareness of his memory difficulties had grown to such an extent that he began to make conscious attempts to compensate for the problems these caused in his daily living. At this stage Jay's sister and father were asked to keep a memory diary of daily memory failures for a period of 2 wk.

THE ASSESSMENT

Jay was assessed on tests of general intellectual functioning, naming, memory, perception, executive skills, and reading. His general intellectual functioning was in the superior range and his scores on all tests of naming, visuospatial and visuoperceptual functioning, reading and executive skills were all above average. It was only on tests of memory where his scores gave cause for concern. Like Jack in the previous chapter, Jay had all the characteristics of a pure amnesic syndrome. The main neuropsychological test results can be seen in Table 4.1.

One interesting aspect of Jay's assessment was his almost complete lack of retrograde amnesia. On tests of famous events, as well as on the *Autobiographical Memory Interview*, Jay was able to recall events and details for the time period immediately predating his hemorrhage. Indeed, he was able to recall being at the tutorial when he collapsed. When asked about this he said, "I can remember the night before and I can remember what I wrote 5 minutes before—it was about Land Law Reform. I can remember right up until the time of the hemorrhage, about 5:05 P.M." Thus any RA that might have been present in the early days appeared to have resolved. In all other ways Jay had the characteristics of a pure amnesic syndrome: his immediate memory was good, he had problems after a delay or distraction, he had difficulty learning new information, and his cognitive skills (apart from memory) were good.

Table 4.1. Jay's Main Neuropsychological Test Results

1986

Wechsler Adult Intelligence Scale

VERBAL SUBTESTS	AGE SCALED SCORES	PERFORMANCE SUBTESTS	AGE SCALED SCORES
Information	15	Digit symbol	13
Comprehension	16	Picture completion	8
Arithmetic	13	Block design	17
Similarities	13	Picture arrangement	8
Digit span	14	Object assembly	17
Vocabulary	16		

Verbal IQ	124	(Superior)
Performance IQ	115	(High average)
Full scale IQ	121	(Superior)

Wechsler Memory Scale

Logical memory $\left\{ \begin{array}{l} \text{Immediate recall} \quad 8 \quad \text{(Normal)} \\ \text{Delayed recall} \quad 0 \quad \text{(Severely impaired)} \end{array} \right.$

Rivermead Behavioural Memory Test

Screening score   = 1 (Maximum 12) $\left. \right\}$ (Severely impaired)
Standardized profile score   = 5 (Maximum 24)

Recognition Memory Test

Words   Age scaled score < 3   (Very impaired)
Faces   Age scaled score < 3   (Very impaired)

The Autobiographical Memory Interview

	PERSONAL SEMANTIC		AUTOBIOGRAPHICAL INCIDENTS	
Childhood	19/21	(Normal)	8	(Normal)
Early adult life	20	(Normal)	9	(Normal)
Recent (past year)	14	(Abnormal)	2	(Abnormal)
Total	54	(Normal)	19	(Normal)

Immediate Memory Span

Corsi blocks	7	(Good average)
Forward digits	8	(Average)
Backward digits	6	(Average)

Rey-Osterreith Complex Figure

Copy	32/36	(Average)
Recall	1/36	(Severely impaired)
Percentage retained	3	(Severely impaired)

(continued)

Table 4.1. Jay's Main Neuropsychological Test Results (*continued*)

Wisconsin Card Sorting Test (Nelson's Modified Version)

Categories   6 ⎫
Total errors   0 ⎬   (Above average)
Perseverative errors   0 ⎭

Graded Naming Test

26/30   (95th percentile)

Verbal Fluency

F = 21 + 1 perseveration   ⎫
A = 14 + 3 perseverations ⎬   (Above average)
S = 15 + 2 perseverations ⎭

Reitan Trail Making Test

A: 25 sec   (75th percentile)
B: 40 sec   (Above 90th percentile)

Semantic Processing Test (True/False Decision)

Mean time per item = 2.2 sec (Average)
Errors   = 0

Cognitive Estimates

Error Score = 1 (Normal)

National Adult Reading Test

Predicted premorbid IQ = 120 (Superior)

1989

Wechsler Memory Scale-Revised

General memory index	=	69	(Impaired)
Verbal memory index	=	75	(Impaired)
Visual memory index	=	80	(Borderline)
Attention and concentration	=	99	(Average)
Delayed memory index	=	< 50	(Severely impaired)

Rivermead Behavioural Memory Test

Screening score   =   1   (Maximum 12) ⎫
Standardized profile score =   5   (Maximum 24) ⎬ (Severely impaired)

OUTPATIENT REHABILITATION

During the first 6 mo of his outpatient rehabilitation Jay began helping in his father's shop, so some of the strategies investigated during our sessions were put into practice in the work situation. With regard to treatment strategies investigated during June to December 1986, we concentrated on (1) external aids, (2) mnemonics, (3) rehearsal strategies, and (4) chaining. A summary of the treatment report of December 1986 reads as follows:

1. *External aids:* Jay uses his diary and notebook efficiently although he is likely to write the same thing twice. I gave him some information about the Casio® databank wristwatch and I understand his father is going to get one on approval.
2. *Mnemonics:* Jay is able to benefit from first letter mnemonics and from the face–name visual imagery procedure in an experimental setting. He claims to use the face–name method to help remember people when he is serving in his father's shop. I am sure the mnemonics are of limited value in everyday life but if he needs to learn certain limited pieces of information, mnemonics may help.
3. *Rehearsal:* I compared Jay's ability to recall verbal material using a. the PQRST method (Preview, Question, Read, State and Test; Robinson 1970[1]), and b. Rote rehearsal. He was able to learn some material with both methods. Neither was superior to the other. It would be worth investigating the method of expanding rehearsal (Landauer and Bjork, 1978).
4. *Chaining:* i.e., breaking a task down into small steps and teaching one step at a time. This method was used successfully to teach Jay short routes.

The conclusion to the 1986 report was as follows:

> Jay still has considerable memory problems although he retains some information reasonably well. For example, he gave a good and fairly detailed account of a recent trip to the USA but he repeated segments of the account during the same conversation and gave me the same account twice more during the same session. He still shows evidence of everyday memory difficulties. For example, he learned where my room was situated during July. In August I moved to another room further along the same corridor but Jay never learned the way to this room and still waits outside the original room. Obviously it is going to be enormously difficult for him to resume his studies. I am not sure if Jay and his father are aware of how handicapping his problems are. I have spoken to Mr. C. (SR.) on several occasions but I am not sure whether he is ready to be told that Jay is extremely unlikely to complete his degree. One of my difficulties is that I do not know what message the neurosurgeon has given the family. Perhaps the rather gloomy outlook should be broached by the neurosurgeon? Anyway, I am sending him a copy of this letter and will leave it in the hands of the Cambridge team to advise. I am willing to contact the family again if you think this is best.

[1]This is described more fully in the next chapter.

Jay went on to do well. He is now self employed, making cane furniture, and lives independently. This success has been achieved through heroic organization, hard work, intelligence, and sensible support from his family, in particular his aunt. Jay's system centers around a number of external memory aids of which the most important are his dictaphone, his personal organizer, and his alarm watch. The development of this very efficient system has taken years to perfect and even now, 10 yr after the hemorrhage, Jay is still modifying and refining his system. A summary of the natural history of Jay's compensation system follows.

THE DEVELOPMENT OF JAY'S SYSTEM

For the first few months after the hemorrhage Jay expected and hoped to get better and recover his memory functioning. By the end of the year however, coinciding with his outpatient rehabilitation with me, he realized the need to compensate for his damaged memory rather than expect memory recovery.

During the last 3 mo of 1986 Jay used a notebook that he kept in his shirt pocket together with a watch alarm that sounded every hour. Whenever the alarm sounded Jay noted what he was doing. Each evening he transferred this information to a journal but did little in the way of forward planning.

In January 1987 Jay devised his "Grand Plan." He had a weekly sheet of paper on his desk and a daily card, which he filled in with details from the weekly sheet and one-off appointments from his diary. He decided to write down *all* appointments as he had been somewhat careless about this procedure. In addition he decided to keep his daily card in his diary, place a written list of all his daily and weekly tasks on his desk, and check each evening that the weekly or one-off appointments were transferred to the daily card for the following day. His aunt or one of his sisters agreed to prompt him each evening to carry out the transfer of tasks. Jay says at this point he changed from thinking about loss of memory for the past to forward planning.

Soon afterwards he obtained a dictaphone to record ongoing events. Each evening he listened to his recordings and transcribed the information to a journal. He continues to do this today. At the beginning of this strategy Jay's aunt saw him almost every day to prompt, help, advise, and think of solutions to problems.

The next major step was for Jay to leave his parents' home and start up in his own flat, further along the same road. He removed his old front door key from his key ring so that he would not go to the old home by mistake. At this stage it was 19 months since the hemorrhage. Jay was living independently but with considerable support from his family.

The following month, in an attempt to solve another problem, one of Jay's sisters gave him a small loose leaf diary similar to a thin date book/personal organizer. Jay found that he would look through his diary to find some information but forget what it was he was looking for. Being able to remove a loose leaf page seemed to help. In January 1988 this loose leaf diary was replaced by a full-sized personal organizer. Jay still missed some appointments however because he forgot to set his watch alarm. This gradually improved over the next few months. At this stage Jay's aunt was seeing him three times a week.

In July 1988, Jay learned to type. He appears to have found little problem with this new skill, presumably because it depended on implicit learning, which is intact or relatively intact in people with amnesia. He learned to type because he wanted to see if he could use a computer to help him retrieve stored information. Although he continued toying with the idea of a computerized diary system, this ambition petered out after a few months because, I suspect, it was not portable enough for Jay's needs.

Not only had Jay learned to type but he had also discovered he had a practical ability. He said, "practical skills were developed without me being aware of how this came about. I could do things without being able to explain how." He decided to apply for a course at a college of furniture. He began in September 1988, just over $2^{1}/_{2}$ yr after his hemorrhage. He had maps showing him how to get to the college and kept a note handy telling himself to get on at the front of the train so that he would use the right exit at the station. Initially Jay went to college 3 days a week and then 4.

The following February Jay was given a new watch for entering messages and reminders. Instructions for putting information into the watch were written on a sheet of paper in his personal organizer. It took him 6 wk to memorize these instructions. He still uses the watch alarm regularly but finds it difficult to explain *how* to program it. Nevertheless he can program it without difficulty, presumably again because implicit learning is involved.

By April 1989 Jay's system was running fairly smoothly. He used his coat as a "base" when away from home, and in it he carried his dictaphone and personal organizer, and together with his alarm watch. These external aids enabled him to survive fairly independently. He used his dictaphone to plan his course work and found it was best to do the planning at the end of each lesson. His college folder had different sections for different skills.

Jay wanted to complete a 2nd yr at the college of furniture and for this he needed an application form. At his aunt's prompting he made a note on his dictaphone. In the evening he listened to the tape and wrote a note in his personal organizer about the need to request an application form. At the same time he set his watch alarm to sound at a suitable time when in college to remind him to look in his personal organizer. The alarm duly sounded, Jay looked in his personal organizer, saw the note, and spoke to his tutor. The tutor's response was recorded onto the dictaphone, Jay went immediately to fetch the form, and noted this on his dictaphone. Later that evening he took the forms to his regular meeting with his aunt and the two of them discussed the form, filled it in, and photocopied it. A note to this effect was recorded on the dictaphone. On returning home he filed one copy, placed the other with his college work, and set the alarm on his watch to remind him to hand in the form. He was duly accepted for a 2nd yr at college.

In September 1990 Jay began his new course. He used a London street map while traveling on the bus so that he would know when to alight. After 20 journeys he no longer required the street map. He also had a map of the college grounds to enable him to find the workshop and another to help him to make his way to an annex in another part of the grounds. He kept notes on bus numbers and positions of bus stops. His visits to his aunt now dropped to once a week.

The following year Jay refined his system still further having made a date with a girlfriend. The notes made on the dictaphone during the evening were put onto a yellow sheet with her name at the top. This sheet was placed in his organizer, and was called the *social sheet*. More sheets were added about his girlfriend, followed by sheets for other people. One colleague had nine social sheets with non-current ones placed in a reserve file. Jay put sticky backed notes on the sheets with suggestions and ideas for future joint activities, when to telephone again and so forth.

As the yellow social sheets were so successful Jay began using different colored sheets for different aspects of his life. Green sheets were used for work on his apartment, so, for example, he had a sheet for the plumber who was called regularly to clean the pilot light on the boiler. Details of what needed to be done were written on a note and stuck to the social sheet so that Jay knew what to say when he telephoned the plumber. Completed work was written up on the social sheet.

Red sheets denoted restaurants with their names, telephone numbers, addresses, and directions as well as information about favorite dishes. Pink sheets denoted leisure pursuits such as swimming pools, holidays, and so forth. Blue sheets were for work and will be described in more detail below.

Since 1992 Jay has been self employed as a French polisher and maker of cane chairs. Potential customers telephone and a job sheet is opened in his organizer. A job number is written on the sheet as well as details about the customer, type of work, date work commenced, deadline for completion, price quoted, and any other relevant details. The job number corresponds to a page in a book with duplicate sheets.

During the telephone call Jay takes the customer's details and agrees to a time when he will provide a quotation. He makes a note on the relevant daily sheet, "To job 122." He also sets his watch alarm to make sure he will leave in good time. He provides the quotation for the job and leaves the top copy from the duplicate book as a record of what has been agreed. Jay and the customer also agree when the completed work is to be collected or delivered. Jay notes on his daily sheet in the organizer when he will carry out the work and also sets the watch alarm to remind him to do this. He notes how long he spends on the work and enters this information in the job book and on the job sheet. He also notes the cost of the materials. When the customer pays this is recorded in the job book and the job sheet in the organizer is discarded.

The colored sheets provide a cross referencing capability and a capacity to retrieve information, which Jay feels is of more value than a computer because (1) several sheets can be viewed at a time, (2) the system is more portable, (3) it is less prone to theft, and (4) the colored sheets are very easy to find in his personal organizer.

Since his hemorrhage Jay has needed to eat regularly or else he gets very short tempered. From 1988 he has used a system to ensure he has a balanced diet and eats seasonal foods. For this he uses a menu chart that is planned every few weeks for the meals he eats alone or with friends. He cross references the menu chart with his organizer, noting when he will be eating out and when friends will be coming over. The menu chart is kept in the kitchen. He also uses sticky-backed notes to remind him to make his packed lunch or to remind him that he has already made his lunch. These notes are kept on a cupboard in the kitchen ready for use.

In addition to the menu chart Jay uses other kinds of lists for such purposes as shopping—he writes down information as food or household items begin to run out. He also attaches a check to the shopping list if he needs to go to the bank. There are also telephone lists in which he logs all calls to make sure they are not duplicated. He puts a note in his organizer to remind himself to make a call and he enters this onto the watch alarm. Once he has made a call he checks the note so he knows he has made it, he enters details of the call on to the appropriate social sheet or job sheet, and he makes a recorded note on the dictaphone.

Although the main strategies have been described here there are others that Jay uses in certain situations. For example, when leaving his seat on a train or an airplane he repeats continuously something like "Fourth row on the right, " or whatever. In his flat he always keeps everything in the same place and returns things to their rightful place after use. He follows certain routines to avoid errors. For example, he always follows the same procedure when going to or getting up from bed. When he is with other people he firmly asks for space to process information straight away, before he forgets. Thus when seeing me in Cambridge he interrupts regularly to record what we are discussing. These recorded messages are transcribed into a journal in the evening. The journals are kept in a locked trunk.

JAY TODAY

At the time of writing in 1997 Jay is independent and visits his aunt only when something difficult occurs such as having to deal with bureaucratic problems. He has in the past gone through times when he has felt very low and sad about his life. He was expecting to be a lawyer with a good income and has instead become a craftsman with just enough to live on. However, by and large his mood remains good. He is very active in a local self-help and support group for people with memory problems following brain injury. He has appeared on television and radio in documentary programs about amnesia and has come to gain self-esteem through realizing the extent of his achievements in the face of severe organic memory impairment.

Jay once said to me, "I try to make the system foolproof. It's like a web, it's hard for anything to slip through the system. If I miss it with one thing, I'll pick it up with another. I've individualized the system. It's constantly developing and I'm constantly refining and correcting it."

Although Jay's system is not absolutely foolproof there is no doubt that he has developed an extremely effective compensatory method that enables him to live independently and earn his own living. This is a monumental achievement for someone with such severe memory impairment.

Finally, we must ask why it is that Jay has succeeded when most others in a similar situation would fail? Wilson and Watson (1996) made some predictions about the successful use of compensations by memory impaired people. They found that being younger than 30 yr of age at the time of insult was associated with independence, and Jay was 20 yr old at the time of his hemorrhage. They found that memory impaired people without additional cognitive deficits were more likely to compensate adequately and be more independent than those with more widespread problems, and of course Jay has a pure amnesic syndrome. A magnetic resonance imaging (MRI) scan was carried out recently and from this it can be seen that his lesions are restricted to the hippocampal area, with minor damage caused by the surgery performed to clip his aneurysm (Fig. 4.1).

Wilson and Watson (ibid.) also noted that people obtaining at least 3 screening points on the Rivermead Behavioural Memory Test were more likely to compensate and be independent than those scoring 2 or less. Although this was not true of Jay, who scored only 1 on the test each time he was tested, it would seem that this discrepancy can be explained by Jay's superior intelligence. As noted earlier, Jay's frontal lobes were not affected at all by the hemorrhage and, by his own account, he was always extremely well organized, even as a small child. Thus the combination of youth, intelligence, organized behavior, determination, lack of additional cognitive deficits, and of course a fully supportive and imaginative family who worked with him at every stage of his progress, goes a long way in explaining Jay's achievements. He also had several months of rehabilitation, both as an inpatient and outpatient. Although the effect of this cannot be measured, there is some evidence to suggest that people receiving rehabilitation do better in the long run than those who do not (Brooks 1991; Cope et al., 1991; Greenwood and McMillan 1993; McMillan and Greenwood 1993).

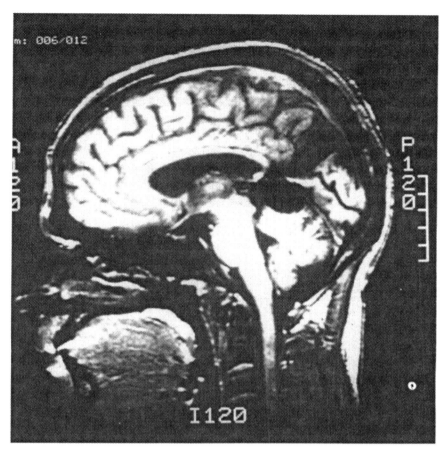

Figure 4.1. Jay's MRI Scan.

An interesting comment made by Jay in his account of his system was that he learned practical skills without knowing how he learned them. In common with other amnesic people, Jay's implicit memory appeared normal and he was undoubtedly using this intact memory system when learning some of the skills he demonstrated in his daily routine. His aunt notes that he learned to type without consciously being aware of how he achieved this skill, and this is a good example of procedural or implicit learning. The fact that Jay successfully completed a course at a furniture college is probably due in part to the fact that he was able to bring his implicit memory into play. Jay himself feels that his ability to learn practical skills was a big advantage. He also said that he considered it a big step forward when he started to do things twice, as this proved "the system was beginning to work." He then had to refine procedures to prevent himself from repeating things. As I said earlier, the system is not perfect and he finds, for example, that at times he telephones people twice with the same information. Nevertheless, he has achieved an impressive level of independence in the face of a severe amnesic syndrome.

While most other memory impaired people may be less intelligent than Jay, and less fortunate in that most are likely to suffer more general damage involving cognitive skills other than memory, Jay's success shows what can be achieved by patience, ingenuity, and commitment, as exhibited by himself and other members of his family. Although the degree of sophistication reached by Jay in his use of compensatory memory aids may be beyond the level likely to be achieved by less gifted individuals, his efforts can at least be emulated in treatment programs that of necessity will require more intensive rehabilitation and support along the way.

5

ALEX: SOME RECOVERY, RETURN TO WORK, AND MARRIAGE FOLLOWING ANOXIC BRAIN DAMAGE

BACKGROUND

Alex was the oldest of three boys born to a family in the West of England. On leaving school he decided to spend a few months in Australia before taking up a university place. Although the details are not clear, it appears that while vacationing on the Queensland coast, Alex, then aged 19 yr, went to a barbecue beach party and engaged in some heavy drinking. The following morning he went on a diving trip and almost drowned. One report states that he was resuscitated on the beach for a period of 10 min or so before any spontaneous breathing occurred. He was admitted to the intensive care unit of a nearby hospital where he was placed on a ventilator. On the very first day there he was, apparently, only extending his arms to pain, suggesting fairly severe brain damage. However, a CT scan showed no significant abnormality. The following day Alex opened his eyes and obeyed simple commands. As a result of this improvement he was taken off the ventilator approximately 56 h after the accident. Soon after this he was able to speak to his parents who, having heard the news of the accident, had traveled out from England on the first available flight. They found Alex to be excited, hyperactive, and with a memory span of only a few seconds.

As far as we know from reports at the time, when Alex first recovered consciousness he had a retrograde amnesia, that is a memory gap, of about 3 mo.

55

This gradually shrank until he was able to remember the barbecue on the beach that took place the night before the diving accident. He was reported as being in post-traumatic amnesia for about 3 days, although it is unclear how this was established given the persistence of his memory problems.

Why did the accident occur? There is some suggestion that Alex had developed epilepsy prior to his visit to Australia. At the age of 17 yr he is believed to have sustained an epileptic seizure while watching television. He fell off the chair and was unconscious for a few minutes. There was no incontinence and no tremor. One of his brothers witnessed the attack. Epilepsy was considered a possibility and anticonvulsants were prescribed. Alex's parents also reported that 2 mo prior to the near drowning, Alex had been admitted to a hospital in Australia after he had become ill following a party. On this occasion he remained in the hospital overnight. From these reports it would seem possible that the heavy drinking at the barbecue party triggered off a seizure that occurred while Alex was swimming in the sea the next day. Some Australians present at the diving expedition wondered if Alex had been hyperventilating prior to his dive. This widely used technique among divers to increase their time under water can also aggravate epileptic tendencies.

A few weeks later, Alex returned to England with his parents and was assessed by various people. At this time he was assisting his parents in their farming activities. He was referred to me in September 1985 and I saw him as an outpatient in October of that year, that is 4 mo after his accident.

THE ASSESSMENT

When I first saw Alex, he had recently seen a psychologist who had administered some neuropsychological tests. The subsequent report suggested Alex's predicted premorbid IQ was in the superior range of ability, his forward digit span was above average, although his backward digit span was poor. He also did poorly on the Rey Auditory Verbal Learning Test, suggesting that he would find academic work difficult.

I saw Alex on five occasions between October and December. Two of these were for assessment and three were to discuss treatment strategies. One or both of his parents accompanied him on the long car journey to London where I was then working. Alex was assessed on the Wechsler Adult Intelligence Scale, The Rivermead Behavioural Memory Test, the Recognition Memory Test (Words and Faces), the Rey-Osterreith Complex Figure (Copy and Recall), Corsi Blocks, the Semantic Processing Test, the Modified Wisconsin Card Sorting Test, and Verbal Fluency ("s," "v," and "animals"). The results can be seen in Table 5.1.

These results suggested that Alex's verbal IQ was above average and fairly

Table 5.1. Alex's Main Neuropsychological Test Results

Wechsler Adult Intelligence Scale

VERBAL SUBTESTS	AGE SCALED SCORES	PERFORMANCE SUBTESTS	AGE SCALED SCORES
Information	14	Picture competitions	11
Digit span	10	Picture arrangement	10
Vocabulary	14	Block design	11
Arithmetic	15	Object assembly	5
Comprehension	9	Digit symbol	7
Similarities	11		

Verbal IQ	114	(Above average)
Performance IQ	92	(Low average)
Full scale IQ	105	(Average)

Rivermead Behavioural Memory Test

Screening score	3/12	(Moderately)
Standardized profile score	12/24	(Impaired)

Recognition Memory Test

Words	Age scaled score	4	(Below 5th percentile)
Faces	Age scaled score	2	(Below 5th percentile)

Rey-Osterreith Complex Figure

Copy	31/36	(Low average)
Recall	8/36	(Impaired)
Percentage retained	25.8	(Impaired)

Immediate Memory Span

Corsi blocks	5	(Average)
Forward digits	7	(Average)
Backward digits	4	(Low average)

Prose Recall

Immediate	4	(Low average)
Delayed	0	(Severely impaired)

Semantic Processing Test

Number completed in 2 min	36
Age scaled score	6
Mean time per item	3.33 sec
Errors	1

(Below average for speed of information processing)

(continued)

Table 5.1. Alex's Main Neuropsychological Test Results (*continued*)

Modified Wisconsin Card Sorting Test

Categories   =   6 ⎤
Total errors =   3 ⎦   (Normal performance)

Fluency

"S"   90 sec   13   plus 1 perseveration
"V"   90 sec   6
"Animals" 90 sec   24
(Within normal limits)

close to the predicted IQ from the earlier psychological assessment. The big discrepancy between an age-scaled score of 9 for comprehension and 15 for arithmetic implies, however, some cognitive decline as a consequence of the anoxic episode. The performance IQ was below average and this, together with the large verbal-performance discrepancy of 22 points, is further evidence of cognitive impairment as a result of the near drowning incident.

The major area of difficulty for Alex was, without doubt, memory. Despite a normal immediate memory span he had considerable episodic memory difficulties for both recall and recognition, and for both visual and verbal material.

In addition to the formal tests Alex and his mother were asked to rate Alex's everyday memory problems using the adapted Kapur and Pearson (1983) rating scale. Alex rated his major problems as being (1) remembering the day of the week; (2) remembering things he had been told; (3) remembering where he had put things; and (4) remembering how to get to somewhere he had been to only once or twice previously. His mother agreed with him on the day of the week and where he had put things but felt, overall, he was only slightly worse now than before his accident. From a maximum rating of 24 (with 0 being equal to no more difficulty now than before the accident), Alex's self rating was 13 and his mother's was 9. It is unusual for relatives to rate lower than brain injured people themselves and this may mean that Alex's mother was trying to deny the severity of her son's everyday memory problems.

When asked what strategies he was using to help overcome the difficulties, Alex and his mother reported six: a diary, a personal organizer, a notebook, a calendar, a memo board, and repetition and rehearsal.

On the basis of the assessment, the family was offered three sessions to discuss ways of helping Alex to by-pass or compensate for his memory problems. Although this was not considered ideal, the family lived a long way away and it was not realistic to see them weekly or fortnightly, as we were able to with Jack (Chapter 3) and Jay (Chapter 4).

EARLY TREATMENT

The aims of the three therapy sessions were twofold: first, to find ways of helping Alex by-pass his memory problems, and second, to find ways of improving learning. We tried to meet the first aim by considering available external aids. We looked at particular aids, discussed advantages and disadvantages, and encouraged Alex to practice using some of them. He was reasonably successful at using his diary, personal organizer, and so forth but was not particularly systematic or efficient.

With regard to the second aim, improving learning, a number of mnemonic strategies were demonstrated to Alex and his mother. In particular, we used (1) PQRST, (2) first letter cueing, (3) method of loci, (4) the Crovitz Story Method, and (5) Face–Name Association Procedure. These are described briefly below.

1. *PQRST* is an acronym for *Preview, Question, Read, State, and Test,* which comes from the field of study techniques. Robinson (1970) was probably the first person to describe PQRST. A similar method is known as SQR3 (Rowntree, 1983) which stands for *Survey, Question, Read, Recall, Review.* In practice, the stages of both techniques are virtually identical. The procedure in PQRST is as follows:

   a. PREVIEW: Preview the material to be remembered, that is, skim through it briefly.
   b. QUESTION: Ask important questions about the text.
   c. READ: Read the material thoroughly in order to answer questions.
   d. STATE: State the answers. If the answers to key questions are not clear, read through again until they are.
   e. TEST: Test at frequent intervals for the retention of information.

   In 1987 I described a number of studies (Wilson, 1987d) comparing rote rehearsal with PQRST. In each case PQRST was the superior method.
2. *First letter cuing* uses initial letters to act as retrieval cues and is commonly used in everyday situations. Gruneberg (1973) points out that 53% of undergraduates use the method for finals revision. Higbee (1978) reminds us that first letter cueing may be used for learning the names of the cranial nerves: the rhyme begins "On Old Olympus Towering Tops." Rawles (1978) also reports that this method was used by Royal Air Force pilots during the second world war to enable them to remember action drill.
3. *The Method of Loci* or "place method" is an ancient one that can be extremely complex. Rawles (1978), for example, describes a scheme devised in the Middle Ages by Petrus Ravennas, in which 100,000 different loci were used.

4. *The Story Method* was based on Crovitz's (1979) "Airplane List" in which the 10 words to be remembered are embedded in a story. Crovitz (1979) attempted to train three brain injured patients to produce their own bizarre stories, and concluded that "bizarreness" was not a crucial feature. Gianutsos and Gianutsos (1987) also used the story method to improve recall of brain injured people. Cermak (1980) describes a similar procedure to remember an unusual name, and the example he gives is turning *Chowmentowski* into a phrase, *Show men to ski.* A colleague once described to me the way he used the story method to remember directions for getting to a particular place in London. The streets involved were *Cannon Street, Queen Victoria Street, Threadneedle Street,* and *Broad Street.* His story was as follows: "A cannon was fired at Queen Victoria who was threading a needle to mend her drawers before going abroad."

5. *Visual mnemonics* have been employed for many centuries (Yates, 1966) and have been adapted for use in memory therapy. One commonly used mnemonic is the simple procedure of turning a word or name into a picture. "Neil Kinnock" for example, can be drawn as a kneeling king knocking at a door. Although one should not expect an amnesic person to use this method spontaneously, it is useful for teaching that person a few names of those with whom s/he comes into daily contact.

   Gruneberg et al. (1991) used visual mnemonics with people who had developmental learning difficulties. The value in the method is that people learn more quickly using it than they do when relying upon repetition or rote rehearsal (see Wilson, 1987d for research findings concerning this procedure).

6. *Face–Name Association* is a more sophisticated version of visual imagery to learn names and involves four stages: (a) selecting a distinctive feature of a person's face (e.g., large ears); (b) transforming the name to one or more common nouns (e.g., "Mr. Crosley" could be imagined as a cross leaf or a leaf on a cross); (c) linking the distinctive feature with the transformed name (e.g., imagining the cross leaf sticking out from large ears); and (d) when needing to remember the person's name, searching the face for the distinctive feature to be reminded of the image that should help recall of name.

Mnemonics are successful in assisting learning because (1) they encourage a deeper level of processing, and, as Craik and Lockhart (1972) demonstrated, deeper processing results in better recall); (2) previously isolated items are integrated with one another (Bower, 1972); and (3) they provide inbuilt retrieval cues in the form of initial letters, locations, or pegs.

Alex also did better in experimental situations when remembering stories or lists of words with a strategy was compared to learning without a strategy. All the mnemonics described above resulted in more material being retained than when simple repetition was employed. I have argued elsewhere (Wilson, 1992) that mnemonic strategies are difficult for amnesic people to use spontaneously in new situations. Their main advantage is that *therapists* and *relatives* can use them with memory impaired people to speed and enhance learning. Thus, in December 1985, at the end of the three therapy sessions, suggestions were provided for Alex and his parents so that his parents could try them out with Alex.

Alex's rehabilitation, then, was far more superficial than that provided for Jack in Chapter 3, but like Jay in Chapter 4, contact was maintained with the family and advice given at intervals over the following years.

1 YEAR AFTER THE ACCIDENT

In June 1986 Alex came back for a reassessment of his memory. His RBMT score had increased slightly: his screening score had moved from 3 to 4, and his standardized profile score from 12 to 14, both still remaining in the moderately impaired band. On the Rey-Osterreith Figure, Alex's score for the copy was also a little better, he now scored 33, well in the average range, while his recall had increased from 8 to 13. The recognition memory test for faces also showed a little improvement and his age scaled score was now a fairly respectable 8. There was no change however on his recognition memory score for words. The semantic processing test result suggested his speed of information processing had increased. He was now able to complete 56 items in 2 min, that is, a mean time of 2.14 sec per item, with no errors and an average score for someone of his age. He had also shown a marginal improvement on the digit symbol subtest of the WAIS.

The main concerns for Alex and his family at this stage, however, were driving a car and further education. Both of these issues arose in the discussion following his assessment.

Driving

Alex had obtained a full driving licence when he was 17 yr old but some months later, after his suspected seizure had occurred at home, he was diagnosed as having epilepsy and prescribed sodium valproate, an anticonvulsant. Because British law requires people with epilepsy to have 2 yr free from seizure before being allowed to drive, Alex had to return his driving licence and refrain from driving.

The sodium valproate was stopped at the end of 1985 and no further seizures followed. In June 1986 I put Alex in touch with a center specializing in driving assessments for people with disabilities. I also referred him to a consultant specializing in epilepsy and driving, and in my letter to the consultant I suggested that from a cognitive point of view there was no reason for Alex not to drive. In September Alex and his mother went to see the consultant who arranged for an electroencephalogram (EEG) that indicated that Alex did indeed have epilepsy. This meant that Alex was legally required to remain seizure free for 2 yr before his driving licence could be returned. Alex fulfilled the conditions and his driving licence was returned in 1987.

Further Education

Alex obtained a place at a college to read for a degree in environmental biology. I was asked to contact the college to explain the nature of Alex's difficulties and to find out if the counseling service would "keep an eye on him." I wrote a brief outline of Alex's recent history and described his problems. I indicated that Alex would find a degree course harder than he expected and, although capable of learning new things, his learning was slower than his general intellectual ability would imply. Nevertheless, it would be wrong to conclude, as does sometimes happen with memory impaired people, that Alex's slow learning was the result of laziness or carelessness. I also pointed out that Alex had lost his self-confidence as a result of the anoxic episode, so needed someone to take a special interest in him. Needless to say, I offered to provide further information and keep in touch as requested.

Alex took 2 yr to complete his 1st yr, and as a result of all the difficulties he faced during those years, never managed to complete the degree course. He considered a number of options before finding work as a salesman, first in a bookshop and later in a department store.

FOLLOW-UP

For a while I had regular news about Alex from his mother. In 1987 Deborah Wearing and I founded the *Amnesia Association* (Wearing, 1992), and Alex's mother became an active member. At each meeting she passed on news of her son and sometimes asked for advice about his memory problems and career. In March 1988 she asked if I would see him again to discuss his future plans so I met him in April of that year, when he was still at college although considering changing his course. When asked how things were progressing he said there were high and low spots and that the former were connected with the people he met while the latter involved the taking of examinations.

I readministered the Kapur and Pearson (1983) rating scale, which showed that his own rating of his everyday memory problems was identical to the rating he gave in 1985. Of the total score of 13 out of a maximum of 24, there were two slight changes in composition: (1) he now rated his ability to remember the date as being a little worse than before the accident (rather than a lot worse) because he now used a watch with the date on it; and (2) he now rated his ability to remember things he had seen as a lot worse than before (rather than a little worse). In general Alex's memory appeared to be better although I did not give him any formal memory tests. The fact that he achieved the same score on the rating scale might suggest he had better insight in 1988.

We discussed Alex's course and I learned that he had to pass two further modules before the end of the year in order to remain at college. He wanted to switch to a course in hotel management and catering but this course was not offered at his college. He had also considered the army and the tourist industry but no real decisions were possible at this meeting in which I acted as a listener. He felt that he would not get a degree but would be able to get through the first yr in order to gain a certificate.

In July 1989, just over 4 yr since his accident, I saw Alex again as part of a follow-up study of memory impaired patients. By then he had moved to another town and was working in a bookshop. He had worked in several jobs prior to this position, including work as a college handyman and work in a festival box office.

In reply to a question of mine about his problems, he said: "The main one is making arrangements and forgetting to keep them. That's always happening." When asked if he had other problems he replied: "I also haven't got to grips with writing things in the same place. I write everything down but it's all in different places." He said he either did not have further problems, or, if he did, he could not remember them.

He had a steady girlfriend named Liz, and was of the opinion that he participated in a reasonable social life and was therefore not lonely. He was using nine strategies to help with his memory problems, these being an alarm clock, a watch with the date, a personal organizer, a daily journal, a notebook, lists of things to do, a wall calendar, mental retracing (that is, trying to remember what he did or where he was earlier when he had lost something), and asking other people to remind him to do things.

In the follow-up study (Wilson, 1991b), I found that memory impaired people using six or more strategies were significantly more likely to be independent (defined as either "in paid employment," "living alone," or "in full time education"). Viewed in this way, Alex could be regarded as independent. His RBMT assessment had jumped from a screening score of 4 to 10, and his standardized profile score from 14 to 22, thus putting him in the normal range. A probable explanation for this score at a normal level is that Alex employed compensatory strategies during the assessment. The RBMT is, to a large extent, a measure of coping skills, and predicts independence in everyday life (Wilson, 1991b). Alex, as we know, was independent and thus able to succeed in this everyday memory test.

Alex was also assessed on the Wechsler Memory Scale-Revised and his results were as follows: general memory 91 (low average); verbal memory 86 (low average); visual memory 103 (average); attention and concentration 97 (average); and delayed memory 76 (impaired).

My conclusions about Alex at this time were that although he had shown some recovery his ability to retain information after a delay was still poor. Nevertheless he had managed to hold down a job, was able to engage in a stable relationship, and could certainly be regarded as one of the successes in my follow-up group.

ALEX TODAY

I heard little of Alex for several years until a call came from his mother one weekend. Alex, now married and with a baby daughter, was finding life stressful. His mother wondered whether I could suggest anyone who might be able to see him for some counseling. I mentioned a colleague who worked close to Alex's home, who had worked closely with brain injured people for a long time and was sensitive and sensible. Later a meeting was arranged between this colleague and Alex and his wife. It was clear at the meeting that Alex was exhausted with the efforts required to cope with a full-time job and a family that included a young child. Alex was encouraged to take a break from his work and then return to part-time work. Fortunately his employers were sympathetic and agreed to these changes. They had in fact been informed of Alex's history when he first joined the company but as time passed, and Alex seemed to be coping very well, they had forgotten about his problems. As a result of the change to part-time working, Alex and his family appeared to benefit from a reduction in stress.

Soon after this I visited Alex, in June 1996, 11 yr since the near drowning. We met at the railway station and walked to his house about 10 min away. If I had not known his story I would have thought that there was nothing wrong with Alex. He was a polite, sociable, and likeable person who hid his problems well. I met Liz, his wife, and their delightful baby daughter who was 16 mo old at the time. I wanted to know how he felt about the original accident and about his life today. The following is a transcript of the conversation between Alex, Liz, and myself.

BAW: How do you think you have changed as a result of the accident?

ALEX: Before going to Australia I was more confident and more sociable. This has changed quite a lot. My confidence is down and that affects every-thing.

BAW: I know you won't remember but what do you understand about the accident?

ALEX: I'd been holidaying up the coast and there'd been some heavy drinking. The next morning I went out to clear my head and I blacked out. The next thing I remember is mum and dad coming into my room. I'd had the kiss of life, the person I was with was a trained life saver. There was a doctor there knowledgeable about my type of injury. I was in a coma and they were trying to bring me out and he said, 'No, not yet.'

BAW: You were probably sedated.

ALEX: Every time my mother came in, even if she'd only gone out for a few minutes, I said, 'What are you doing here?' That soon loses its appeal. I probably did this for several weeks. After some time, I don't know how long, I came back (to England) with my parents.

BAW: What happened after you came back?

ALEX: For a while I was around the farm, then I did a computer course, I don't know when and for how long. After I saw you in London I helped to build a barn. That was probably before the computer course—it was for some neighbors. It was fairly simple stuff and good for a while. Then I went on a B. Tech (Bachelor of Technology) course I was not officially on the course but I was allowed to sit in.

In 1986 I started at the Polytechnic. It was frustrating that I didn't do well. It wasn't that I *couldn't* do it but I *didn't* do it. I forgot the assignments. Liz was in the same hall of residence doing history.

LIZ: I went into Alex's room for coffee. I thought what an awful mess, it was amazingly untidy and chaotic. I felt sorry for the woman who would ever marry him. The next year we shared a house. Alex's mother said, 'You'll probably have to remind Alex to pay his bills.' I thought what a funny thing to say. When I told Alex later, he said, 'That's because of my memory problems. I just thought he was scatty.'

ALEX: I didn't finish the course. I took 2 yr to pass the 1st yr. It was a modular course so I could have stayed and got a poor degree and that wouldn't have helped. I left the Poly and carried on living in the same city. I did a number of jobs and still lived in the same house. My friends were doing their finals. Then we moved to this town and I started working in the book shop when it first opened. Liz had got a college place to do her Post Graduate Certificate of Education and that's why we moved here. My parents helped with the house. In 1990 Liz started teaching and the following month I changed jobs to a department store.

LIZ: We got married in August 1991. Emily was born in 1995.

BAW: Tell me a bit more about the work situation.

ALEX: I worked in fairly menial posts and then as a sales assistant. They don't think I would be good management material. They don't see me as someone with memory problems.

BAW: Do you see yourself as someone with memory problems?

ALEX: Yes, I still get frustrated. The main thing is confidence. I can't say, 'I'll be there then.' I have to say, 'I'll try to be there then.' Liz does most of the reminding.

LIZ: He needs an awful lot of sleep, he gets very tired and very cross with himself. He repeats questions a lot. If we're going to do something he forgets. For example, some friends came, we were going to take their little boy to the park. Alex went to put the rubbish out and got sidetracked and started doing something else. It was very irritating. Recently we tried to come to terms with it. Alex kept forgetting to help, to do little things and it's very hard with a new baby. Then we saw your colleague as a result of Alex's mother telephoning you. It was a big relief when the employers were told about Alex's memory problems. It was on file but they'd forgotten. We went to see their doctor and they've been incredibly understanding. Why didn't we do this earlier?

ALEX: If we're going out and Liz says, 'Where shall we go?' I can't remember the options but I wouldn't say this until recently. I can't remember routes. I have to drive to the middle of town to look at the signposts because that's where they are although it's often quicker to go another way.

LIZ: Since I understand more Alex hasn't been so tired. I'll take the lead, for example, about when it's time to go back to our car. He's working part time now and that's much easier. S...(the colleague who had provided counseling) gave us permission not to cope. She understood. She told us to take time off.

BAW: Can you tell me a bit about your coping strategies?

ALEX: I try to write everything down.

LIZ: Every night we talk through the day and what we're both doing the next day. We pin it up in the bedroom so Alex can go and check up if I'm not here. He'd forget to ask me. If, for example, I'd been to the doctor, he'd forget to ask me how it went. Now it's more organized I do all of the driving unless Alex particularly asks, so he's fresh when we get somewhere and he can shut his eyes when we're in the car.

Alex can lead a normal life but at a gentler pace now, without rushing things and knowing it's not going to be impossible. We don't arrange more than one thing in a day. We spread it out really. It's a hidden problem so people expect Alex to be 100% normal like when his brother and girlfriend came.

ALEX: Those 3 hours of being normal were totally exhausting.

LIZ: People don't realize that things get worse if Alex is anxious or tired.

BAW: Is there anything else you'd like to say?

ALEX: Because I've got a bad memory it doesn't mean I'm intellectually impaired. People talk down to me, they see the handicap and not the person.

LIZ: The biggest thing is your confidence in yourself is low. It's an immense frustration, particularly in the work situation. He's stuck in menial jobs. Intellectually he's much more capable but organizationally he isn't able.

We always put things in the same place or there's a major panic. The diary is by the phone. He has a piece of paper for the day.

ALEX: I can't carry my personal organizer at work, it doesn't fit into my pocket. I phone Liz every day at lunch time to see what I should be doing and I take a mobile phone with me when I'm going out.

BAW: We've been investigating a paging system in Cambridge. It's called *NeuroPage®* and was designed by the father of a young man with memory problems following a head injury. The father is an engineer. He designed the system with a neuropsychologist. You simply wear a pager on your belt. We work out with you what messages you need to receive and at what time. We put the messages onto a computer and at the right time the message comes to your pager. It beeps, you look down and see the message. You can clear the message by pressing the one button on the pager and you can get the message back again by pressing the button once more. If the beeping is inappropriate at work we can set it so the pager vibrates instead. It just might be the answer for you. I'll arrange for one of my colleagues to come down so you can try it out.

On my return to Cambridge I arranged for my colleague Hazel Emslie to see Alex and sort out the pager for him. Alex is currently trying the *NeuroPage®* system (Hersh and Treadgold, 1994; Wilson et al., 1997), and it appears to be helping him with some of his problems.

Although Alex and Liz have some frustrations and stresses caused by the memory impairments, there is little doubt that Alex has achieved an enormous amount. He holds down a job, has married, and has become a father since his accident. Relatively few brain injured people achieve all of these things. It is an enormous effort for him to cope with everyday life, which explains his phenomenal need for sleep. Despite the frustration caused by difficulties arising from her husband's memory impairment, such as listening to the same questions over and over again, Liz has succeeded in taking on many more responsibilities than other wives. I can appreciate the difficulties they face in their daily lives, and sympathize with the stress they experience as they try to come to terms with the extra burdens they carry. Nevertheless, from a neuropsychological point of view, Alex has done extraordinarily well. He is a credit to his parents, his wife and, above all, to himself. It is up to individuals and groups within Alex and Liz's community to recognize these extra burdens (as indeed his employers seem to have done) and make the necessary adjustments required to see the intelligence and indeed the person behind the handicap.

.

MEMORY AND OTHER COGNITIVE PROBLEMS

Most memory impaired people have additional cognitive problems such as impaired attention, word-finding difficulties, slowed thinking, and poor reasoning or judgment. It is much harder for these people to compensate well because skills needed to find ways around difficulties are compromised along with memory skills.

Efficient use of external memory aids such as that shown by Jay in the previous section, is virtually impossible because using an aid not only involves memory but also planning and organization. For aids to be beneficial they must be very simple to use (for example, the pager described in the chapter about Alex), and even then may not be sufficient to solve the problem. Lorna (Chapter 8), for example, once tried our paging system but was unable to act upon the message she received.

People with widespread difficulties can often only benefit from environmental adaptations, i.e., structure or organize their environment in order to avoid or by-pass memory problems. Another way to think about this is that the environment provides the cues to remember. Environmental organization or adaptation is the simplest way to help people with cognitive problems. For example, memory impaired people can be provided with kettles, electric lights, and cookers that turn themselves off after a certain interval and thus avoid dangers and risks. People who forget where things are kept or forget where the bathroom is may be helped if closets and doors are labeled or painted a very distinctive color. A line may be drawn on the floor to help someone remember the way from the kitchen or to the bathroom. Signposts may be erected directing them to the bedroom and the garden. Positioning objects so they cannot be missed or forgotten is another helpful strategy. Examples include clipping a key ring to the memory impaired person's belt and using a neck cord to prevent spectacles being lost. It is sometimes possible to eliminate or reduce constant questioning by identifying the verbal trigger that elicits the repetition and avoiding its use. Two of the patients in this section benefited from this approach—Clive (Chapter 6) and Martin (Chapter 7).

Even people with numerous and widespread problems can learn some new information or skills under certain circumstances. One useful strategy to enhance their learning is to avoid trial-and-error approaches. In order to benefit from our mistakes we need to be able to remember our mistakes. If we cannot remember our errors we cannot learn from them. Errorless learning, described in the next section, has also helped the people described in this section.

Included here are four people: Clive who survived encephalitis 12 yr ago; Martin who sustained a head injury followed by a blood clot and later a brain infection; Lorna who has a slowly progressive condition; and Jason who also survived encephalitis, which left him with memory and reading difficulties. Three of these people live in residential care and none are independent but all have learned some skills and information.

6

CLIVE: THE MAN WHO CONTINUES TO HAVE JUST WOKEN UP

BACKGROUND

At the age of 46 yr Clive was an outstanding musician, a gifted musical scholar, and one of the world's leading authorities on Renaissance music. Wilson and Wearing (1995) describe the enthusiastic and exhaustive manner in which Clive would conduct his research, the excitement he obtained from his musical studies, and the manner in which he was able to pass on this excitement to others. Historians of music agreed that Clive's concerts of early music were researched in the minutest detail and were considered to be the "next best thing to going back in time." For example, Clive would investigate all aspects of the original performance, including local pronunciation, the manner in which voices carried in the concert room, and the tones of voice used by singers. With the aid of dictionaries and tracts he translated whatever he required, from medieval church Latin as pronounced in Renaissance Bavaria to sixteenth century Neapolitan dialect. For his part in the British Broadcasting Company's wedding day celebration of Prince Charles and Lady Diana Spencer, Clive chose to reconstruct the 1568 wedding of Duke Wilhelm of Bavaria: he unearthed the original music, translated a contemporary account of its performance, and edited the original score.

Prior to joining the national radio's classical music station in 1983, Clive was for 25 yr a freelance conductor, musicologist, and singer. While continuing his exhaustive studies he still found time to sing daily at Westminster Cathedral. He typically worked 7 days a week until late at night, rarely taking breaks or vacations. Everything he undertook was carried out rigorously, in great depth, and with integrity. Then, just as his career was reaching a peak, he was struck down with an illness that robbed him of virtually all of his memory functioning. For several months he had suffered from exhaustion and increasing headaches until one Saturday afternoon he asked his wife, who had begun to play her violin, to stop because the pain in his head was so intense. This headache became even more acute over the next few days and he developed a high fever and photophobia. Two doctors diagnosed influenza.

Clive had great difficulty sleeping because of the intense pain in his head, then on Wednesday morning, having a very high temperature, he became confused and unable to answer the simplest questions. Once again the local doctor was called, said the confusion was due to lack of sleep and prescribed sleeping tablets. Clive's wife was told to expect her husband to be "out for 8 hours." She was due to give a lecture that afternoon and, expecting Clive to remain asleep, decided to honor her commitment. On returning home however she found her husband was missing. She called the police who began a search. Meanwhile a taxi driver had taken Clive to a police station. It appeared that while his wife was away Clive had woken up, gone out, and hailed a taxi. As he was unable to give an address, the taxi driver took Clive to the police station where his identity was established through a credit card in his wallet. The police telephoned Clive's wife who then hurried to the police station and brought him home.

When Clive arrived home he did not recognize his apartment. Two doctors visited and maintained their diagnosis of influenza with "meningitis-like" symptoms. Clive slept for most of the following day. By Friday morning the 6th day of the headache, his temperature had fallen but his wife became increasingly alarmed at Clive's odd behavior: he failed to identify the toilet in his own bathroom and his physical movements became very disorganized. A doctor arrived just before 8.00 A.M., called the emergency services, and left. Clive was admitted to the hospital at 9.00 A.M. Eleven hours later, a diagnosis of herpes simplex virus encephalitis (HSVE) was confirmed. He was treated with acyclovir, an antiviral drug, which probably saved his life but left his brilliant mind full of holes. A computerized tomography (CT) scan indicated an area of low density, particularly in the left temporal lobe extending into the inferior and posterior frontal lobe and into the right medial temporal lobe.

Clive's consciousness fluctuated over the next few days. Two days after admission to hospital he had a grand mal seizure. Several days of confusion and disorientation followed with Clive wandering about the hospital and climbing into other patient's beds. His comprehension appeared to be very limited, he repeated meaningless phrases, and was dysphasic, repeatedly using, for example, the word "chicken" to refer to any object. A speech therapy assessment carried out over the next 2 to 3 wk noted Clive's extreme distractibility, poor auditory comprehension, inability to understand single words, and difficulty defining written words that he could read with 100% accuracy. At this time, Clive's mood was euphoric and he appeared unconcerned by his plight. As his wife said, "he was too confused to be confused." However, as his dysphasia decreased, despair began to set in and for about 2 months Clive spent most of each day crying. On one occasion his wife passed him a notebook and pen during such an episode and asked him to write down why he was crying. Clive wrote "I am completely incapable of thinking."

By July 1985 Clive was writing compulsively. He began recording the time, date, and the fact that he had just "become conscious" or had "just woken up." On July 7th he wrote "awake first time." This theme has been repeated throughout the 12 years of his amnesic state and continues to this day. An illustration from one page of his 1990 diary can be seen in Figure 6.1.

Other features first appearing at this time were episodes of belching, jerking, and shaking. After an acute bout Clive might vomit and then fall asleep. A psychiatric report from July 1985 described an episode of marked shaking and frequently repeated burping sounds. An EEG was carried out indicating that the noises and movements were epileptic in origin. This report also described Clive as having (1) severe organic memory deficit, (2) severe depressive reaction in the presence of some insight, and (3) retention of many cognitive abilities such as language and music.

Soon after this his wife noted object recognition difficulties. She reported that Clive could not tell the difference between jam, honey, and marmalade although he "knew" he preferred honey. He tried to spread cottage cheese on his bread thinking it was honey, he could not tell which of several bottles and tubes in the bathroom was toothpaste, he gave his wife talcum powder when she requested soap, and had mistaken his wife's sweater for his shirt.

Another characteristic of this time (July–November 1985) was Clive's attempt to work out reasons for his illness. Sometimes he assumed someone wanted to "shut him up" because he had uncovered an international conspiracy. He typically attributed the explanation to whatever was on the front page of the Times newspaper that day. King Hussein of Jordan, the "secrets-for-sex" trial at the Old Bailey, Sir Geoffrey Howe a Conservative politician and Mrs. Victoria Gillick mother of 10 and a Catholic with outspoken views on contraception were each blamed in turn for causing his illness. He frequently searched the hospital corridors looking for a policeman to whom he could tell his story.

From the earliest days of his illness Clive has confabulated. The hospital notes from April 1985 record his conversation as marked by confabulation and perseveration. By July he had begun on his most consistent confabulation, insisting that he was employed in whichever hospital he happened to be a patient at the time. He would say he worked in the hospital when he was a university student

15 Thursday
Week 7 · 46-319

4.40am   I WAKE U/ FOR THE FIRST TIME   ALL SYSTEMS SO

5.30am   I AM ~~TOTALLY~~ AWAKE FOR THE FIRST TIME   PATIENCE BE

6.02am   I AM ~~REALLY~~ AWAKE FOR THE FIRST TIME.   PATIENCE.

6.12 am   TIME FOR FIRST ~~CONSCIOUS~~ STROLL

6.19am   PATIENCE CONTINUES.

6.34am   I AM ~~PERFECTLY~~ AWAKE (FIRST TIME)   PATIENCE.

7.41am   I AM ~~COMPLETELY~~ AWAKE (FIRST TIME)   PATIENCE

7.47am   I AM ~~TOTALLY~~ AWAKE (FIRST TIME). I LOVE DEBORAH FOR EVER. WAL

8.42 am   NOW I AM ~~SUPERBLY~~ AWAKE (FIRST TIME). FIRST ~~~~ STROLL

9.38 am   NOW I AM ~~PERFECTLY~~ AWAKE (FIRST TIME). ~~~~ STROLL

9.45am   I RETURN AND AM ~~COMPLETELY~~ AWAKE (FIRST TIME). I PLAY THE PIANO

10.18 am   I SEARCH FOR A DRINK

10.35am   NOW I AM ~~PERFECTLY~~ AWAKE (FIRST TIME)   PATIENCE

11.05am   NOW I AM ~~REALLY~~, ~~PERFECTLY~~ AWAKE (FIRST TIME). ~~FIRST CONSCIOUS~~ STROLL.

11.17am   NOW I AM ~~REALLY~~ ~~COMPLETELY~~ AWAKE (FIRST TIME).

11.38am   NOW I AM ~~SUPERHUMANLY~~ AWAKE (FIRST TIME)   PATIENCE (

11.46am   FIRST ~~CONSCIOUS~~ STROLL.

12.06pm   NOW I AM ~~PERFECTLY~~ AWAKE (FIRST TIME). I LOOK FOR LUNCH

12.56p   NOW I am ~~REALLY~~ ~~TOTALLY~~ AWAKE (FIRST TIME). PATIENCE.

4.00pm   NOW I AM ~~SUPERLATIVELY~~ AWAKE (FIRST TIME). PATIENCE

4.25p   FIRST ~~CONSCIOUS~~ STROLL

4.32p   SECOND ~~CONSCIOUS~~ STROLL — FIRST EVER CONSCIOUS STROLL.

4.54p   NOW I AM PERFECTLY AWAKE (FIRST TIME). PATIENCE FOR DIN

5.17p   NOW I AM ~~COMPLETELY~~ ~~REALLY~~ AWAKE (FIRST TIME).

5.19p   FIRST ~~EVER~~ ~~CONSCIOUS~~ STROLL   RETURN 5.28p TOTALLY AS AS

5.30p   SECOND ~~TOTALLY~~ ~~CONSCIOUS~~ STROLL.

6.21pm   DINNER IS OVER AND NOW I AM ~~PERFECTLY~~ AWAKE (1st TIME)

6.40pm   PATIENCE STARTS TO BE SEEN AT LONG LAST.

—"—   I AM ~~PERFECTLY~~ AWAKE (1st TIME)

Deb came in better but a bit weak

Clive made w feel a lot better as only
he knows how ((

8.18pm   ALL MY SYSTEMS WORK — I AM ~~PERFECTLY~~ AWAKE 1st TIME)

8.19pm   PATIENCE ~~STARTS TO BE SEEN~~ — FIRST TIME

8.22pm   BLOOD PRESSURE IS TAKEN. THEN PATIENCE RESTARTS

9.54p   NOW I AM ~~PERFECTLY~~ AWAKE (1st TIME). ~~PATIENCE~~ .

   PATIENCE STARTS TO BE SEEN — FIRST TIME

10.18p   I RETURN AFTER TAKING 1st MODELINE. TIME FOR LOO + BED

10.21p   I AWAKE AT THE LOO. TIME FOR BED

February | Thu Fri Sat Sun | Mon Tue Wed Thu Fri Sat Sun | Mon Tue Wed Thu Fri Sat Sun | Mon Tue Wed Thu Fri Sat Sun | Mon Tue Wed
         | 1 2 3 4 | 5 6 7 8 9 10 11 | 12 13 14 15 16 17 18 | 19 20 21 22 23 24 25 | 26 27 28

Figure 6.1. Illustration from one page of Clive's 1990 diary.

many years before. He claimed he organized fellow students to work in the hospital during vacation times when the doctors and nurses were on holiday. Sometimes he added that he did this for the whole country. Occasionally he saw a nurse who had worked on his ward for several months and pointed her out as someone who worked there at the time he himself was working there.

INITIAL ASSESSMENT

Clive was referred to me in October 1985, having been previously assessed by several neuropsychologists all of whom noted his severe amnesia. Clive's wife arranged for me to see him for the assessment and to obtain advice on the management of his memory difficulties. He was seen as an outpatient and came once a month between November 1985 and May 1986. He was always accompanied by his wife, although sometimes he was seen alone while his wife was interviewed by a colleague (Alan Baddeley). Clive was not an easy man to assess. He interrupted regularly to tell me he had just woken up. He usually said something like, "This is the first time I've been awake, I don't remember how I got here but now I'm awake, I'm conscious for the first time. This is the first sight I've had, the first sound I've heard, it's like being dead." Every few minutes he interrupted to tell me again that he had just woken up. Sometimes he became very angry and testing had to be abandoned. For example, on one occasion I gave him the Seashore Test of Musical Abilities (Seashore et al., 1960), thinking it would be good for his morale to be faced with a task that would not be too demanding. Instead he became furious, feeling very insulted that a musician of his caliber should be asked to discriminate between pitches. The test he appeared to enjoy the most was the block design subtest of the Wechsler Adult Intelligence Scale (WAIS; Wechsler, 1955). Despite the difficulties involved in testing Clive, his eventual cooperation enabled us to obtain what we thought were reliable results.

The confabulation observed earlier by his wife was also noted. In October 1985, when seen at a hospital we are fairly certain he had never visited before, he said he used to run the hospital during the summer vacation when the doctors and nurses were on holiday.

During the initial assessment Clive was tested on the Wechsler Adult Intelligence Scale, the Rivermead Behavioural Memory Test (RBMT), the Logical Memory subtest of the Wechsler Memory Scale, the Rey-Osterreith Complete Figure, the Prices Test of Retrograde Amnesia (Wilson and Cockburn, 1988), the Autobiographical Memory Interview (AMI; Kopelman et al., 1989), tests of immediate memory span, the Semantic Processing Test (Baddeley et al., 1992), the modified Wisconsin Card Sorting Test (WCST), Verbal Fluency (S,V and Animals), and the National Adult Reading Test (NART). His results can be seen in Table 6.1.

Table 6.1. Clive's Neuropsychological Test Results

Wechsler Adult Intelligence Scale

VERBAL SUBTESTS	AGE SCALED SCORES	PERFORMANCE SUBTESTS	AGE SCALED SCORES
Information	11	Digit symbol	8
Comprehension	11	Picture completion	12
Arithmetic	13	Block design	14
Similarities	9	Picture arrangement	11
Digit span	10	Object assembly	10
Vocabulary	12		
Verbal IQ	105	Performance IQ	106

Rivermead Behavioural Memory Test

Screening score	0/12	(Severely impaired)
Standardized profile score	0/24	(Severely impaired)

Logical Memory (Prose Recall)

Immediate recall	1	(Severely impaired; some confabulation
Delayed recall	0	noted on immediate recall)

The Rey-Osterreith Complex Figure

Copy	33/36	(Normal)
Delayed recall	0/36	(Severely impaired)

The Prices Test of Retrograde Amnesia

Score	18	(Severely impaired)
Mean score for normal controls	0	
Mean score for Korsakoff patents	18	

The Autobiographical Memory Interview

	PERSONAL SEMANTIC	AUTOBIOGRAPHICAL INCIDENTS
Childhood	6/21 (Abnormal)	2 (Abnormal)
Early adulthood	4/21 (Abnormal)	1 (Abnormal)
Recent	0.5/21 (Abnormal)	0 (Abnormal)
Total	10.5/63 (Abnormal)	3 (Abnormal)

Immediate Memory Span

Digits forward	6	(Normal)
Digits backward	4	(Normal)
Corsi blocks	6	(Normal)

(continued)

Table 6.1. Clive's Neuropsychological Test Results (*continued*)

Semantic Processing Test (Baddeley et al., 1992)

Mean time per sentence	4.8 sec	(Abnormal)
Errors	6	(Abnormal)

Modified Card Sorting Test

Categories	4	(Consistent with frontal lobe damage)
Total errors	21	
Perseverative errors	8	

Verbal Fluency

"S" (90 sec)	12	(Plus 7 perseverations and 2 rule breaks)
"V" (90 sec)	3	(Plus 7 perseverations, 2 rule breaks, and 2 neologisms)
"Animals" (90 sec)	12	(Plus 8 perseverations and 2 rules breaks)

(Abnormal scores consistent with frontal lobe damage)

National Adult Reading Test

Predicted premorbid IQ	122 (Superior)

Clive's assessment is commented on in some detail in Wilson et al., (1995). It can be seen from Table 6.1 that on the WAIS, all Clive's age scaled scores were within the normal range, from a low of 8 on the Digit Symbol subtest and a high of 14 on the Block Design subtest. Although his IQ results were within the average range, they are without doubt much lower than one would predict from his pre-morbid occupation and status. Even the NART, which gave him a predicted pre-morbid IQ of 122, is almost certainly an underestimate given that Clive was a very gifted musical scholar. The NART requires subjects to read and pronounce a range of orthographically irregular words ranging from common to rare. Although Clive made only seven errors, it was later discovered that he has a degree of surface dyslexia for low frequency words, that is, he has problems with less common irregularly spelled words. This probably accounted for his errors on the NART.

On the two tests of frontal lobe functioning Clive's responses were poor with a high number of errors on the Modified Card Sorting Test and many perseverations and inappropriate responses on verbal fluency. For example, when asked for as many animals as possible within a 90 sec interval he said "dog, sausage, camel, hump." His neologisms included "strick, spitch, strungle, and swingle." His basic perceptual skills were intact as suggested by his relatively good performance on the WAIS performance subtests and his good copy of the Rey-Osterreith Complex Figure. Nevertheless, his wife's description of his object recognition difficulties suggested some visual semantic memory deficits that were not investigated in any detail until several years later.

With regard to episodic memory functioning, Clive's problems were more severe than anyone I have ever seen. Despite a normal immediate memory, he not only failed to recall anything after a brief delay he vehemently denied being tested earlier. "I have only just woken up," he said, "how could I have seen anything?" "Just guess," I would ask. "No, I never saw (or heard) anything before. I have just woken up now for the first time." On the two very simple recognition memory tests from the RBMT, he denied seeing any of the stimuli earlier, consequently there was no point in administering the more difficult Recognition Memory Test (Warrington, 1984).

Clive showed evidence of confabulation on the immediate recall of the Logical Memory Prose Passages. In the Anna Thompson story he claimed, "There was an interview at the police station with a girl about a case. They asked her a number of questions." The second story about an American liner is told as follows:

> The American liner, New York, struck a mine near Liverpool, Monday evening. In spite of a blinding snowstorm and darkness, the sixty passengers including 18 women, were all rescued, though the boats were tossed about like corks in the heavy sea. They were brought into port the next day by a British steamer.[1]

When asked for immediate recall of the story, Clive said, "A crash—people were thrown off a ship and picked up by another ship. There was chaos because of the speed the boats were traveling. It was a question of timing. Information was by no means clear and children were screaming."

Clive's autobiographical memory was extremely impaired. He was given the Autobiographical Memory Interview in 1985 (prior to publication). The AMI asks subjects about their childhood, early adult life and recent times (i.e., the past year). For each time period the subject is tested on both factual questions (e.g., "tell me the name of your first school") and on autobiographical incidents (e.g., "tell me about an incident or event that happened to you in your first job"). Clive's scores were in the very impaired range for each time period. The previously described confabulation about working in the hospital was also elicited during administration of the AMI. Clive had lost a great deal of his autobiographical knowledge, he knew he had studied music at university, he knew where he had lived as a child, he knew his wife, although could not remember his marriage, and he knew he was employed by the national broadcasting company. Very little else remained however. It was hard to establish the length of Clive's retrograde amnesia because he did not recognize famous events or famous people, either from earlier decades or from the present time. When shown a photograph of Queen Elizabeth II and Prince Philip, he thought they might be members of his choir. He was many years out of date on the Prices test of retrograde amnesia

(Wilson and Cockburn, 1988) when he was asked to estimate the current price of 12 common objects such as a first-class stamp and a pint of milk. The mean error score for control subjects is 0 and for Korsakoff patients it is 18. Korsakoff patients typically have a lengthy RA (Parkin, 1984). Clive's score was 18.

Clive was also slow at making true/false decisions. On the semantic processing test where subjects have to decide as quickly as possible whether each sentence in a series of short sentences is true or false, he was very slow in comparison to controls and made far more errors than control subjects.

REHABILITATION

Autobiographical Memory

Like other memory impaired patients, Clive and his wife Deborah were provided with information and explanations about the nature of memory impairment. However, Deborah had already undertaken a great deal of research into memory impairment and knew a considerable amount about the anatomical and cognitive aspects of memory. In collaboration with a colleague, Alan Baddeley, we decided to attempt to improve Clive's autobiographical memory by reteaching him autobiographical information. We had already noted that people with poor autobiographical memory tended to be anxious, irritable, agitated, and difficult for carers to manage (Baddeley and Wilson, 1986). We suggested that this difficult behavior might be due to the fact that in order to have a sense of one's self, one needs a past. Without a past, one might lose one's identity and sense of integrity as a person. Thus, the rationale for focusing on autobiographical memory was first to see if it would be possible for Clive to relearn autobiographical information and second to see if this led to a reduction in his agitated behavior.

The procedure agreed with Deborah was as follows: First, she would work out a set of 20 questions and answers for each of four different episodic events in Clive's recent life from 1980 onwards. She would work on one set of questions at a time. On day one she would go through all 20 questions and record Clive's answers. We assumed that (1) Clive had originally known the answers because they were personally important events to him and (2) he could no longer remember the answers because of his retrograde amnesia. Following this preassessment Deborah would take every alternate question and practice the answers with Clive using the Socratic method of prompts, hints, and cues. This procedure would be followed for 5 to 10 min each day for 7 days, after which all 20 questions would be administered again. Then Clive and his wife would work on another set of 20 questions in the same way and so on. Thus we expected to have a control set and a tested set for each of the four time periods. The episodes selected were Clive's conduction of Thérèse in 1980, a holiday in Spain in 1982, singing for the Pope in 1982, and an Italian Choir Tour in 1984.

After working hard at drawing up 80 appropriate questions and answers, Deborah planned to start questioning in January 1986. Immediately she felt daunted. She wrote, "If I even try to break out of the cyclic dialogues of obsessive stock questions and stock answers I always get a catastrophic reaction. The fitting is now much worse and always occurs when he feels exposed. Last night fitting was almost nonstop until dawn."

By the following month Deborah felt able to start the questioning, which she audiotaped. However, the whole process was so difficult for her in view of the distress it was causing Clive that the procedure was abandoned. Part of the taped conversation is reported below and is offered as evidence of why our first attempt failed.

Wife: Do you remember with Thérèse, whether you had any intervals or whether you just performed it all in one chunk?

Clive: No, I can't remember, my memory's gone—my knowledge of what's happening to me.

Wife: In fact, with Thérèse you performed it all in one chunk, it wasn't that long, I think it lasted less than 2 h, but there was no natural break because he conceived the whole in such a large structure which couldn't be divided, there was no way it could be divided, so there was no interval. It was just about the right length for people dying to go to the loo or get a cup of coffee, so it worked.

Clive: As far as I am concerned, this is the first conversation I have yet had for something approaching what must be between 18 months and 2 years to me. I have not been speaking to anybody. I know nothing about what's happening, I know nothing at all of what's supposed to be happening to me or what is happening around me to anybody else. I've been completely disconnected, and my life has been an absolute bloody misery all the bloody time. Why haven't the doctors been able to do anything?

The Amnesia Association

Through conversations with Deborah, it became apparent that there was nowhere in the United Kingdom that could offer appropriate rehabilitation for Clive. This unsatisfactory state of affairs inspired us to do something ourselves so in September 1986 we established the Amnesia Association. Our aims and objectives were as follows:

1. To provide support and information to memory impaired people and their families.
2. To promote the interests of memory impaired people.
3. To urge for provision of appropriate rehabilitation and care facilities.

4. To offer information seminars and workshops to health service professionals engaged in the care of brain injured people.
5. To encourage research into the management of memory impaired people.

The Amnesia Association provided a focus or a platform as it were for memory
impaired people, their families, and health service professionals to come together
to offer support and advice to each other. A number of local groups became established and Jay the young man described in Chapter 4 is still very active in his
local Amnesia Association Group.

Some Later Rehabilitation Strategies Tried with Clive

In 1991, Avi Schmueli, a clinical psychology trainee at the time, carried out an
analysis of Clive's repetitious statements and episodes of belching and jerking.
Avi Schmueli discovered that a repetition, belch, or jerk was far more likely to
occur following a change in activity such as moving position from sitting to
walking, or moving from one task to another such as from playing cards to playing the piano. With two or more changes of activity in a 10 min period, there was
a 70% chance of a belch, jerk, or repetitious statement. These results can be seen
in Figure 6.2.

I noticed when testing Clive in 1991 that changing from one test to another
produced an outburst of belching and jerking. Although it was not possible to
prevent all changes in activity, Avi Schmueli's observations suggested that Clive
was calmer when there were as few changes as possible.

Other strategies found to help Clive were gradually developed over time and
were almost entirely of the environmental adaptation kind described in Chapter 2
whereby problems are avoided or by-passed. In other words, rather than expect
the patient to change his behavior, other people have to change theirs, or modify
the environment to prevent problems occurring. In Clive's case, addressing him
in a formal way caused him less distress than using his first name, which is more
often done on a long-stay ward. This was because to Clive all the staff were always strangers, he never remembered meeting them before and was uncomfort-
able with (to him) inappropriate familiarity. Coffee was found to be reinforcing
and often used to encourage compliance with the ward routine. Sympathizing
with his plight over having just woken up led to an increase in the repetition of
the phrase and to an increase in agitation. A change in conversation, however,
often avoided this accelerated repetition. Temper outbursts were best avoided by
a nonconfrontational approach. If one tried to persuade Clive that he had not just
woken up and that in fact he must have been awake to record his previous diary
entries, he became angry and would at times appear quite frightening. It was simpler to avoid discussions of this type. Finally, when testing Clive it was fatal to
ask permission. If I said, "Would you mind reading this passage?" he would

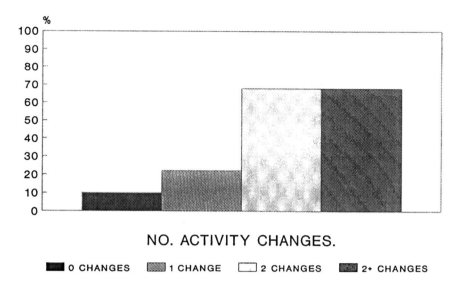

NO. ACTIVITY CHANGES.

■ 0 CHANGES   ▨ 1 CHANGE   ☐ 2 CHANGES   ▨ 2+ CHANGES

Figure 6.2. An analysis of Clive's repetitious statements and episodes of belching and jerking.

rarely agree, say he had just woken up and become agitated. Although, if I said, "What does this passage say?" he would read it without fuss.

In short, people interacting with Clive modified their behavior and found better ways to manage and to interact with him. Clive became calmer over time probably because others had learned strategies that preempted some of the earlier difficulties. As far as memory functioning was concerned, however, Clive showed virtually no change over the next few years.

FOLLOW UP

Clive was seen on several occasions between 1989 and 1992 for follow-up assessments. He had an MRI scan in 1991 arranged by Narinder Kapur of the Wessex Neurological Centre in Southampton (see Fig. 6.3).

A report on this scan said there was *marked* abnormality in both hippocampal formations, both amygdalas, both mamillary bodies, both temporal poles, the substantia inominata on both sides, the left fornix, the left inferior temporal gyrus, the anterior portion of the left superior temporal gyrus, and the left insula. In addition, there was *mild* abnormality in the posterior portion of the left middle temporal gyrus, the left medial frontal cortex, the left striatum, the right insula, the right fornix, and the anterior portion of the right inferior temporal gyrus. The third ventricle and both lateral ventricles were dilated. The thalamus both on the

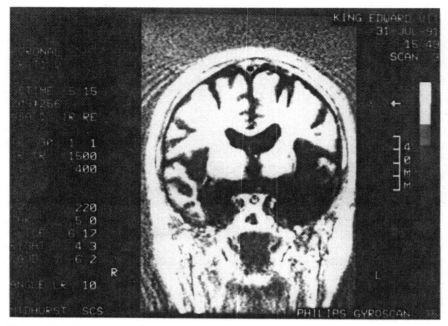

Figure 6.3. Clive's magnetic resonance imaging (MRI) scan.

left and the right was considered to be intact and, apart from the left medial frontal abnormality mentioned above, no other frontal lobe abnormality was detected. Thus, Clive has very extensive brain damage affecting both temporal lobes and the diencephalon. Amnesia can follow damage to either of these regions, few patients have such severe lesions in both areas.

Clive's memory functioning showed no obvious improvement between 1985 and 1992. His immediate memory span remained as before, 6 digits forward, 4 backwards and a Corsi block/visual tapping score of 6 on each of three occasions tested. His RBMT score was 0 on each occasion; he failed to recall anything of the logical memory passages both in the immediate and delayed conditions although he no longer confabulated. His Rey-Osterreith delayed recall score also remained at zero with his copy score at follow-up being 33/36, identical to that obtained in 1985. In 1989 Clive was given the revised version of the Wechsler Memory Scale (Wechsler, 1987). His index scores on general memory, verbal memory, visual memory, and delayed memory were all below 50, the lowest possible index score. On the remaining index, attention, and concentration, he scored 105, in the average range. On the visual reproduction subtest he scored 17 (4th percentile) on immediate recall and 0 on delayed recall. The density of Clive's amnesia is further illustrated by the fact that of a group of 10 postencephalitic patients tested by Kapur et al. (1994), none were as severely impaired as Clive.

Clive's autobiographical memory was reassessed in 1992. There was marginal improvement, particularly in recall of factual, personal semantic information from childhood although his score was still in the impaired range. The recall of autobiographical episodes or incidents was essentially unchanged.

To investigate his retrograde amnesia a modified version of Kapur's Retrograde Amnesia Test (Kapur et al., 1989) was administered to Clive in 1989. On this test subjects are asked to indicate whether famous people are dead or alive and, if dead, when and how they died. Clive scored 1/20, correctly stating that Elvis Presley was dead. He said he had never heard of people such as John Lennon, Lee Harvey Oswald, or John F. Kennedy. He claimed he had vaguely heard of Margaret Thatcher, Mohammed Ali, and Cliff Richard but was unable to say anything about them or guess whether they were alive or dead.

Clive had improved on a few tests at follow-up. His performance on the modified WCST was without error in 1992 and he made fewer perseverations on verbal fluency. However, when asked to name as many musicians as possible within a 60 sec period, he mentioned only four (Mozart, Beethoven, Bach, and Haydn), omitting Lassus the composer for whom he had been considered the world expert prior to his illness.

Clive had also improved on the semantic processing test. In 1985, he took an average of 4.8 sec for each sentence (controls take about 2 sec per sentence) and he made six errors (controls rarely make more than one or two). Clive's errors included "Dragonflies have wings." marked as false and "Forks have a lot of industry." as correct. His reading aloud of these sentences was fast and accurate, indicating his difficulty was not due to reading problems. By 1992, however, Clive averaged 2.44 sec per sentence, an improvement of almost 100%. He made only one error and therefore was no different from normal control subjects.

In contrast, Clive's performance had deteriorated on parts of the WAIS and the NART. In 1992, the revised WAIS (Wechsler, 1981b) was administered. This typically estimates both verbal and performance IQ's to be 7 to 8 points lower than those obtained on the old WAIS. Even allowing for this, however, Clive's verbal IQ of 92 would appear to have deteriorated a little. The quality of his responses was poorer in 1992. For example when asked to define "reluctant" in 1985 he said, "unwilling." In 1992 he replied, "Not overpersuaded." Similarly when asked, in 1985, "In what way are North and West alike?" he replied, "part of the compass." In 1992 he replied, "at right angles to each other." Clive's NART score dropped from 7 errors in 1985 to 20 errors in 1992. One explanation for the declining scores on the WAIS and the NART is that Clive is slowly forgetting his general knowledge as time passes and he has less opportunity to practice or rehearse this information and less exposure to conversation, newspapers, radio, and television.

A more detailed examination of Clive's semantic memory was carried out in 1991 and 1992. In retrospect there was considerable evidence of semantic memory disorders as far back as 1985. The speech therapist's report of 1985 noted that Clive complained, "words have changed their meaning." Deborah described his confusion about jam, honey, and marmalade and about bathroom furniture and clothing. This was all consistent with impaired information about the world both for visual and verbal material. In 1991 Clive was given the Graded Naming Test (McKenna and Warrington, 1983). He scored only 2 out of 30 (Kangaroo and Radius). Although some of his errors were obviously due to word finding difficulties such as "a swimming tortoise" for "turtle," some of his errors appeared to be due to recognition difficulties e.g., to the picture of a scarecrow he replied, "a worshipping point for certain cultures." Later when asked "What is a scarecrow?" he replied "A bird that flies and makes funny noises."

On a semantic memory battery (Hodges, et al., 1992) Clive exhibited a discrepancy between living and nonliving items, matched for frequency, with his performance on living things being poorer and worse than people with mild to moderate Alzheimer's disease. His scores on three subtests of this battery can be seen in Table 6.2.

CLIVE TODAY

Clive lives in a small group home in the grounds of a private hospital. He appears to be reasonably calm and certainly less agitated than I have known him in the

Table 6.2. Scores on naming pictures, naming to description, and recognition of pictures for living and nonliving items obtained by C

	LIVING		NONLIVING
Naming Pictures Total	11/24		20/24
Land animals	9/12	Household items	9/12
Water creatures	1/6	Vehicles	5/6
Birds	1/6	Musical instruments	6/6
Naming to Description Total	2/12		8/12
Land animals	1/4	Household items	3/4
Water creatures	0/4	Vehicles	3/4
Birds	1/4	Musical instruments	2/4
Recognition of Pictures Total	17/24		24/24
Domestic animals	6/6	Electrical items	6/6
Foreign animals	4/6	Household items	6/6
Water creatures	2/6	Vehicles	6/6
Birds	5/6	Musical instruments	6/6

past, probably because of better management and interaction from those caring for him, although he still persists in claiming he has just woken up. He still belches and jerks, particularly when anxious or challenged, and persists in his confabulation about working in hospitals.

A new development, which began around 1990, was the experience of an auditory hallucination. Clive appears to hear a tape of himself playing in the distance. In his diaries he refers to this as a "master tape." If asked to sing what he can hear, he picks up the tune in midphrase and is puzzled that no one else can hear it. If asked again after a delay to sing what he can hear he usually sings the same tune but sometimes in a different style as if the tune were being played in variations.

Although Clive's musical skills have not been formally assessed since his illness, his wife believes there has been virtually no change in his ability to sight-read, although his pianistic skills may have declined. She feels he is less confident when playing and plays some pieces at a speed beyond his present capacity. Premorbidly of course he could have played them at that speed with ease. She also says Clive now restricts his playing to straightforward pieces from the sixteenth to the twentieth centuries and no longer attempts anything obviously difficult. To the untrained ear Clive is still as skillful and competent as ever.

In conclusion, Clive still lives in a sheltered environment within a hospital setting. The major improvements have been in environmental and behavioral management approaches aimed at reducing the likelihood of temper outbursts and distress. Clive himself remains profoundly amnesic with a retrograde amnesia extending back for much of his life. He has semantic memory deficits for both visual and verbal material. Yet despite the great extent and severity of his memory difficulties his musical skills appear to be intact.

7

MARTIN: A MORE COMPLETE HUMAN BEING

BACKGROUND

Martin was described by his parents as "laid back, quite modern, long hair, flower-power, very peaceful, kind, and gentle". He did not like sports, having been hit on the cheek by a cricket ball when he was a boy and thereafter unwilling to play. He loved animals and abhorred fox hunting. After he left school, Martin went to work as an animal technician in the laboratories of a nearby university. He enjoyed it there as he was looking after the animals' welfare. After a time he went for an interview at a bigger animal laboratory in Huntingdon. He became very upset at what he saw and decided he no longer wanted to be an animal technician.

Martin became interested in looking after children and went to work in a home for maladjusted children in the southeast. He did well and was highly regarded. As a result of this work he became accepted on a course in Newcastle-on-Tyne, leading to the Certificate of Qualified Social Workers, with probation work as his main focus. He decided to go to Newcastle because his sister lived nearby in Sunderland at the time. At the age of 24 yr, while celebrating his final examinations and a friend's birthday, Martin had an accident that was to change his life forever.

At 6:20 A.M. one morning in June 1980, his parents were woken from sleep by the telephone ringing. It was the Neurological Hospital in Newcastle saying that Martin had been admitted. Apparently, there had been some horseplay at the party. Someone took his legs from underneath him. Although no one was quite sure what actually happened, Martin fell backwards and hit his head. His parents never learned the full story and felt people at the party were covering up for one another.

Martin had fallen against the fireplace. At first he appeared dazed then he lost consciousness for a few minutes. When he regained consciousness, he could not put his boots on and his pupils were dilated. His girlfriend, a qualified nurse, realized something was seriously wrong and sent for an ambulance. Because of the party and cans of beer lying around, the ambulance men thought he was drunk. Martin was taken to the Accident Hospital where he was examined by a doctor who realized neurological expertise was required. Martin was transferred to the Neurological Hospital where he was put to bed with suspected concussion.

Meanwhile Martin's girlfriend, who had not been allowed to travel with him in the ambulance, had gone first to the Accident Hospital and then to the Neurological Hospital. She described the accident to the consultant. Realizing Martin needed urgent help, and that 4 h had now passed since the initial injury, the consultant examined Martin and discovered a blood clot had formed on his brain.

His parents gave consent to operate over the telephone, found friends to look after Martin's younger brother, and set off by car to Newcastle—a journey of about 4 h. Unable to wait for the news, Martin's father telephoned halfway through the journey. He was told to go straight to the ward when he arrived. He felt the nurse he spoke to was hiding something from him and he did not dare ask if Martin was still alive. "We feared by then he was dead," said Martin's father, "because of the seriousness of the telephone call and because we didn't know anything about head injury." His parents were told later that had another hour gone by without the operation Martin would have died.

On his way back to the car from the telephone Martin's father said he heard an inner voice saying, "Have faith." Both parents took comfort in that and said they could provide many examples of spiritual support. They arrived at the hospital about midday. They went to the ward and were asked to sit in the waiting room. When the consultant arrived he told them that although the operation was very serious there were "grounds for hope."

Martin remained in that hospital for over 6 mo. He first regained consciousness in September—3 mo after the accident. The sister on the ward took his tracheostomy tube out one day to clean it and Martin groaned and said "Ow." "Did you feel that, Martin?" asked the sister and he said "Yes." He continued to improve from then on. He appeared to know his parents right from the start as he would squeeze their hands but would not squeeze the hand of the consultant (whom he did not know) when requested. His girlfriend spent almost all her off-duty time at Martin's bedside and was devoted to him although she seemed jealous of his parents and would not leave them alone with Martin. She remained devoted for 6 mo and then left, apparently realizing he was not going to make a full recovery and there would be no future in their relationship. She was in touch a few times afterwards but essentially that was the end of the relationship. She wrote a poem for Martin that his parents described as "heartbreaking—a broken-hearted poem."

The sister on Martin's ward was concerned because there was nowhere in the northeast suitable for Martin once he left the hospital. However, a place was found for him at Rivermead Rehabilitation Centre where he was to be admitted in January 1981. Late in 1980 a complication developed concerning Martin's physical state. During the accident he had sustained a depressed fracture of the right tempero–parietal bone. This necessitated removal of part of the bone, which was kept for reinsertion later. This piece of bone (bone flap) was replaced shortly before Christmas. Martin was to be allowed home for Christmas but the bone flap became infected and had to be removed. As a result Martin was too ill to go home and remained in the hospital where he surprised everyone by singing all the carols and knowing all the words.

In January 1981 Martin arrived at Rivermead—minus his bone flap. A special helmet was obtained for him until a synthetic bone flap was made for him at another Oxford hospital towards the end of his stay. Meanwhile he was confined to a wheelchair, not because of the missing bone but because of paralysis in his left leg. In February 1981, I was asked to see Martin for an assessment of his cognitive functioning.

INITIAL ASSESSMENT

I saw Martin six times during the second half of February. He was very slow and frequently asked for questions to be repeated. He was always cooperative although rather facetious. I found he had significant memory and perceptual deficits. These results together with two further assessments, in October 1981 and July 1997, can be seen in Table 7.1.

Martin's verbal IQ was in the average range but his performance IQ was in the retarded range. There was a huge discrepancy between the poorest age scaled score (2 for Digit Symbol) and the best age scaled score (13 for Digit Span). On the National Adult Reading Test Martin made 17 errors. This gave him a predicted premorbid IQ in the above average range. He made perseverative errors on the Modified Wisconsin Card Sorting Test and on the FAS Fluency Test. He failed to recall anything of the Wechsler Memory Scale prose passages or the Rey-Osterreith Complex Figure after a delay. He had problems identifying both unusual views and the objects on the Hooper Visual Organization Test. He had problems with tests of face recognition and omitted items on the left in the Digit Symbol task.

Following this assessment Martin was offered help with his cognitive problems by the clinical psychologists. In particular we offered attention training and
memory therapy.

INITIAL REHABILITATION

Attention Training

The strategy used here was basically practice in two paper-and-pencil tasks and
one electronic task believed to be dependent on attention. Although at the time of
writing I no longer believe in the cognitive exercise or drilling approach (Wilson,
1997a), this belief was not so strongly held by me in 1981. I was still experiment-
ing with a number of strategies, particularly with attentionally impaired patients.
Attention problems were less clearly thought out prior to the theoretical developments in the 1980s and 1990s (Sohlberg and Mateer, 1989; Ponsford and Kinsella, 1992; Robertson et al., 1996).

Martin practiced three tasks three or four times a week for 4 weeks. These
tasks included (1) the Coding subtest from the WISC, (2) a simple reaction time
task, and (3) a letter cancellation task. Results were as follows:

TASK	INITIAL SCORE	FINAL SCORE	COMMENTS
Coding	25 in 2 min	33 in 2 min	Neglect of left side frequent. Marginal improvement
Simple reaction time	19.5 sec per response	6.36 sec per response	Improved
Letter cancellation task	15 Omissions	Mean of 6 omissions	Improved

Of course there was no way of knowing from these results whether Martin's
improvement was due to the specific practice or to natural recovery. Nor were we
able to say whether the improvements on these tasks generalized to everyday life.

Memory Therapy

Martin attended the memory group five times a week for 6 wk. He followed the
syllabus described in Wilson (1984). Although he enjoyed the group activities
and was popular with the other people attending, there was no evidence that he
improved or used any strategies as a result of group therapy.

We had limited success with other strategies. Martin did not use external aids or employ any internal strategies. Always cheerful, charming, sociable, and polite, Martin managed to hide some of his problems. For example, if he heard someone saying, "Good morning, Barbara" to me, he always said, "Good morning, Barbara" too, despite the fact that he found it impossible to recognize a photograph of me as being the person sitting in front of him. I decided to see if I could teach him to retain my name through the use of expanding rehearsal. Initially, he appeared to retain the name "Barbara" for 30 sec. I told him my name and asked him, "What is my name?" at intervals ranging from 6 to 60 sec. He was invariably correct if the interval was 30 sec or less but almost never correct if the interval was more than 30 sec. Next I set a timer to sound at 20 sec, 30 sec, 40 sec, and so forth. Each time the timer sounded Martin was asked, "What is my name?" Through gradually increasing the interval in this way, Martin was able to recall my name without error after 10.5 min. I then asked him, "What is my name?" without the timer sounding. He returned to baseline levels here, i.e., he could only recall my name, once told it, for a maximum of 30 sec. However, if I imitated the timer and said, "beep" he replied, "Barbara." Thus he had learned to pair "Barbara" with the beep but could not recall the name without this prompt. When asked the names of his therapists or other patients at Rivermead, he reliably recalled three. When asked, "Who is your OT [occupational therapist]?" he said, correctly, "Anne." His physiotherapist he knew was Sue and his psychologist he knew was Barbara. However, he could not name these people when he saw them. He would tell me his psychologist was Barbara, but did not know that Barbara was sitting in front of him. When given the initial letter of my name (or Sue's or Anne's), he produced the correct name.

Martin himself said that when he saw photographs of faces they seemed confusing, they were pictures that did not mean anything. He said this was due to his brain damage. His tendency to repeat the same question over and over gradually decreased and by the time of his first discharge from Rivermead in October 1981, his repetition was restricted to repeating the same responses to certain questions. For example, when I was working with him, in order to get his attention I would say, "Are you ready, Martin?" He always replied, "Ready, willing, and disabled." Initial amusement soon gave way to irritation after numerous repetitions of this joke but the solution was simple. I had to change my behavior to avoid eliciting this response. Instead of saying "Are you ready, Martin?" I substituted, "We are going to start now, Martin," and the problem was avoided.

Martin was competent at getting around in his wheelchair in the sense that he could manipulate it without difficulty. Nevertheless he was frequently lost due to his memory and visuospatial problems. He tried to get through locked doors or went into rooms he had no need to enter. When asked how he saw the future, he said he thought he would get back to normal and return to work. His parents, however, were well aware that this would not be possible. They were pleased to note that Martin, at that time an agnostic, came to believe in God during his first stay at Rivermead. He used to go home every weekend with his parents. They came to collect him every Friday evening. One Friday evening Martin, still in his wheelchair, said "By the way, I now believe in God and if I forget will you remind me?" His parents went on to say "He never forgot and he never once wavered. Every time we saw him—every weekend for a year or so—he told us of his belief. Then it became normal. For 3 weekends in particular, the first words he said were "By the way, have I told you, I now believe in God?" Although pleased, his parents did not enthuse too much knowing Martin was brain damaged and they did not want to push too far. One weekend his mother said, "How do you mean you now believe in God?" Martin replied, "Well God came to me in the night. He came and stood by my bed and told me to put all my care on him and I have." His father, many years later, said, "Martin worries about nothing at all because his heavenly father is looking after him."

SECOND ASSESSMENT

Just before Martin's first discharge in October 1981, I reassessed him on the tests administered 8 mo earlier (see Table 7.1). My conclusions in October were:

1. Martin has shown noticeable improvement since his assessment in February 1981.
2. In particular his visuospatial and perceptual skills are less impaired than they were.
3. His reasoning skills also appear to be better.
4. Not surprisingly there are still signs of cognitive problems associated with right temporo-parietal damage.
5. Unfortunately Martin's memory remains severely impaired.
6. Few techniques appear to be of benefit despite some intensive training. The most useful strategies are (a) providing Martin with a first letter cue and (b) asking him to record information in a notebook. Even then he needs reminding to use his book. He is also likely to lose the book so it should be attached to his wheelchair.
7. Further assessment will be carried out when Martin returns after Christmas.

Martin returned home from October 1981 to January 1982 and then returned to Rivermead for a further 6 wk "top up" period of rehabilitation.

THIRD ASSESSMENT

I saw Martin three times in January 1982 to administer a few more tests. I wrote that he was cheerful and cooperative and appeared to be more alert. There was, however, little change on his test scores since October 1981.

Unlike earlier, he was now consistently correct when asked the year. He always used to answer correctly when asked, "What is the name of the place we are in now?" In January 1982, he thought he was in a day center near his home. Whenever I said, "No, you are at Rivermead," he always replied, "I thought I'd left you." Martin came to the memory group for part of his stay and performed much as he had previously. He did not stay long this time and returned home after a few weeks. I wrote to a clinical psychologist in Martin's home town, who had agreed to see Martin, to tell her about the program and his progress.

FOURTH ADMISSION: TEACHING THERAPISTS' NAMES

In November 1982 Martin came back to the rehabilitation center for a further period of rehabilitation. This time he stayed (with a break for Christmas) until February 1983. The main focus of his psychological intervention this time was to teach Martin the names of his therapists and others at the rehabilitation center. We also repeated a few of the tests, the results of which can be seen in Table 7.1.

As before, Martin could recall the names of three therapists if asked (1) what is the name of your (OT/physiotherapist/psychologist)? or (2) given the first letter of each of these three names. A fourth therapist named Anita told him that he would be able to remember her name because she had "*a neater* way of doing her hair," whereupon she shook her hair. From then on Martin reliably recalled the name "Anita" provided she shook her hair as a cue. The trouble with this was that any woman who shook her hair would be called "Anita!" Nevertheless, because of Martin's ability to associate a movement with a name, we decided to try to use this as a mnemonic to help him learn names. Twenty names of therapists, patients, or other members of staff were selected, all of whom knew Martin well. It was hard to say if *he* knew them because of his face recognition and his memory difficulties. Half the names were randomly allocated to the motor movement condition and half to a visual imagery condition.

In the first session Martin was shown a photograph of his physiotherapist and asked for her name. He could not do this so was told, "Her name is Sue. We are going to try to think of a sign to help you remember Sue. What sign could we use? What does Sue make you think of?" Martin replied, "soup" and mimed the action of eating soup with a spoon. A second photograph was shown of the nurse on Martin's ward. Again Martin could not supply the name so was told, "His name is Mike, we are going to try and draw a picture to help you remember his name, what does Mike make you think of?" Martin suggested a microphone and a picture of a man holding a microphone was drawn for Martin on a white card with a black felt tip pen. This procedure was followed for the first eight names on the list, four from each condition.

After each name, Martin was tested on the names already covered. Thus, following the first name he was shown the sign for Sue and asked, "Who is this?"

After the second name he was shown the picture of the microphone and asked, "Who is this?" He was then shown the sign for Sue again. After the third name all three names were tested in random order and so forth. The following day began with a 24 h recall with signs and pictures shown to Martin one at a time and Martin asked to supply the name that accompanied the sign or the picture. Two new names were then added. The results can be seen in Table 7.2.

A sign test (comparing the number of names successfully recalled in each condition on 11 test occasions) was applied to the results. On 10 of the 11 occasions more names were recalled under the motor movement condition than under the visual imagery condition ($p = 0.01$). However, although this meant that Martin could produce the correct name significantly more often when he was shown a motor movement than when he was shown a drawing, in practice this did not help a great deal as he never learned to match the appropriate movement to each face.

A shaping procedure was adopted in an attempt to overcome this problem. The first photograph (Sue) was shown, the sign (eating soup) made, and Martin replied, "Sue." The photograph was removed for 3 sec, shown again, and Martin recalled "Sue" without the sign. The photograph of Mike was shown next and Martin saw the accompanying drawing before replying "Mike." Mike's photograph and picture were removed for 3 sec, the photograph shown again, and once more Martin recalled "Mike." Then the two photographs were shown together and the same procedure followed. Once again Martin was able to retain both "Mike" and "Sue." Then a third photograph, Anne, was added, Martin was shown the three together and asked to point to the picture of Sue. He made an error and continued to make errors for the next few trials. After 17 trials he made three consecutive correct responses successfully pointing on each trial to Mike, Sue, and Anne (following each trial the photographs were removed for several seconds and replaced in a different order). Three consecutive correct responses were the most Martin achieved. He never achieved four consecutive responses after a delay of 15 sec even with these three names. The face recognition problem was such that Martin did not recognize the photograph of me placed in front of him even though I was testing him. When I said, "This is a photograph of me," he said, "So it is." He said this each time I told him. After 85 trials, attempts to match names to faces were abandoned.

FOLLOWING RIVERMEAD

Martin came back in 1984 for a brief visit and then I lost touch with him for 4 yr. In 1988, his parents invited me to speak to the local branch of the National Head Injuries Association where Martin's father had been chairman since 1983. I went

Table 7.1. Martin's Test Results

TEST	FEB. 1981	OCT. 1981	JAN. 1982	NOV. 1982	APR. 1989	JUL. 1997
Wechsler Adult Intelligence Scale			Not administered	(Only three subtests given)	WAIS-Revised administered here (gives a lower estimate than old WAIS)	Not administered
Verbal IQ	96	108			94	
Performance IQ	56	80			70	
Full scale	77	96			82	
WAIS Subtests	**Age Scaled Scores**				**Age Scaled Scores**	
Information	6	7			4	
Comprehension	10	14			13	
Arithmetic	5	7			6	
Similarities	10	13			11	
Digit span	13	13			12	
Vocabulary	11	12			9	
Digit symbol	2	5			4	
Picture completion	4	8		7	6	
Block design	5	8		8	7	
Picture arrangement	4	6		8	4	
Object assembly	4	7			5	
National Adult Reading Test						
Predicted premorbid IQ	114 (Above average)	117 (Above average)	—	—	— —	117 (Above average)

Ravens Standard Progressive Matrices

Percentile	Below 5th	Below 5th	7th	—	—	—
Raw score	22	28	35	—	—	—

Wechsler Memory Scale

Personal & current information	1/6	1/6	1/6	1/6		
Orientation	2/5	2/5	1/5	1/5		
Mental control	4/9	9/9	9/9	9/9		
Logical memory						
Immediate recall	3	3	6	6		
Delayed recall	0	0	0	0		
					Wechsler Memory Scale-Revised administered here	
General memory index						71
Verbal memory index						76
Visual memory index						56
Attention & concentration						95
Delayed recall						Well below 50

Corsi Span

	6	6	—	6		6

Rivermead Behavioural Memory Test

Screening score	0 / 12 ▼	0 / 12	0 / 12	0 / 12 Severely impaired	1 / 12	1 / 12 ▲
Unusual Views	4 / 20 ▼	13 / 20	14 / 20	15 / 20 Impaired	14 / 20	12 / 20 ▲
Usual Views	11 / 20 (Impaired)	17 / 20 (Impaired)	17 / 20 (No change)	17 / 20 (Essentially same)	17 / 20 (No change)	18 / 20 (Normal)

(continued)

Table 7.1. Martin's Test Results (*continued*)

TEST	FEB. 1981	OCT. 1981	JAN. 1982	NOV. 1982	APR. 1989	JUL. 1997
Rey-Osterreith Figure						
Copy	16 / 36	19 / 36	26 / 36	22 / 36	—	24 / 36
Recall	0 / 36	6 / 36	6 / 36	3 / 36	—	0 / 36
	(Impaired)	(Impaired)	(Impaired)	(Impaired)		(Impaired)
Recognition Memory Test						
Words	—	—	32 / 50 (Raw)	—	36 / 50 (Raw)	—
			0 (Age scaled score)		4 (Age scaled score)	—
			(Impaired)			
Faces	—	—	23 / 50 (Raw)	—	25 / 50 (Raw)	—
			0 (Age scaled score)		0 (Age scaled score)	—
			(Impaired)		(Impaired)	
Same / different faces	—	—	15 / 20	12 / 20	11 / 20	15.20
			(Just within normal limits)	(Impaired)	(Impaired)	(Just within normal limits)
Famous faces Naming					5 / 30	
Famous names Identifying					22 / 30	
Mooney's Closure Faces	25 / 44	26 / 44				
	(Impaired)	(Impaired)				
Benton & Van Allen Face Recognition					39 (Borderline)	
VOSP* (Prepublished version)						
Fragmented letters	18 / 20	18 / 20	—	20 / 20	—	20 / 20
	(Within normal limits)					

(continued)

Test						
Position discrimination	14 / 20 (Impaired)	17 / 20 (Borderline)	12 / 20 (Impaired)	—	15 / 20 (Impaired)	12.20 (Impaired)
Cube analysis	7 / 10 (Just within normal limits)	7 / 10 (Just within normal limits)	10 / 10 (Normal)	—	—	6 / 6 (Normal)
Hooper Visual Organisation Test	12.5 / 30 (Severely impaired)	17.5 / 30 Moderately impaired	17.5 / 30 Moderately impaired	16 / 30 Moderately impaired	18.5 / 30 Moderately impaired	16 / 30 Moderately impaired

Behavioural Inattention Test

Conventional tests

Line crossing	36 / 36	
Letter concellation	40 / 40	
Star concellation	49 / 54	(Impaired)
Figure & shape copying	4 / 4	
Line bisection	7 / 9	(Impaired)
Representational drawing	3 / 3	
Total	139 / 146	
Picture scanning	4 / 9	(Impaired)
Telephone dialling	9 / 9	
Menu Reading	9 / 9	
Article reading	9 / 9	
Telling and setting time	8 / 9	
Coin sorting	7 / 9	(Impaired)
Address and sentence copying	9 / 9	

Table 7.1. Martin's Test Results (*continued*)

TEST		FEB. 1981	OCT. 1981	JAN. 1982	NOV. 1982	APR. 1989	JUL. 1997
Map navigation						9 / 9	—
Card sorting						9 / 9	—
					Total	73 / 81	—
					slight evidence of neglect on 4 subtests		
Modified Wisconsin Card Sorting Test							
Categories		4	6	—	—	6	—
Total errors		17	2	—	—	1	—
Perseverative errors		9	1	—	—	0	—
		(Poor)	(Normal)			(Normal)	
Speed of Information Processing		—	—	—	Mean time per item 5.7 sec (Impaired)	Mean time per item 4" (Impaired)	Mean time per item 4.4" (Impaired)
Fluency							
"S"	Raw score	17		18		21	19
	perseverations	(2)		(8)		(9)	(0)
"A"		—		—		—	19
							(0)
"F"		—		—		—	17
							(0)
"Animals"	Raw score	12		18		17	10
	perseverations	(2)		4		0	(1)

* VOSP, Visual object and space perception battery.

Table 7.2. Number of Names Successfully Recalled by Martin after a Delay of 24 h

DATE	MOTOR MOVEMENTS	IMAGES
11.25.82	4/4	4/4
11.26.82	5/5	1/5
11.29.82	5/6	4/6
11.30.82	7/10	5/10
12.1.82	8/10	5/10
12.3.82	10/10	7/10
12.6.82	10/10	7/10
12.8.82	10/10	4/10
12.9.82	9/10	4/10
12.13.82	10/10	9/10
12.14.82	9/10	4/10

along and met Martin once more. He was looking well, he was cheerful, and appeared to know me. The following year I saw Martin for several hours as he agreed to take part in a long-term follow-up study (Wilson, 1991b). By now Martin was living in a Cheshire Home for physically handicapped people. I learned a little about what had happened to Martin since his discharge from Rivermead in 1983.

For a while Martin went twice a week for outpatient physiotherapy at the nearby General Hospital. After 6 mo he was told that he would never walk again. He then had private physiotherapy and began going to day centers and to a club for physically handicapped and able-bodied people (Phab). Martin did learn to walk independently but he sometimes fell and caused anxiety for those around him.

His parents had arranged for him to go to various groups for people with disabilities. He had somewhere to go almost every day of the week. At first his father drove him to all of them but then the local authority arranged for Martin's transport. His parents found this helpful but continued to accompany Martin every now and again so they could keep in touch with his day-to-day activities. Martin, of course, could not remember how he spent his day.

He attended day centers at Groby and Quorn, the latter called SPLATS (special people's laughing and talking society), a Dry Sports Club, a physically handicapped and able-bodied club, and went swimming. His father invented a mnemonic to enable him to remember which group he attended each day:

Monday, Groby:dry;

Tuesday, Quorn or SPLATS;

Wednesday, home;

Thursday, Phab;

Saturday, have a splash;

and he always added, "Sunday, go to Church."

A second mnemonic was devised to help Martin remember the names of the villages between Loughborough and Leicester. The mnemonic was *QUERY MR B*. This stood for Quorn, Mountsorrel, Rothey, and Birstall. Martin learned what these letters stood for and still retains this information at the time of this writing in 1997.

In 1983 Martin's father became chairman of the local branch of the National Head Injuries Association known as Headway. One of the Headway members wanted to find a residential home for her son who had sustained a head injury as a child and was now becoming impossible to manage at home. Martin's father helped this woman obtain a place in a Cheshire home not too far from their home town. Cheshire Homes were founded by Leonard Cheshire and were established to offer choice and opportunity for people with disabilities. The Leonard Cheshire Charter's mission is "to assist people with disabilities throughout the world, regardless of their color, race or creed, by providing the conditions necessary for their physical, mental, and spiritual well-being." While visiting the Cheshire Home, Martin's parents talked to the matron about Martin, not with any idea of Martin living there but simply to explain their involvement in Headway. The matron liked the sound of Martin and offered him a place. After talking it over with Martin who wanted to go, and a family conference with Martin's brothers and sister, they decided to take up the offer. The local authority needed some persuading that they should fund Martin but eventually it worked out and Martin finally went to the Cheshire Home in October 1988.

Earlier Martin had spent 6 wk at an employment rehabilitation center for a work assessment but all his parents were told at the end of it was, "He's not serious enough." His parents however, feel Martin's sense of humor is an essential part of Martin. They admire it and feel it has helped him to cope with his head injury and his brain damage.

I saw Martin in 1991 when he agreed once more to take part in a research project. This was the errorless learning project described in Chapters 9 (Jason) and 12 (Ron) (Baddeley and Wilson, 1994). In addition I usually spoke on the telephone or wrote to his parents once a year.

MARTIN TODAY

I last saw Martin in July 1997 at the Cheshire Home where he still lives. His parents were there and we spent several hours together. Over the past few years Martin has had several falls so the staff preferred him to remain in a wheelchair. He was mobile and independent in his chair but I felt his parents were saddened by

the fact that he no longer walked independently although the physiotherapist exercises him by walking with a walking frame, and he walks using a stick on his visits home. I reassessed Martin on a number of tests. Although there appeared to be very little change on the standardized tests, his parents feel Martin has changed in a number of ways. They describe his conversation as being more serious and less euphoric. They feel he is more likely to refer to something that happened earlier in the day than he did a few years ago, although if questioned directly about an episode or event his mind "goes blank."

They told me that right from the time Martin regained consciousness he kept his brain active by counting marks on the ceiling above his bed or in the pattern of his wallpaper. Then when his parents brought him home at weekends from Rivermead in the winter when it was dark, he counted the headlights of oncoming cars. While some might interpret this as perseverative behavior, Martin's parents interpret it as an attempt to keep his mind busy.

Although the early days were painful, Martin's parents were supported by their faith and seem to have felt no bitterness. His father said, "Our prayers for Martin's full recovery were not answered in the way we wanted but in real terms I feel they were answered because Martin is more of a complete human being now than he was before his accident. Then he was certainly an agnostic (if not an atheist) and yet he came to have faith."

All three feel that the Cheshire Home is a good place to be. His parents said, "It is the best thing for him there's no doubt about it. He's with his peers. He's one of the top dogs. He doesn't feel inferior. He hasn't got mummy and daddy around. He gets on with the staff. The staff enjoy talking to him. He never whines, never has a tantrum, he's never tired but when the light's off he's out like a light. He's never hungry but eats a good meal."

I asked how Martin spent his day and was told, "It's difficult to know, he can't remember to tell us. They have music sessions, reading the newspaper sessions, occupational therapy, swimming. They work and get certificates and go on outings. They go on holiday but not Martin because he comes with us."

"What would you like me to put in this chapter?" I asked Martin. He said, "Where there's life, there's hope." His father said, "The paramount need in rehabilitation is for the patient to be surrounded by love. In spite of the worst prognosis, there is always grounds for hope, never give up, maintain a loving happy atmosphere, and surround the one injured by prayer and love."

I will let Martin's mother have the last word. She said, "It isn't the disaster you might think because he's so lovely."

8

LORNA: COGNITIVE DECLINE AND MYOTONIC DYSTROPHY

BACKGROUND

Lorna was born in May 1954, the younger of two sisters. She was a normal child, did reasonably well at school, and had an active social life. She liked sports, particularly horseback riding, squash, walking, and tennis. When she was 18 and working as a secretary she came home one day for lunch and tried to remove a plug from the wall. She found she had difficulty letting go of the plug. This began to happen more often, she just could not immediately let go of things she was holding. Her parents, thinking there was a trivial explanation, asked their general practitioner to see Lorna. He sent her to a specialist.

Lorna was diagnosed as having myotonic dystrophy, a genetic autosomal dominant disorder. Dystrophy means weakening and wasting of the muscles whereas myotonia refers to an inability to relax the voluntary muscles after activity. Thus myotonic dystrophy is characterized by progressive weakness of the muscles together with impaired muscle relaxation. Other systems are often affected too. For example, cataracts are common, so too are heart problems. Hair, bone, gonads, and insulin metabolism may also be affected (Harper, 1989).

The disorder is also likely to appear progressively earlier in successive generations usually with increasing severity. This phenomenon is known as anticipation. In Lorna's case she inherited the condition from her father whose only symptoms were stiffness of the neck and cataracts developing later in life. The two main forms of myotonic dystrophy are the congenital form, which is invariably inherited from the mother (Hageman et al., 1993), and late onset form, which can be inherited from either parent. Although there is great variability in the age of onset, it most often appears between the ages of 20 and 40 years. Lorna's older sister (by 4 yr) was not diagnosed as having the disorder until she was 28 yr old. She had no symptoms until following the birth of her daughter when she noticed weakness in her legs. She has never been incapacitated by her condition however.

Following Lorna's diagnosis, life went on as normal. Her sister married and had a daughter. Lorna worked as a receptionist in a general practitioner's office. She continued to ride, to play tennis, and to go on long walks. She had a steady boyfriend. When she was about 25 yr old memory problems began. She had difficulty remembering what she had done at work, she had several disagreements with a colleague at work and lost her job. She also began having trouble with her boyfriend and they terminated their relationship. Her parents put the memory problems down to stress and depression. One weekend Lorna's parents went to visit friends, leaving Lorna alone in the house, something they had done many times before. When they returned, however, they found Lorna very distressed and upset. She had been unable to cope. Soon after this Lorna and her parents went on holiday to Canada where Lorna did some hang gliding. On one occasion when she landed she fell back and lost the feeling in her legs. On return to England she went to see a neurologist who referred her to a psychiatrist. After 3 mo of outpatient treatment, the psychiatrist said Lorna was fit for work. Lorna went for an interview and was told she would hear the result in a few days. Three days later she woke up and said, "I can't remember anything." Later the same day the telephone rang and Lorna was offered the job although she was never able to take up the offer.

The memory problems continued and Lorna was referred for further neurological investigations. She had a computed tomography (CT) scan that showed cerebral atrophy, i.e., shrinking of the brain, but was told the cerebral atrophy and the myotonic dystrophy were unrelated.

Lorna also had a neuropsychological assessment when she was 28 yr old. As a result of this assessment both her verbal and performance IQ were estimated to be in the low-average range and she performed in the impaired range on tests of memory. The assessment was repeated shortly before Lorna's 30th birthday and again when she was 31 yr old. The results from these three assessments were virtually identical showing no change over this 3 yr period.

In 1986, when Lorna was 32 yr old she was referred to me for assessment and advice about her memory problems that, by now had persisted for 7 yr. I saw Lorna six times between July and early October 1986 to complete an assessment and make some suggestions to her parents. Her parents brought her on each occasion—a journey of about 2 h each way. I spent about 2 h each time with Lorna.

INITIAL ASSESSMENT

Lorna was assessed on the Weschler Adult Intelligence Scale (WAIS), the National Adult Reading Test (NART), and the Raven's Matrices, together with some tests of memory, executive functioning, language, and perception. The results can be seen in Table 8.1. Lorna was always friendly and cooperative although somewhat superficial and she showed little concern at any failures.

My conclusions at this time were that premorbidly Lorna had been functioning in the average range. The evidence for this came from (1) her scores on the NART, a reasonably good test for estimating premorbid ability, and (2) her vocabulary subtest result from the WAIS on which she achieved an age scaled score of 9 (9–11 can be considered average). She still achieved an average nonverbal IQ on the Raven's Matrices, so her nonverbal reasoning skills were adequate. Despite these normal results, Lorna showed evidence of widespread cognitive impairment in the domain of memory, language, executive functioning, and perception.

Her immediate verbal memory as assessed by digit span was 5 forwards, just within the normal range, although her age scaled score on the total number of forward and backward digits on the WAIS was well below average. Her immediate recall of a prose passage was extremely poor. She only managed one item and could recall nothing after a delay. On the paired associate learning test from the original Weschler Memory Scale (WMS), she could learn only a few easy pairs.

Lorna's visual memory was slightly better. Her Corsi span was 5 (normal range) and her 40 min recall of the Rey-Osterreith figure resulted in a score of 7/36, which although very impaired, was not as bad as her verbal recall.

On the Rivermead Behavioural Memory Test (RBMT) Lorna's total screening score was 4/12, i.e., in the moderately impaired range. She passed the delayed route, delivering a message, remembering one name, and picture recognition. Lorna had great difficulty with all tests of remote memory, suggesting a long period of retrograde amnesia.

As far as language was concerned, Lorna showed quite a marked anomia. She scored only 5/30 on the Grade Naming Test (GNT). The majority of her failures were due to word finding difficulties, for example, for the sundial she said "It's—oh God—a clock thing in the garden."

Lorna's executive functions were assessed with the modified version of the WCST (Nelson, 1976), verbal fluency, and a speed of information processing task (Baddeley et al., 1992). On the short WCST, she achieved only 2 of 6 categories and made a total of 25 errors of which 13 were perseverative errors. These

Table 8.1. Lorna's Neuropsychological Test Results

General Intellectual Ability

National Adult Reading Test (Nelson, 1982)

	OCT. 1986	JUL. 1991	JAN. 1992	OCT. 1995	DEC. 1995	MAR. 1997
Errors	25	31	28	32	33	32
Predicted IQ	107	102	105	101	100	101

Raven's Standard Progressive Matrices (Raven, 1960)

	OCT. 1986	MAR. 1996
Raw score	41	26
IQ equivalent	100	89

Spot-the-Word (from SCOLP, Baddeley et al., 1992)

	JUL. 1995	SEP. 1996
Raw score	38/60	38/60
Age scaled score (percentile)	4 (1–5)	4 (1–5)

Wechsler Adult Intelligence Scale (Wechsler, 1981b)

	JUN. 1982	JAN. 1984	AUG. 1985	OCT. 1986	JAN. 1996	STUSS ET AL.'S SS MEAN(SD)*
Performance IQ	83	84	80	79	57	80.7 (10.0)
Verbal IQ	81	89	81	78	71	93.4 (17.1)
Full-scale IQ				78	61	86.6 (12.6)

Wechsler Adult Intelligence Scale Subtests

AGE SCALED SCORES	OCT. 1986	JAN. 1996	STUSS ET AL.'S SS x̄(SD)
Information	6	2	10 (2.8)
Comprehension	5	0	
Arithmetic	6	3	
Similarities	8	5	
Digit span	6	4	7.7 (1.2)
Vocabulary	9	4	11.7 (3.1)
Digit symbol	8	5	
Picture completion	8	8	
Block design	7	4	6.8 (2.0)
Picture arrangement	6	6	
Object assembly	5	4	5.9 (1.6)

*Results (Means and Standard Deviations) from a study by Stuss et al. 1987.

(continued)

107

Table 8.1. Lorna's Neuropsychological Test Results (*continued*)

Executive Functions

Wisconsin Card Sorting Test (Nelson's 1976 modified version)

	OCT. 1986	MAR. 1996
Categories	2	0
Total errors	25	22
Perseverative errors	13	3

Reitan Trail Making Test (time in sec) (Apr. 1992)

	STUSS ET AL.'S SS X̄(SD)*
A = 102″	50.4 (30.9)
B = 329″	144.3 (117.5)

*Verbal Fluency***

	OCT. 1986	FEB. 1992	APR. 1992	MAR. 1994	AUG. 1994	DEC. 1995	MAR. 1996	MAY 1996
"F"		6 (1p)		3 (1p)		0		
"A"		3 (2p)		2 (1p) (2e)		1		
"S"	12 (1p)	7 (1p)		1		4	2 (3p)	
"Animals"	17	9				4 (3p)	5 (3p)	
Boys' Names			5 (3p)		6 (2p)		6 (e)	4 (1p)
Girls' Names			6		6		5 (p)	6 (1e)

Cognitive Estimates (Shallice & Evans, 1978)

APR. 1992			NORMAL RANGE	ERROR SCORE
P.O. tower	How high?	12′	100–300	3
Race horses	How fast?	1 mph	15–40	3
Best paid job	in UK today	Doctors	Pop star, Queen, Head of Corporation	1
Age	of oldest person in UK today	60	104–113	3
Spine	of average man	24″	19–47	0
Height/woman	of average British woman	5′	5′3″–5′8″	3

*Results (Means and Standard Deviations) from a study by Stuss et al. 1987.
** p = perseveration; e = error.

(continued)

Table 8.1. Lorna's Neuropsychological Test Results (*continued*)

Cognitive Estimates (*Shallice & Evans, 1978*)

APR. 1992			NORMAL RANGE	ERROR SCORE
Population	of UK	1000	11–499 million	3
Pint of milk	How heavy	1 lb.	1 lb. 1 oz.–2 lb. 19 oz.	1
Largest object	in house	Table	—	1
Camels in Holland	How many	10	Few in zoos	0

Total 18 (Controls = 3.60) [SD 1.92]

Language

Graded Naming Test (*McKenna & Warrington, 1983*)

	OCT. 1986	APR. 1992	JAN. 1993	OCT. 1995	DEC. 1995
Raw Score	5	0	3	1	0

Semantic Processing (*from SCOLP, Baddeley et al., 1992*)

	OCT. 1986	DEC. 1995	SEP. 1996
No. completed	23	15	14
Errors	5	7	7

Pyramids and Palm Trees (*Number Correct*) (*Howard & Patterson, 1992*)

VERSION	OCT. 1992	JAN. 1993	JUL. 1996
3 pictures	47		32
3 words		43	35
1 word/2 pictures		35	

Exceptional/Regular Words (*Patterson, unpublished*)

	OCT. 1992	DEC.1992	JUL. 1996	AUG. 1996	NOV. 1996
Errors	18	24	60	60	57
Total correct	234	228	192	192	195

Memory

Rivermead Behavioural Memory Test (*Wilson et al., 1985*)

	OCT. 1986	MAR. 1987	JUL. 1991	JAN. 1997
Screening score total (Max = 12)	4	2	1	0

(*continued*)

Table 8.1. Lorna's Neuropsychological Test Results (*continued*)

Rey-Osterreith Complex Figure (Bennett-Levy, 1984)

	OCT. 1986	JAN. 1996
Copy	34	27
Recall	0	0

Corsi Span

	OCT. 1986	OCT. 1995
	5	5

Visuo-Spatial/Perceptual

Unusual/Usual Views (Warrington & Taylor, 1978)

	OCT. 1986	MAR. 1996
Unusual	13/20	3/21
Usual	20/20	13/21

The Visual Object and Space Perception Battery* (Warrington & James, 1991)

	APR. 1992	MAR. 1996
Screening	18 (P)	18 (P)
Incomplete letters	15 (P)	20 (P)
Silhouettes		6 (F)
Dot counting	9 (P)	10 (P)
Position discrimination	10 (F)	18 (P)
Number location	7 (P)	7 (P)
Cube analysis	8 (P)	8 (P)

Famous Faces (Hodges, unpublished) May 1993 (Date of Assessment)

Faces	0/50
Names	0/50

High Frequency Famous Faces May 1993

3 (or 4)/50:	Margaret Thatcher
	Prince Charles
	Prince Philip
	("Esley" = Elvis Presley)

Same/Different Faces (Warrington and James, 1967)

	OCT. 1986	DEC. 1995
Number correct	18/20	12/20

*P, pass; F, fail.

(*continued*)

Table 8.1. Lorna's Neuropsychological Test Results (*continued*)

Facial Expressions (Eckman & Friesan, 1997)

Happiness	2/10
Surprise	2/10
Fear	5/10
Sadness	1/10
Disgust	2/10
Anger	3/10

Motor

Grooved Peg Board

	SEP. 1996		DEC. 1996		TIME SUMMED *two* HANDS*
	TIME	DROPS	TIME	DROPS	
Right Hand	323″	0	317″	0	185.06
Left Hand	378″	3	562″	5	58.43

*Results (time in sec) from a study by Woodward et al., 1982.

scores are in the impaired range. On verbal fluency she managed 12 "S" words (plus 1 perseveration) in 90 sec and 17 "animals," also in 90 sec. These are borderline scores. On the speed of processing test where Lorna had to decide whether short sentences were true or false, she managed only 23 in 2 min with 5 errors. Most people of her age would complete about 50 sentences in 2 min, with very few (certainly no more than 2) errors.

Lorna was also impaired on Warrington and Taylor's (1978) unusual views test where she scored 13/20. This is consistent with right parietal damage. She scored the maximum 20 on usual views so her result was not due to poor vision or her anomia.

Despite these problems there was no evidence of cognitive decline and Lorna's results on the WAIS were almost identical to those achieved in 1982.

REHABILITATION

Apart from some explanations and suggestions to her parents, I felt that there was little I could do for Lorna's memory difficulties and that she would not benefit from specific memory therapy strategies. I demonstrated that she was able to learn certain tasks, especially if these were broken down into stages and Lorna was taught a little at a time. For example, she was able to learn how to do a nine step wooden maze if she were taught in three stages (each comprising three steps). She also improved over time with a 12-piece children's jigsaw puzzle.

One area where Lorna's mother requested help was independence. Lorna rarely went out alone and her mother wanted her to be able to do this. We set up a behavior program incorporating goal setting and shaping. The nearest large town to Lorna's home was about 20 min away by bus. Our long-term goal for Lorna was for her to go into the town alone on the bus, buy some items from a shop, and meet her parents for the return journey home. The first short-term goal was for Lorna to walk to the bus stop alone. At first one of her parents followed closely behind, but gradually increased the distance and finally let her do it alone. Then she was to board the bus and pay for her fare. At first she was closely supervised and someone traveled with her. The amount of supervision was gradually decreased. Lorna soon learned to travel independently.

By now it was the end of 1986 and I was about to move to another job. I referred Lorna to a clinical psychologist near to her own home for continuing therapy.

Meanwhile, Lorna and her parents joined the Amnesia Association (described in Chapters 6 & 9) and, like Jason's mother, became active in their local group.

FOLLOW-UP

I saw Lorna a few times between 1987 and 1989 for discussion sessions with her and her parents. Occasionally we did a few tests but few formal assessments were carried out. These were really opportunities for Lorna's parents to voice their concerns and ask questions. I met them occasionally at meetings of the Amnesia Association and so kept in touch. Lorna appeared stable.

In late 1990, I moved to Cambridge, only an hour's car journey away from Lorna's home. Her parents wanted me to see her regularly as they felt Lorna enjoyed the sessions with me and found them stimulating. Since 1991 I have seen Lorna seven or eight times each year.

In the summer of 1991, Lorna was reassessed by the Clinical Psychology department at her local hospital. At that time Lorna was looking after her daily needs and doing much of the housework without being prompted. She spent two afternoons a week as a volunteer helper in a local charity shop and one afternoon in a local primary school listening to children reading. She could go out alone in her own neighborhood and could still use the bus to get into the local town. She was reluctant to use a diary or notebook but agreed to attend an outpatient memory group at the local hospital.

Lorna attended the group with her mother for an hour each week for 6 wk. The group aimed to (1) help people identify everyday problems caused by memory difficulties, (2) learn to find ways to minimize the effects of these problems, and (3) share with other members of the group ideas and experiences that might help overcome their problems.

Both Lorna and her mother reported that the group had been very useful. On a feedback form Lorna wrote that she had learned "to look into my life and more every day to look into the next day and see everything you want to do." When asked what aspects were most helpful she wrote, "to use my diary more." Her mother wrote she had learned, "that Lorna can improve with further guidance and help but we need to have a lot more patience with her and aim to do things repetitively to get results." For the most helpful aspects, Lorna's mother said, "Meeting people who have the same problems and sharing with them and learning ways of coping with these problems unthought of by us."

Between 1991 and 1997, I spent many hours with Lorna. We spent part of each session discussing Lorna's needs and problems. This extended to discussing the needs of her parents and her sister. Genetic testing was arranged by Dr. John Hodges in the Neurology department at Addenbrooke's Hospital to confirm the original diagnosis and to determine whether Lorna had inherited the myotonic dystrophy from her mother or father. The diagnosis was confirmed together with paternal inheritance. Lorna's niece, now a young adult, was found not to have the disorder. Lorna's father was very distressed on learning his daughter had inherited the disease from him. His physical health deteriorated after receiving this news. He stopped driving and developed cataracts that were successfully treated early in 1997. Much of the therapy then could be considered counseling.

We also spent some time investigating Lorna's ability to learn during this period and monitored her cognitive performance, which was showing evidence of deterioration.

NEW LEARNING

Because of my interest in errorless learning that grew out of joint research with Alan Baddeley (see Chapter 9), I wanted to see whether Lorna would benefit from an errorless learning procedure. She was included as a subject in a study funded by the European Community (Evans et al., in press) in which three tasks were administered in each of three different ways. The first task was teaching names of unfamiliar people from photographs, the second task was learning to program an electronic organizer and the final task was learning a diagrammatic route around a room (see Fig. 8.1). The three teaching methods were: (1) demonstrating the task (or telling the correct name) and then asking Lorna to complete the task (or say the name) after me with feedback; the task was repeated again in the same way and so on for a given number of trials (the errorful condition); (2) removing steps gradually, for example with names, the full name, PEGGY, was presented, then presented with one letter missing, PEGG_, and Lorna had to write in the last letter; PEG__ was presented next and Lorna had to write in the last two letters and so on; (3) following written instructions for a given number of

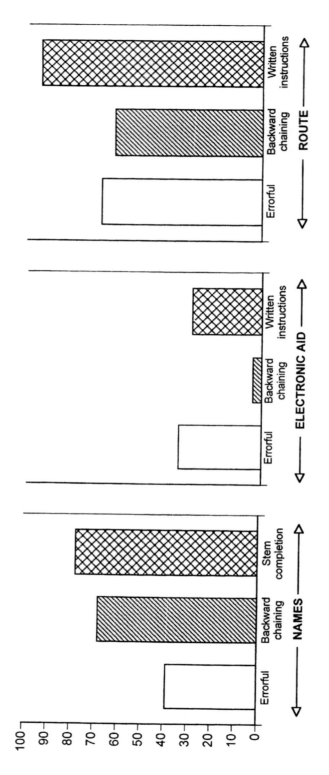

Figure 8.1. Percentage success for learning three tasks under three different methods for each task.

trials before attempting the task alone (or in the case of names, saying the name, providing the initial letter, and asking Lorna to complete the name). Conditions 2 and 3 were both errorless learning conditions. Lorna showed a variable pattern as can be seen in Figure 8.1.

We discussed the implications of these findings for real life tasks. Lorna seemed to show reasonably good learning of the route under all three conditions and her parents agreed that she seemed to be able to learn routes when traveling by car. She could learn people's names if the first letter was provided although had great difficulty if it was not provided, a similar result to that reported earlier by Glisky et al., (1986). If Lorna needed to learn a simple six-step task, she might be better with several demonstrations rather than breaking the task down.

One of the positive results from this study was the effect on the morale of Lorna's parents. Lorna herself appeared to forget after a few seconds that which had gone before although she was pleased at the time when told she was correct. Her parents, however, were delighted to hear of any achievement.

Observations of Lorna's performance during her route learning suggested that she might do better if (1) she were given regular breaks between trials, and (2) a chunking procedure were used as she appeared to remember the route in short sections or chunks of three or four steps. I decided to test out this hypothesis. I took the original eight-stage route and added another step in order to make three chunks of three steps each. The drawing of the route can be seen in Figure 8.2.

The first chunk was taught and learned rapidly. The second was taught and also learned rapidly. Chunks one and two were then demonstrated and taught as a whole. Chunk three was taught next before being added to the combined one–two chunk. In addition to the chunking, regular breaks were built in. Not only did Lorna learn the whole route with few mistakes but she retained it a month later with very few prompts. The results can be seen in Figures 8.3 and 8.4.

The principles of chunking and distributed practice were then applied to teach Lorna (1) another mock route using doll's house furniture, and (2) a route through a maze comprising 20 squares. She learned these with similar ease to the original route. Indeed with the doll's house furniture she showed incidental learning by pre-empting me on one occasion when I started to place the furniture in the pre-arranged locations. Lorna took the box from me and put the nine pieces of furniture out herself—and in the correct places. Unfortunately, I was unable to teach her verbal information such as names of objects using the same principle.

By now (1994–1995) it had become clear that Lorna had declined cognitively, her word finding was very poor, and her reading, which had shown no signs of impairment in 1986, was becoming more surface dyslexic (see Chapter 14). She had problems with semantic memory tasks and her episodic memory was very impaired.

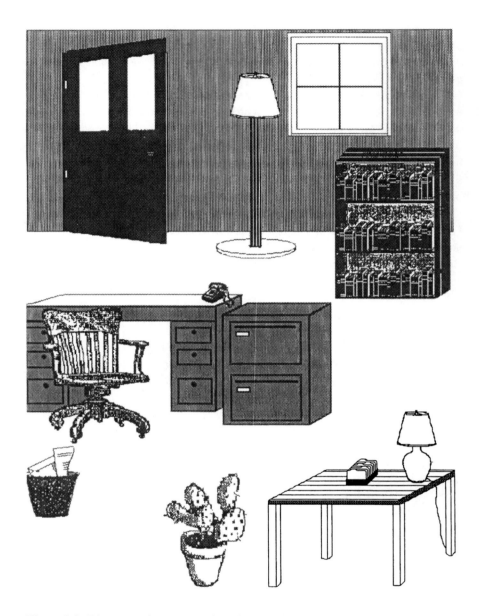

Figure 8.2. Diagrammatic representation of a room for a route learning task.

Chunks	A			B			C		
Stages	1	2	3	4	5	6	7	8	9
Places	Door	Desk	Table	Book case	Window	Lamp	Chair	Plant	Bin
3 demonstrations of these 3 steps provided									
	✓	✓	✓						
	✓	✓	✓						
	✓	✓	✓						
Four second break									
	✓	✓	✓						
	✓	✓	✓						
	✓	✓	✓						
Three demonstrations of			these 6 steps provided						
	✓	✓	✓	✓	X	X			
	✓	✓	✓	✓	✓	✓			
	✓	✓	✓	X	stopped here				
One demonstration of these 6			steps provided						
	✓	✓	✓	✓	✓	✓			
	✓	✓	✓	✓	✓	✓			
	✓	✓	✓	✓	✓	✓			
Four second break									
	✓	✓	✓	✓	✓	✓			
	✓	✓	✓	✓	✓	✓			
	✓	✓	X	✓	✓	✓			
Ten second break									
	✓	✓	✓	✓	✓	✓			
3 demonstrations of these 3 steps and 3 demonstrations of all 9 steps									
	✓	✓	✓	✓	✓	✓	✓	Reversed these 2 steps	
	✓	✓	✓	✓	X	✓	✓	Reversed these 2 steps	
3 demonstrations of these 3 steps									
	✓	✓	✓	✓	✓	✓	✓	Reversed these 2 steps	
3 more demonstrations of these 3 steps									
	✓	✓	✓	✓	✓	✓	Telephone rang at this point		
	✓	✓	✓	✓	X	✓	✓	✓	✓
20 second break									
	✓	✓	✓	✓	X	✓	✓	✓	✓
One demonstration of all 9			steps						
	✓	X	X	✓	✓	✓	✓	Reversed these 2 steps	
Two minute break									
	✓	✓	✓	✓	Reversed these 2 steps		✓	Reversed these 2 steps	
One demonstration of all 9			steps						
	✓	✓	✓	✓	✓	✓	✓	✓	✓
	✓	✓	✓	✓	✓	✓	✓	✓	✓
Four minute break									
	✓	✓	✓	✓	✓	✓	X	✓	✓
	✓	✓	✓	✓	✓	✓	✓	✓	✓
Two demonstrations of all 9			steps						
	✓	✓	✓	✓	✓	✓	✓	✓	✓
	✓	✓	✓	✓	✓	✓	✓	✓	✓
One minute break									
	✓	✓	✓	✓	✓	✓	✓	✓	✓
	✓	✓	✓	✓	✓	✓	✓	✓	✓
Four minute break									
	✓	✓	✓	✓	✓	✓	✓	✓	✓
	✓	✓	✓	✓	✓	✓	✓	✓	✓
Five minute break									
	✓	✓	✓	✓	✓	✓	✓	✓	✓
	✓	✓	✓	✓	✓	✓	✓	✓	✓
Fifteen minute break									
	✓	✓	✓	✓	✓	✓	✓	✓	✓
				END OF SESSION					

Figure 8.3. Route learning through errorless learning, chunking, and distributed practice.

117

Date - 4/4/95

				Stages				
1	2	3	4	5	6	7	8	9
Door	Desk	Table	Bookcase	Window	Lamp	Chair	Plant	Bin
1 demonstration provided of these 3 steps (1 chunk)								
✔	✔	✔						
✔	✔	✔						
✔	✔	✔						
			1 demonstration provided of these 3 steps (1 chunk)					
			✔	✔	✔			
			✔	✔	✔			
			✔	✔	✔			
1 demonstration provided of			all 6 steps (2 chunks)					
✔	✔	✔	✔	✔	✔			
✔	✔	✔	✔	✔	✔			
✔	✔	✔	✔	✔	✔			
						1 demonstration provided of these 3 steps (1 chunk)		
						✔	✔	✔
						✔	✔	✔
						✔	✔	✔
Break of 2 minutes								
✔	Lamp	✔	✔	✔	✔	✔	Bin	Plant
✔	✔	✔	✔	✔	✔	✔	✔	✔
✔	Bookcase	✔	abandoned - in danger of making errors					
1 demonstration provided of first 3 steps								
✔	✔	✔	✔	✔	✔	✔	✔	✔
Break of 5 minutes								
✔	✔	✔	✔	✔	✔	✔	✔	✔
✔	✔	✔	✔	✔	✔	✔	✔	✔

Figure 8.4. One month relearning of route.

NEUROPSYCHOLOGICAL CHANGES 1986–1997

All tests administered in 1986 were readministered in 1995–96 together with various other tests. The main results can be seen in Table 8.1.

The old WAIS was employed rather than the revised version in order to have a direct comparison. Lorna's performance IQ had declined from 79 (Oct. 1986) to 57 (Jan. 1996). Her verbal IQ had declined to a lesser extent from 78 to 71 over the same period. Her fluency for animals had declined from 17 in 1986 to 3 (with 2 perseverations) in January 1997. Her Raven's Standard Progressive Matrices

(SPM) score had held up reasonably well and she was still functioning in the low-average range.

Her RBMT screening score, which was 4/12 in 1986, dropped to 2/12 in March 1987, to 1 in July 1991, and when last tested in January 1997 she failed to score. She had declined on the Rey-Osterreith figure too, only scoring 27/36 on Copy (compared to 34/36 in 1986) and remembering nothing after a delay.

On the semantic processing test Lorna's score had dropped from 23 completed in 1986, to 15 in 1995, and 14 in 1996, furthermore she made 7 errors on these last two occasions. She was unable to name anything on the GNT in April 1992, but increased her score to 3 in January 1993 following additional speech therapy, 1 in October 1995 and 0 in December 1995.

All in all there was marked evidence of cognitive decline. How abnormal was this? Lorna's family and I had been told by more than one neurologist that the cognitive decline and the cortical atrophy were unrelated to her myotonic dystrophy. Heather Balleny, a clinical psychology student working with me during 1996 and I decided to look into this a little further.

HOW DOES LORNA COMPARE WITH OTHER PEOPLE WITH MYOTONIC DYSTROPHY?

Over the past 100 years or so since myotonic dystrophy (MYD) was first described, there have been numerous observations of decreased mental capabilities in patients with myotonic dystrophy and it is fairly well established that the congenital form is associated with mental retardation (Harper, 1989). However, relatively few neuropsychological studies using standardized tests have been carried out (Stuss et al., 1987). One of the earliest reports comparing control subjects and people with myotonic dystrophy was that of Woodward et al. (1982). They administered the Halstead-Reitan Battery to 17 patients and 25 controls and found the MYD group worse than normal controls on nearly every measure of the battery. They also reported that there was no relationship between the neuropsychological test results and (1) degree of weakness, (2) myotonia, and (3) muscle atrophy.

The following year Bird et al. (1983) published the results of a study in which 29 MYD patients from 14 families were assessed on the WAIS. Approximately one third of the patients had WAIS IQ scores below 80 and 7% had WAIS scores above 120. The majority therefore performed in the average range. Bird et al. (1983) also found that females had poorer cognitive function than males and that limited cognitive ability was associated with maternal inheritance and severe physical handicap, although the authors noted there were individual exceptions to this. Verbal and informational skills tended to be least affected in this group with poorest performance found on tasks involving immediate recall, abstraction, spatial manipulation, and orientation. Finally they found no evidence of intellectual decline with time and signs of cerebral atrophy on CT scans were uncommon.

Lorna was atypical of the Bird et al. subjects in at least three ways: (1) she inherited the disease from her father yet had marked cognitive impairment, (2) she showed decline over time, and (3) cerebral atrophy was noted as long ago as 1982.

A more detailed study by Stuss et al. (1987); appeared in 1987. This study compared 19 MYD subjects with 19 controls matched for age, sex, education, and WAIS-R full scale IQ. The MYD subjects, as a group, performed in the low-average range overall although there was a wide range of abilities suggesting that MYD subjects do not form a unitary group. Stuss et al. (1987) found no evidence of aphasia, apraxia, or agnosia and no evidence of specific problems in slowed information processing once the effects of IQ and motor impairment were partialed out. Stuss et al. (1987) noted that age of onset and duration of disease were important variables influencing cognitive impairment although they recognized that there were problems in determining both of these. Myotonic dystrophy patients may not be diagnosed, for example, for several years after the first symptoms appear. The authors concluded that MYD patients do not appear to have a cortical dementia.

Three years later, Malloy et al. (1990) looked at 20 MYD patients and 20 controls. They found that MYD subjects performed significantly poorer on both motor and cognitive functions particularly those assessing spatial functions. Like Bird et al. (1987), Malloy and his colleagues (1990) suggested that cognitive deficits are relatively stable over time in MYD patients and do not progress with age.

One of the earliest positron emission tomography (PET) studies by Mielke et al., appeared in 1993. They looked at three patients, two males aged 42 and 50 years and one female aged 59 years. An impairment of regional cerebral glucose metabolism was found in all cortical and subcortical regions particularly in the frontal cortex and lentiform nucleus. The metabolic pattern seen was similar to that observed in normal aging but was qualitatively more severe suggesting that MYD is a progeric (i.e., rapid aging) disease.

Another imaging study published in 1993 was that of Chang et al. who looked at neuroimaging and neuropsychological changes in 22 MYD patients and 10 normal control subjects. Their results suggested neuropsychological abnormalities in visual perception, constructional ability, and visual memory. These deficits were strongly correlated with decreased cerebral blood flow (CBF) in the right temporal and right frontoparietal regions. Magnetic resonance imaging (MRI) scans revealed no white matter lesions or histories suggestive of progressive dementia. Single photon emission computer tomography (SPECT) investigations found significant differences in CBF between MYD patients and control subjects.

In the same year, 1993, a Finnish study reported on 35 MYD patients. Five of these were of congenital onset and all had moderate or mild mental retardation. All 30 adult-onset patients had a normal IQ and memory quotient (MQ). The authors found no effect of paternal or maternal inheritance. The reason this study found no effect of paternal or maternal inheritance (unlike several other studies) is no doubt because all subjects had normal cognitive functioning. This in itself is unusual and one wonders whether the sample was biased in some way. Of the adult-onset Finnish patients, 16 were followed up after a mean interval of 12 yr and no severe cognitive decline was found over this time span.

A further MRI study was carried out by Censori et al. (1994). They scanned 25 MYD and 25 control subjects. The results were different from those of Chang et al. (1993). Censori et al. found 81% of MYD subjects had white matter hyperintense lesions compared to 16% of controls. The lesions involved all cerebral lobes. Furthermore 28% of the MYD subjects showed particular white matter, hyperintense lesions at the temporal poles. This is interesting in light of Lorna's semantic memory impairment given that the temporal neocortex is involved in patients with semantic memory disorders (Patterson and Hodges, 1995).

Censori et al. also found the MYD subjects had significantly more cerebral atrophy than controls. Although the abnormalities were not related to clinical or cognitive parameters, MRI brain abnormalities were almost always found in MYD patients. This is in contrast to the absence of abnormalities on CT scans as noted by Bird et al. (1983).

The final study to be reported here is that of Palmer et al. (1994) who studied 7 MYD patients with maternal inheritance, 14 with paternal inheritance, and 10 normal control subjects. They found that the group with paternal inheritance had a normal neuropsychological profile apart from slowed information processing whereas the group with maternal inheritance had abnormal scores on measures of intelligence, visual construction, and some frontal lobe measures.

Thus, apart from general agreement about the congenital form of MYD, there are conflicting findings about the extent of cognitive impairment in the late onset form. By and large most studies agree that maternal inheritance results in a greater likelihood of cognitive problems and that there is little evidence of severe decline over time. Lorna, in contrast, inherited the condition from her father and did show considerable decline over time.

LORNA TODAY

Lorna had an MRI scan in 1993. It showed generalized focal cerebral atrophy without focal involvement. There was no obvious progression since her previous scan in 1985 although it was difficult to be sure on this point given changes in technology over time.

Lorna continues to live at home with her parents. She sees her sister and niece every now and again. Physically she has deteriorated a little. She walks with the aid of a stick and her mother needs to help her in and out of a chair. The myotonia is minimal and there is no obvious sign of muscle wasting. She appears to be stiff and ungainly rather than weak. Until 10 yr ago, she went on long walks but now can walk only short distances.

As described earlier, she has declined cognitively. She stopped using buses and going out alone 3 to 4 yr ago. She helps her mother a little in the house by doing some dusting and setting the table.

Her mother seems optimistic about Lorna and appears not to see much deterioration. In part this might be because Lorna has improved in some areas. For many years she had choking and vomiting spells and could eat only a small amount of food. If she ate larger amounts, particularly bread and potatoes, she would regurgitate the food. Her parents always worried when they took her to a restaurant and always carried a plastic bag with them. She was also giddy when she first got up in the mornings. About 2 yr ago, they saw a new young doctor at the general surgery. She diagnosed anemia and prescribed iron. She also thought Lorna had asthma and gave her an inhalant. In the last year there has been no giddiness and very few choking spells. Everyone can relax when they go to a restaurant. Because the myotonia and weakness has not worsened, the specialist is pleased with Lorna and reduced her check-ups from every 6 mo to every 8 mo. Lorna also had "petit mal" for a number of years but these have now almost ceased.

Even with the cognitive problems, Lorna's parents appear to think she is managing. I asked Lorna's mother why she thought Lorna had memory problems and her sister did not. She said Lorna's sister "always had a good memory and Lorna didn't. She [Lorna] was a perfectionist. She worked hard and checked everything, so kept up at school and at work. Her sister had an excellent memory and didn't have to worry."

I asked Lorna's mother what she thought caused the problems. She said she thought it was stress: "Stress at thinking she should leave home, trouble at work, and trouble with her boyfriend. She also had a fall from her horse. She fell on to her back onto some concrete. She was winded and may have lost consciousness for a moment or two. She had back problems after that but maybe the fall had made her memory worse."

Although one can be fairly certain that the stress did not cause the cerebral atrophy, it is possible that the fall from the horse (and perhaps the fall at the hang gliding landing) contributed to Lorna's memory problems. It would appear more likely, however, that she has atypical myotonic dystrophy in (1) having severe cognitive impairment and paternal inheritance together with late onset and (2) marked decline over a 17 yr period. Perhaps if other MYD patients were studied so extensively over so long a period, others like Lorna would be found.

9

JASON: LEARNING TO BE INDEPENDENT AFTER ENCEPHALITIS

BACKGROUND

In July 1982, I had a telephone call from Alan Baddeley asking for advice on how to respond to a letter he had received from the mother of a young man, Jason, who had sustained viral encephalitis over 2 yr previously. I suggested that Alan should ask the mother to request a referral to our center for an assessment to see if her son was suitable for our memory rehabilitation program. Alan later sent me a copy of the letter so that I would know the background. Jason's mother wrote:

> Dear Sir,
> After following the "Human Brain" programmes I wrote to the B.B.C. hoping they might appeal to families of patients suffering from memory problems to write to me and that we might be of some mutual help. My son contracted Virus Encephalitis $2^1/_2$ year ago, he is now 26. I had a reply from the B.B.C. (Dick Gilling), who thought that you might be the one person who could be interested enough to give me some help and advice, as your main interest was memory. So far I have not been able to get any help, there are no organisations who know of people like Jason, I have written to so many. It is always the same, there are so few cases and there is no centre of information. Jason cannot remember much of his life before his illness, just facts, like the name of his school, name of his University, but has no recognition, when taking him to the University he did not know it or the way around. He has a Degree in Electronic and Electrical Engineering but has forgotten all he ever learnt

as far as I can ascertain. He does not recognise friends by face, but remembers names. He only knows his father, brother and sister and me, his mother. He does not recognise most animals, on pictures nor does he know which food he eats, all that memory has gone. He seems to be able to learn some things, like facts, after constant repetition, but remembers quickly anything emotional. My mother died last week and he knows without any reminders. He is a very unhappy boy, as he worries about his future, what is going to happen to him when we die, we are nearing 60, and he knows he would live longer than we could. He worries about meeting strangers, won't open the door in case he does not know who it might be. He cannot go out alone only round the block with the dog as he has forgotten the way if it is further. He was a good swimmer and swam for Great Britain in the World Student Games in Mexico 1979, he can still swim as well as ever, but does not want to, he says, 'what is the use of winning if I cannot remember the feeling of it afterwards'. He leads a very negative life as friends drop off when he does not recognise them, I think they get embarrassed. I had hoped that there were other people whose families were similarly affected and we could be of mutual help, but it seems that is not feasible either.

Please is there anything you could suggest that might help to get him to lead a more happy life any suggestions as to what might make him remember or learn again? I bought him some tablets in the USA which are called IQ Plus, they consist of: 500 mg. L-Glutamine, 100 mg Phenylalanine, 100 mg. L-Lysine and 1000 mg. Choline (in 1 tablet). He takes 4 of these per day, I think he seems brighter to absorb information, but don't know yet if it is my imagination or hopefulness. Please is there anything you could do to help? There just is no-one else. All I have ever been told is, 'He won't get any better', 'Put him in a Home'. I cannot give up just like that, please try to help if you can.
Yours sincerely,
M.... B....

The encephalitis developed when Jason was 23 yr old. In January 1980, he woke up one Saturday morning and said he had a bad headache. He thought he had influenza and so did his parents as several of their acquaintances had influenza at the time. Later that day Jason even went swimming but on his return felt very ill. The following day he could not do anything and felt wretched. On Monday his mother called the doctor who could find nothing wrong. He prescribed antibiotics and pain killers. On Monday evening Jason had a seizure and was taken to the hospital. At first he was thought to have meningitis and was taken to another hospital where he remained for 2 days before being taken to a hospital specializing in neurological diseases. Here Jason was found to have herpes simplex encephalitis. By now Jason was virtually comatose. He showed little awareness of his surroundings.

Jason remained in the specialist hospital for 2 mo. A CT scan was performed, which showed widespread attenuation maximal in both temporal lobes. At first his parents were told the encephalitis would leave Jason with a poor memory. His parents were not too concerned thinking he would have to repeat his final year at the university where he was due to take his final exams in June 1980. At the end of March, Jason's father went to talk to one of the hospital staff and said, "Jason doesn't seem to be getting any better." He was told, "Oh no, his memory is impaired for life you should put him in a home." At least this is how Jason's parents remember being given the information that their son would never recover. Jason's mother said they had great difficulty accepting this information. They had never heard of encephalitis before Jason became ill.

At the beginning of April, Jason was transferred to a local general hospital where the staff found it very difficult to manage him. There were not enough staff and they had little expertise in dealing with Jason's particular problems. He kept getting out of the hospital to telephone his parents, desperately pleading to come home. He came home on weekends and was easy to manage until Sunday afternoons when he had to return. Then he became aggressive and created dramatic scenes. Eventually his parents, unable to bear his distress, agreed to let him stay home. He remained at home for 4 yr. He was awarded his degree on the basis of his first 2 yr work even though he never took his finals. He was able to attend the graduation ceremony with his parents. In June 1982, his mother wrote to Alan Baddeley and in October 1982 Jason began attending Rivermead Rehabilitation Centre in Oxford. He came for 2 days a week for a period of 4 mo. Although his father had cancer at the time, he drove him there and back each time, the journey lasting about 2 h. I learned later that it was a huge battle to get Jason in the car for the journey. He wanted to drive and thought that if he could drive he would get his memory back. He ran to the car to try to get there before his father so he (Jason) could get into the driver's seat and force his father into the passenger seat.

INITIAL ASSESSMENT

Before Jason came for his initial one-day assessment, we had a brief neuropsychological report from the specialist hospital he attended over 2 yr earlier. His verbal IQ was in the average range and his performance IQ in the borderline range. He showed average performance on the Raven's Matrices, a nonverbal reasoning test, but was at chance level on recognition memory tests. The most interesting findings from the earlier investigations were Jason's difficulties with recognition of certain classes of objects. He could, for example, recognize manufactured or man-made objects fairly easily but had lost virtually all knowledge of animals, plants, and foods. He was one of the first people to be described with a category specific semantic memory disorder (Warrington and Shallice, 1984).

When I first saw Jason for his one-day assessment I observed a very anxious and frightened young man. He appeared terrified that his father would leave him at the center. His father looked ill and also under stress. I administered some memory tests to Jason, and he saw some other members of staff and at the end of the day. We offered Jason a place at the rehabilitation center for 2 days a week for

the next few months to assess his cognitive and memory functions in more detail
and to see if we could teach him some compensatory strategies. Jason's father
said he could manage 2 days a week although we were somewhat concerned
about this arrangement as he was an elderly and obviously unwell man who was
upset by his son's distress.

Jason was duly assessed and cooperated reasonably well with the testing although he appeared to be suspicious of us. One of the items on the Rivermead
Behavioural Memory Test is "Remembering a hidden belonging." A belonging is
borrowed from the subject and hidden in a drawer. The subject is asked to remind
the tester about the belonging when told, "We have now finished this test." I took
Jason's comb and put it in the drawer, having explained the task to him. Jason
was furious with me and asked for his comb every few seconds. He was so focused on his comb that I had to give it to him in order to ensure he paid sufficient
attention to the other items. At the end of the test when I said we had finished, I
went on to say, "At the beginning of the test I hid one of your items away to see if
you could remember it. Do you know what it was?" But Jason had forgotten. His
amnesia was very severe. His main results can be seen in Table 9.1.

Thus his general intellectual functioning was below average and, without
doubt, far below his premorbid level given that Jason had a degree in electronic
and electrical engineering. These results are essentially the same as those found
during his first assessment in 1980. Both the original report and my report concluded that Jason had a dense global amnesia, a surface dyslexia and dysgraphia,
and an agnosia, particularly for living things.

I discussed Jason's results with Alan Baddeley and we decided to look at
Jason's reading abilities in some detail. As he had a surface dyslexia and a dense
amnesia, we wondered whether his errors would be consistent. He was assessed
on a word list containing irregular and regular words 10 times within a week (five
times in each of two sessions). Jason always denied having seen the list before,
both within and between sessions. Both consistency for some words and inconsistency for other words across testing session were found, as can be seen in
Table 9.2.

Although Jason had particular difficulty with irregularly spelled words such as,
DOUGH, YACHT, and SWORD, he also had difficulty with some regularly
spelled words such as TROUT, which he always read as "TROOT," and sometimes misread words, saying for example, "FLESH" for FLASH or "SPORT" for
SPOT.

Jason's spelling was even more impaired than his reading. This is typical of
people with surface dyslexia, i.e., their dependence on phonetics is even more apparent when they write words. This surface dysgraphia showed itself clearly in
words such as KNOWLEDGE, which he spelled as NOLEJ, and SPAGHETTI,
which he spelled as SBGETEY. Some of his errors however were unexpected
such as GETE for GUILTY and REGRIER for REQUIRE.

Table 9.1. Jason's Neuropsychological Test—Results from 1982

Wechsler Adult Intelligence Scale

VERBAL SUBTESTS	AGE SCALED SCORES	PERFORMANCE SUBTESTS	AGE SCALED SCORES
Information	5	Digit symbol	5
Comprehension	8	Picture completion	7
Arithmetic	6	Block design	12
Similarities	8	Picture arrangement	6
Digit span	6	Object assembly	6
Vocabulary	8		
Verbal IQ	80	(Low average)	
Performance IQ	82	(Low average)	
Full scale IQ	80	(Low average)	

Raven's Standard Progressive Matrices

Raw score	38	
Predicted IQ	93	(Average)

Wechsler Memory Scale

Logical memory	Immediate recall	4	(Below average)
	Delayed recall	0	(Severely impaired)

Rivermead Behavioural Memory Test

Screening score	0	(Max 12)	(Severely impaired)
Standardized profile score	2	(Max 24)	(Severely impaired)

Recognition Memory Test

Words	Age scaled score	< 3 (Severely impaired)
Faces	Age scaled score	< 3 (Severely impaired)

Digit Span

Forward	5	(Within average range)
Backwards	3	(Below average)

Rey-Osterreith Complex Figure

Copy	34/36	(Normal score)
40 minute recall	0/36	(Severely impaired)

Benton Visual Retention Test

Correct	5	(Impaired)
Errors	9	(Impaired)

(continued)

Table 9.1. Jason's Neuropsychological Test—Results from 1982 (*continued*)

Corsi Blocks

Visuospatial span	5	(Normal)

Graded Naming Test

Raw score	0	(Severely impaired)

Usual/Unusual Views

Usual	13/20	(Impaired)
Unusual	13/20	(Impaired)

Same/Different Faces

Raw score	11/20	(Chance level)

Reading

Single letters	Upper case	100%	
	Lower case	100%	
Regular vs. irregular	Regular better	(see Table 10.6)	
Lexical decision	Errors	16 (max 40)	
(selecting words	False positives	13	(Impaired)
from nonwords	False negatives	3	
Reading nonwords		50% correct	(Impaired)

Spelling

Vernon Spelling List	17/80 Correct	(Impaired)

The majority of errors were phonetic (e.g., HUNY for HONEY, YUNG for YOUNG, BUTERFUL for BEAUTIFUL

The quick brown fox jumps over the lazy dog was written:
"The grich brown fox jumps over the laccy dog."

Although I intended trying some remediation strategies for Jason's reading and memory problems, it became clear that Jason's father, who had now told us about his cancer, would not be able to cope with the strain of bringing Jason on a journey lasting 2 h each way. Jason, too, never became comfortable or settled at the center. He was extremely suspicious of all the staff and patients. He thought we intended to keep him there, he could not settle if his father left the room, he would not attend the memory group, and was generally very uncooperative.

The staff met and following a discussion with Jason's father felt attendance at the center was counterproductive. Jason stopped coming and for the next 5 yr I lost touch with him.

AFTER RIVERMEAD

I next heard of Jason and his mother through the Amnesia Association. This was an association set up in September 1987 by Deborah Wearing, the wife of Clive (see Chapter 6) who became amnesic following herpes simplex encephalitis, and myself. Deborah Wearing talks about the founding of the Amnesia Association and other self-help groups in an excellent chapter published in 1992 (Wearing, 1992).

The first meeting of the Amnesia Association was held at Charing Cross Hospital in September 1987 and Jason's mother attended. Local support groups were set up around the country and Jason's mother became active in a local group that met once a month near her home. Jason sometimes attended these meetings and I once went to talk to the group. The format was for everyone to meet together at the home of one of the families involved. After the initial gathering the relatives would go upstairs to talk about their problems and their coping strategies while the memory impaired people would gather downstairs for discussions and for some art therapy with a social worker and a psychotherapist. Everyone would then meet up again before leaving for home.

Although the Amnesia Association ceased functioning in 1990 (due to lack of funds) and became subsumed under the National Head Injury Association, some local groups continue to meet. This includes Jason's group who, at the time of writing in 1997, meet once every 6 wk in the home of one or other of the members.

I learned that Jason's father had died in June 1984. Jason had remained at home until February 1984. His father was too ill to help with his care, his mother was still working and unable to cope with the demands of her son. Jason was admitted to the only hospital that would admit him, a large hospital for people with severe learning difficulties. Jason was in a room with boys and men who had been mentally disabled from birth. He hated it and his mother knew it was not right for him but had no choice.

Meanwhile she and a social worker friend had been fighting to get the local health authority to pay for Jason to go to a private hospital specializing in working with severely brain injured people with behavior disorders. In October 1984, 4 mo after his father's death and 8 mo after going to the large hospital for learning disabled people, Jason was able to go to the private hospital where he has lived ever since.

Jason's mother remembers that time with distress. She said her husband, "couldn't cope with the thought of Jason not getting better and I'm sure that's

Table 9.2. Jason's Responses on Reading Aloud Regular and Irregular Words on 10 Occasions

	11.22.82					11.29.82				
	1	2	3	4	5	6	7	8	9	10
acre	acereal	arch	arch	age	arch	ask	arch	arch	arch	archer
aunt	✓	✓	ayunt	✓	✓	✓	✓	✓	✓	✓
base	✓	✓		✓	✓	✓	✓	✓	✓	✓
blade	✓	✓	bland	blood	bladd	✓	✓	✓	✓	✓
blood	✓	blewed		✓	blewed	✓	✓	blewed	✓	blewed
bowl	✓	✓	✓	✓	✓	✓	✓	✓	✓	blewed
dough	dodge	dog	dooch	doubt	dute	dooge	duel	dooge	duve	dooge
duel	✓	✓	doll	✓	✓	✓	✓	✓	✓	✓
flash	✓	✓	✓	✓	✓	flesh	✓	✓	flesh	✓
gang	✓	✓	✓	✓	✓	✓	✓	✓	✓	✓
glove	✓	✓	✓	✓	✓	✓	✓	✓	✓	✓
love	✓	✓	✓	✓	✓	✓	✓	✓	✓	✓
mile	✓	✓	✓	✓	✓	✓	✓	✓	✓	✓
page	✓	plage		✓	✓	✓	✓	✓	✓	✓
plug	✓	✓	pludge	✓	✓	✓	✓	✓	✓	✓
shrug	✓	✓	scrum	sprawn	shrun	shroog	✓	shurger	✓	✓
spot	sport	sport	sport	sport	✓	✓	✓	✓	✓	✓
steak	✓	✓	✓	✓	✓	✓	✓	✓	✓	✓
sword	sward	sward	sward	sward	sward	sward	sward	sward	sward	sward
trout	troot	troot	troot	troot	troot	troot	troot	troot	troot	troot
turn	✓	✓	✓	✓	✓	✓	wars	✓	✓	✓
vase	✓	vace	wales	✓	ways	✓	✓	✓	✓	✓
wand	wanned	✓	wanned	warned	✓	✓	✓	✓	✓	wanned
yacht	wajarch	watch	wyacht	wyarch	watch	wacht	wacht	wiacht	wacht	wacht

A check mark indicates that the word was read correctly.

why he got cancer." She spent a year battling with the health authority to pay for Jason to go to the private hospital, she said,

> Jason was very aggressive at that time. He wasn't before the illness but the illness made him very aggressive and very demanding, he was threatening and dangerous at times. At one time he pestered me for a suicide tablet. He'd do this maybe a hundred times a day. That was a bad time. Once he got to the private hospital he was still bad. I insisted he came home for Christmas because that was the first Christmas since Jason had been away. The staff said he shouldn't come home but I insisted. I couldn't face Christmas without him. Well, it was an absolute disaster. The staff were right. Two people (a nurse and a driver) came to fetch him back and it was horrendous. He ran through all the rooms and they had to give him an injection to quiet him down. I had to walk round with him promising I'd get him a lawyer to try to get him home. I promised all sorts of things. They (the staff) were so kind—they knew what he was like but I didn't think it would be so hard as that. I didn't have him home for the next 2 years because he was so aggressive and angry. I could take him out for a meal but once he grabbed a waiter and shouted, 'Call the police, they're taking me back to that place and I don't want to go.' It was very embarrassing. I had to say, 'Well let's go for a drive first' so he got in the car but when he saw the signs for the hospital he shouted, 'You're taking me back there.' I said, 'Well we have to get your suitcase.' He went in and as soon as we got in I called one of the staff and said, 'We need help.' Very calmly and gently she said, 'Jason, go and put the kettle on and make a cup of tea,' which he did and I slipped out. I felt so bad because he was so unhappy and wanted to come home and that's so hard. I felt terrible. On the way home we (my friend and I) stopped the car in a bluebell wood and I walked round still crying. I felt so terrible as if abandoning him to a life he doesn't want. And yet that's the only thing you can do.
>
> Now I don't think anywhere could have been so good for him. They taught him things. They taught him to make his own breakfast, they walked with him to the shops so he'd know the way to go. They checked up, without him knowing, to see his behaviour was OK. So he can do his own things, within limits, so he knows when he has to go back and he does that.

FOLLOW-UP

In 1988, I started seeing Jason again for two follow-up studies. One was a follow-up of reading impaired patients (Wilson, 1994) and one was a follow-up of people with severe memory problems (Wilson, 1991b).

I usually saw Jason at home two or three times a year when he was on leave from the hospital. I looked at his memory functioning, his reading skills, and some of his other cognitive abilities. I was able to try out a particular strategy during these sessions to try to teach him some of the things he had forgotten. Thus, although most of Jason's rehabilitation was achieved at the private hospital, I was able to contribute a small amount.

Follow-Up of Reading

I reassessed Jason's reading ability on nine occasions between 1988 and 1989. There was virtually no change since 1982. Thus his reading skills were assessed 19 times altogether (10 in 1982 and 9 in 1988–9). Some errors were very consistent such as "SWARD" for SWORD and "TROOT" for TROUT. Others varied a little such as "BLOOD" which was read correctly on 10 occasions, misread as "BLEWED" on 8 occasions, and "BLODDY" on 1 occasion). Other words were more variable such as ACRE read in 1982 as "ARCH" (six times), "ARCHER," "AGE," "ACEREAL," and "ASK" (once each). At follow-up Jason misread ACRE as "AKREY" on all nine occasions.

Spelling was similarly variable with some words always misspelled in the same way such as RESON for REASON and STRAT for STRAIGHT. Spellings of other words varied slightly while others varied a great deal. There were no effects relating to parts of speech, word length, or imagery.

The most striking finding was the lack of change in Jason's reading and spelling abilities.

Follow-Up of Memory

Episodic Memory

Once again when reassessed in 1989 there was little change in Jason's scores on memory tests and he remained densely amnesic. The results can be seen in Table 9.3.

He still scored 0/12 on the RBMT screening score, 0 on delayed recall of a prose passage, 0 on delayed recall of a complex figure, and below 50 (i.e., minimum score) on the Delayed Memory Index of the Wechsler Memory Scale-Revised.

Semantic Memory

Because of Jason's unusual and intriguing agnosia for living things, observed in 1980, I looked in more detail at his semantic memory functioning between 1989 and 1992. Semantic memory refers to our knowledge about the world. This includes the meanings of words; what things look like, smell like, and feel like; knowledge of social customs, geographical information, and so forth. Jason had lost much of his semantic knowledge about living things whether this knowledge was accessed through pictures or words. Thus, on one occasion I asked him, "What is the name of an animal that gives us wool and says 'baa?'" He replied, "a kangaroo." When shown a picture of a sheep he thought it was a cow. In contrast when asked, "What is the name of a vehicle pulled by cars and people use it to sleep in?" he responded without hesitation, "caravan." He could also name a picture of a caravan.

Table 9.3. Jason's Memory Test Scores at Follow-up in 1989

Wechsler Memory Scale-Revised (WMS-R)

General memory index	= 53	(Very impaired)
Visual memory index	= 60	(Impaired)
Verbal memory index	= 69	(Borderline)
Attention and concentration	= 76	(Borderline)
Delayed memory index	< 50	(Severely impaired)

Prose Recall (from WMS-R)

Immediate recall (A + B)	= 10	(Impaired)
Delayed recall (A + B)	= 0	(Severely impaired)

Rivermead Behavioural Memory Test

Screening score	0/12	(Severely impaired)
Standardized profile score	2/24	(Severely impaired)

Recognition Memory Test

Words	Age scaled score	< 3	(Severely impaired)
Faces	Age scaled score	< 3	(Severely impaired)

Rey-Osterreith Complex Figure

Copy	= 33/36	(Normal score)
40 minute recall	= 0/36	(Severely impaired)

Digit Span

Forward	= 5	(Within normal range)
Backward	= 4	(Within normal range)

Corsi Block

Visuospatial span	= 5	(Average)

Visual Tapping Span (from Wechsler Memory Scale-Revised)

Forward span	= 4	(Low average)
Backward span	= 4	(Low average)

His drawings from memory also reflect his greater semantic knowledge of nonliving things. Figure 9.1, for example, shows Jason's sophisticated drawings of a bicycle and an airplane, which are in contrast to his simplistic and "mechanical" drawings of a bird and a fish shown in Figure 9.2.

In 1990, I gave Jason a semantic memory battery devised by John Hodges (Hodges et al., 1992). This test is designed to assess input to and output from a central store of representational knowledge. One set of stimulus items is used to access semantic knowledge through different sensory modalities. The battery contains 48 items representing 3 categories of living and 3 categories of manufactured items matched for prototypicality. The three living categories are land animals, water creatures, and birds; the three manufactured categories are household items, vehicles, and musical instruments. Knowledge of these items is assessed in several ways, namely fluency, naming, picture sorting, word–picture matching, naming to description, and generation of verbal definitions to the spoken item.

Jason's results from fluency and naming can be seen in Table 9.4, together with mean scores from control subjects and from patients with dementia of the Alzheimer type.

Jason's results are not too dissimilar to those of dementia of the Alzheimer type (DAT) patients with regard to manufactured items but poorer than DAT patients with regard to living items. On the whole, this confirms the earlier findings reported by Warrington and Shallice (1984).

INVESTIGATION OF ERRORLESS LEARNING PRINCIPLES TO HELP JASON LEARN AND RELEARN INFORMATION

In 1991 Alan Baddeley and I posed the question, "Do amnesic subjects learn better if prevented from making mistakes during the learning process?" What prompted this question were findings from (1) errorless discrimination learning studies with (a) animals (Terrace, 1963, 1966) and (b) learning disabled people (Jones and Eayrs, 1992, 1994; Sidman and Stoddard, 1967) and (2) studies from implicit memory and implicit learning with amnesic subjects (Brooks and Baddeley, 1976; Tulving and Schacter, 1990). Prior to our research with amnesic patients (Baddeley and Wilson, 1994; Wilson et al., 1994), errorless learning had not been used, as far as we were aware, in memory rehabilitation. Nor had implicit learning had the effect on rehabilitation expected from the late 1970s and early 1980s. This may be because implicit learning is poorly equipped to deal with errors. A few studies suggested that if errors are introduced into learning, amnesic subjects have difficulty eliminating them (see Baddeley, 1992 for further discussion).

In our first study we used an experimental task to try to answer the question posed above. We devised a list of five-letter one-syllable words and presented these to amnesic subjects, young control subjects, and elderly control subjects in one of two ways. One way—errorful learning—forced subjects to generate guesses (i.e., errors). For example, they were told, "I am thinking of a five-letter word beginning with TH, guess what the word might be." The subject might say

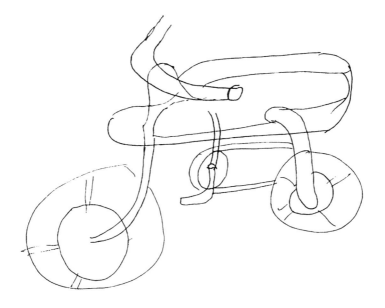

a

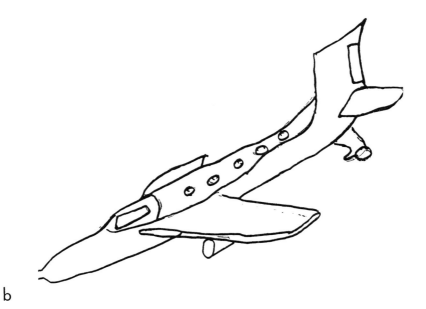

b

Figure 9.1. Jason's drawings of a bicycle (a) and an airplane (b).

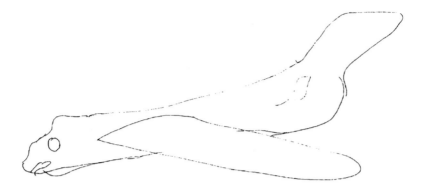

a

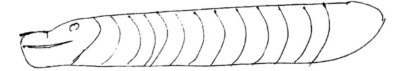

b

Figure 9.2. Jason's drawing of a bird (a) and a fish (b).

Table 9.4. Jason's Scores on the Fluency and Naming Subtests of the Semantic Memory Battery Together with Mean Scores for Dementia of the Alzheimer Type (DAT) Subjects, Elderly Controls (from Hodges et al., 1992), and Young Controls (from Wilson et al., 1997)

SUBTEST	JASON	MEAN FOR DAT SS ($n = 22$)	MEAN FOR ELDERLY CONTROLS ($n = 25$)	MEAN FOR YOUNG MALE CONTROLS
Fluency				
Animals	7	9.9	19.7	21.2
Birds	0	5.4	14.1	16.8
Water creatures	0	4.4	13.0	15.0
Dogs	0	3.2	10.2	12.0
Household items	7	9.1	19.8	21.2
Vehicles	11	6.9	13.9	14.2
Musical instruments	3	6.5	14.0	17.6
Boats	3	4.4	11.6	11.6
Naming	19	35.4	46.5	47.0
Living (max = 24)	5	17.1	23.3	23.0
Land animals (12)	3	8.3	11.6	11.8
Sea creatures (6)	1	4.1	5.9	5.8
Birds (6)	1	4.7	5.8	5.4
Nonliving (24)	14	18.3	23.2	24.0
Household items (12)	8	9.7	11.9	12.0
Vehicles (6)	5	4.9	6.0	6.0
Musical instruments (6)	1	3.7	5.1	5.1

THINK and was told "No, good guess but it's not right—have another go," the next response might be THERE. This would receive the same response from the tester as THINK. After four guesses or 25 sec, the subject was told the correct answer, "The word is THUMB, please write that down." There were 5 words in each list for the amnesic people and 10 words for the control subjects (in an attempt to make it easy enough for the former to get some words right and difficult enough for the latter to get some wrong).

Following three learning trials in which guesses were encouraged but only correct words were written down, each subject was given nine test trials over a 30-min period, i.e., after three trials, there was a 10-min break followed by another three test trials and another 10-min break and then the final three test trials.

The other condition—errorless learning—was carried out as follows: Each subject was told, "I am thinking of a five-letter word beginning with PR and the word is PRICE, please write that down." Other than this the procedure was the same as that described for errorful learning. The only difference between the two conditions was that, in one, subjects were forced to make mistakes, and in the other they were prevented from making mistakes.

Half of the subjects in each group had the errorless condition first and the other half had the errorful condition first. The words themselves were also counterbalanced so that they were in the errorful and errorless conditions an equal number of times. (Baddeley and Wilson [1994] describe this experiment in more detail.)

Every single one of the 16 amnesic subjects did better under the errorless conditions. This included Jason. Of a maximum of 45 correct responses, his score was 32 correct in the errorless condition and 18 correct in the errorful condition. Although the experiment was not like everyday life and in rehabilitation we do not want to teach people lists of words, the results were so strong that I was convinced we should try to avoid trial-and-error learning when teaching new information and new skills to people with severe memory impairments. Indeed I was so convinced that I changed my clinical behavior overnight. Once I had analyzed the results and saw how robust they were (100% of amnesic subjects did better with errorless learning), I stopped asking memory impaired people to guess. Like most of us involved in rehabilitation I would say to patients, "Can you remember my name—No?—Well guess, you might be right," and variations on this theme. No longer do I ask memory impaired people to guess (unless I am administering a test which requires this). Instead I say something like, "Only tell me if you're sure. I don't want you to guess."

Nevertheless we needed to pursue the comparison between the errorful and errorless learning. In particular, we needed to know whether errorless learning was better for teaching real life tasks or information. Alan Baddeley, Jonathan Evans, Agnes Shiel, and I carried out a number of single case experimental designs (Wilson et al., 1994). Once again, Jason was included in our studies.

The question I addressed with Jason was whether he could learn to name pictures of objects better with an errorless or errorful learning approach. It will be remembered that he had a marked semantic memory deficit that included problems with naming pictures (see Table 9.4). Furthermore, Jason's ability to recognize living things was far worse than his ability to recognize nonliving things. Nevertheless, he still had difficulty with some nonliving items and these were selected for treatment.

Jason was given the Renfrew Pictures (Renfrew, 1975), a set of easy pictures to name. He correctly named 17/50, gave incorrect responses to 20 of them (e.g., "teapot" for watering can), correctly described eight others without being able to supply the name (e.g., "things that help you park sea ships" for ANCHOR), mispronounced one ("caddle" for SADDLE), and replied, "don't know," to the remaining four.

Six of the pictures he described without naming and two of the "don't knows" were selected for treatment. I wanted to avoid using pictures for which Jason had made an overt error. Four items were randomly allocated to errorful and four to errorless learning.

The procedure was similar to that described above in that three learning trials were followed by nine test trials in blocks of three. For the errorless condition Jason was shown the pictures one at a time and told, "This is a HINGE (or AN-CHOR, or whatever), please write that down." For the errorful condition Jason was first asked to guess or free associate or say anything the picture made him think of. One of the items for example was LIGHTHOUSE and Jason said he thought it might be a "block of flats." After 25 sec he was given the correct answer and asked to write it down. Once again, only the correct answer was written down and each was written down three times.

The mean number of correct responses during the nine test trials from a maximum of 36 was 19 for the pictures taught in an errorful way and 33 for the pictures taught in an errorless way. Eight of the nine test trials resulted in superior performance for the errorless over errorful trials. A simple statistical test, the sign test, showed these results to be significantly different ($p < 0.005$). Three months later Jason was reassessed. He had retained all four of the names for the pictures taught using errorless learning and the name of one of the pictures taught using errorful learning. The errorless learning procedure was then applied to teach him the remaining names. These results can be seen in Table 9.5.

Further preliminary investigations suggested that errorless learning principles could be used to improve Jason's difficulty with the reading and spelling of irregularly spelled words such as ACHE or DOUGH.

JASON'S LATEST ASSESSMENT

During 1994 and 1995 I reassessed Jason's functioning on a number of cognitive tests partly to see if he had changed and partly to compare his scores with another patient I was seeing with Linda Clare, Andy Young, and John Hodges (Wilson, et al., 1997). The other patient, M.U., had severe visuospatial difficulties and did not know *where* objects were located in space. He could not reach objects accurately although he knew what these objects were. Jason, in contrast, knew *where* things were but not *what* they were. In other words we had one patient, M.U., with good semantic knowledge together with poor visuospatial knowledge and another patient, Jason, with poor semantic knowledge together with good visuospatial knowledge. Jason's scores on these tests can be seen in Table 9.6.

Some of these tests were new for Jason while other tests had been given to him earlier, although he could not, of course, remember any of these. The most striking finding from the repeated tests was the lack of change. Jason's results were virtually identical to those obtained earlier. This confirms the view of many people working in rehabilitation that functional change, i.e., improvements in tasks

Table 9.5. Results from a Study to Teach Jason Object Names

Errorless Vs. Errorful Learning to Teach Jason Object Names

PICTURE	INITIAL RESPONSE	CONDITION ALLOCATED TO	Response to 9 test trials									3 MO LATER
			1	2	3	4	5	6	7	8	9	
Lighthouse	"On the sea-a building."	Errorless	A building	✓	✓	A building	✓	✓	✓	✓	✓	✓
Hinge	"Don't know."	Errorless	✓	✓	✓	✓	✓	✓	✓	✓	✓	✓
Sleeve	"A shirt's right arm."	Errorless	✓	✓	✓	✓	✓	✓	✓	✓	✓	✓
Anchor	"Things that help you park sea ships."	Errorless	Don't know	✓	✓	✓	✓	✓	✓	✓	✓	✓
Igloo	"Don't know."	Errorful	Chimney	Chimney	Chimney	Chimney	Chimney	Chimney	Chimney	Chimney	Chimney	0/9 correct responses
Flame	"Candle fire."	Errorful	✓	✓	✓	✓	✓	✓	✓	✓	✓	9/9 correct responses
Helmet	"Sub aqua hood."	Errorful	✓	✓	✓	✓	✓	✓	✓	✓	✓	9/9 correct responses
Sling	"For broken arm—not plaster."	Errorful	Sleeve	✓	For broken arm	Don't know	Forgotten	Arm thing	Don't know	Arm thing	Arm thing	1/9 correct responses

Errorless learning now used for these pictures

Applying Errorless Learning to Teach Object Names Initially Allocated to Errorful Condition

BASELINE RESPONSE		TEST TRIALS				
		1	2	3	4	5
Igloo	Tent	Candle	✓	✓	✓	✓
Flame	✓	✓	✓	✓	✓	✓
Helmet	✓	✓	✓	✓	✓	✓
Sling	Don't know	✓	✓	✓	✓	✓

Table 9.6. Jason's Latest Neuropsychological Assessment Results

TEST	SCORE TYPE	JASON'S SCORE
Wechsler Adult Intelligence Scale-Revised verbal subtests		
Information	Age scaled score	5
Digit span	Age scaled score	7
Vocabulary	Age scaled score	7
Arithmetic	Age scaled score	9
Comprehension	Age scaled score	6
Similarities	Age scaled score	8
Verbal IQ	Age scaled score	82
Digit span forwards	Span length	5
Digit span backwards	Span length	4
Spot-the-Word Test (Oral presentation)	Age scaled score	< 3
Rivermead Behavioural Memory Test	Screening score	2
Reading single letters-upper case	Raw score	100%
Reading single letters-lower case	Raw score	100%
Reading single words	Raw score	41/50
Spelling single words	Raw score	37/82
Behavioural Inattention Test	Raw score	
Picture scanning subtest	Raw score	6/9
Benton Visual Retention Test		
(Forced-choice version)	Raw score	14/16
Visual Short-Term Memory (Phillips, 1983)	Raw score	23/24
Spatial imagery (Manikin) Test		
(derived from Ratcliff, 1979)	Raw score	26/32
Corsi Blocks	Forward span	6
Visual Object and Space Perception Battery		
(Space Perception Subtests)		
Dot counting	Pass / Fail	10/10 Pass
Position discrimination	Fass / Fail	19/20 Pass
Number location	Pass / Fail	10/10 Pass
Cube analysis	Pass / Fail	10/10 Pass

relevant to everyday life, are not automatically reflected in changes on standardized tests. Thus, despite failure to change on these tests, Jason had learned many tasks and skills that enabled him to be more independent.

On the final assessment session I asked Jason if he could tell me what he considered to be his main problem. He said, "The ability to—after a change in concentration—to remember what was going on prior to that change in concentration. Knowing things are happening but not remembering. It seems to me I'm going to be like this for the rest of my life."

In 1996, Jason had an MRI scan. It showed that his right hippocampus had disappeared entirely together with the anterior part of the left hippocampus. In addition the amygdala was totally destroyed. This explains his severe amnesia. Both temporal lobes were hypointense, i.e., the blood supply to these areas was inadequate. This helps to explain Jason's semantic memory problems.

JASON TODAY

Jason has now lived in the private hospital for 13 yr. A few years ago he moved to a small home attached to the hospital. He attends a sheltered workshop each day and, given the extent of his amnesia, has considerable freedom. In his mother's words,

> He has freedom. He can go out walking and he loves walking. He walks for hours. It gives him a sense of freedom and being able to do things his way. It's always within a structure. For example he does his washing on Wednesdays and Sundays. He's learned to do his ironing, which he never did before. He does his own shopping. He takes a list and he does it all. Within his own limitations he does it well. He doesn't fight any more. If they have patients who don't get on with each other and somebody tries to attack him (as one patient did) then he held this man's wrist to stop him fighting but he didn't fight back. Before he would hit people, he thumped them and caused problems but he doesn't now and that's very helpful for him. He is still quite hostile now, he can't trust people. He's become inhibited and controlled. He knows he has to be or he may lose control and become vicious. He did become vicious once—he attacked a nurse because he wanted to get home.
> He's also become self centered. He used to say, 'I need you, mum,' he never says that now.
> Once, before he went to the mental hospital, he spent some time at a unit in Bristol. I wrote twice asking if I could go and they said no. He went with his father and he was nice while his father was there and then he was left on his own. The next day we had a call to get him back. We don't know how many ructions he caused. He really had been very very bad. When his father went to collect him he had been drugged up to the gills, he slept all the way home from Bristol and still slept when he came home. They didn't take my letter seriously. If I'd been there I could have given him the reassurance. They couldn't foresee he'd be so bad.
> Then later he went to the private unit for a month's trial and they said yes, they could do something for him if we could get the money. They showed us a chart for Jason whereby on the first day he'd been in the 'time out' room 14 times. Over the next fortnight it was two or three times and in the last 2 weeks he didn't go in there at all. So I think the experience was so horrendous, he didn't want to go through it again. With Jason, he's more likely to remember something if it's very emotional whether it's somebody dying or something very happy. It works for him. He seems to know. I only had to tell him once his father died. He knows it. He doesn't refer to it but he knows it. You never have to say it again.

When I asked Jason's mother whether she worried about his future, she said,

> Of course, I'm 72, he's 40 and a very fit young man. He walks a lot. He's fit. He gets the right diet. He's looked after physically as well as mentally. I've been promised he

can always stay there. My friend will always look after his needs. She's promised he can have the holidays he likes if we can fix up a carer he knows.

The private hospital is the only place he can be. He couldn't go to a household. He wouldn't recognize people. He's still always among strangers. It would be devastating for him to move again. When he moved to the small home from the main unit, it was a step up. He has more independence there but it took him about 2 years to get used to it. He'd go into different homes. He'd walk in and sit down and watch television because he thought that's where he belonged. They'd have to go looking for him. That took some while but now it's been over 2 years and he's settled in quite well. He goes to the workshop every day which he enjoys. He likes doing that. The hospital where he lives is good for Jason. It's not for everyone but it's good for him. He needs a structure.

He's fine about going back now. At one point I couldn't stand the tension waiting for the transport to come and asked them to collect him at 10 A.M. rather than 3 P.M., but now he doesn't mind going back, he's content.

My friend will fight for his rights and try to make his life happy. She is a receiver with me in the court of protection so anything Jason has can only be touched with their consent through her and through me at the moment. I trust her implicitly. She is quite determined he will enjoy holidays and enjoy the things he enjoys now.

My final question to Jason's mother at the last interview early in 1997 was, "Is there anything you would particularly like me to say in this chapter?" This was her reply:

I want a cure for him. If they did transplants of brain cells (and I don't believe in that sort of thing) but if there was any possibility of transplanting brain cells for Jason to get his memory back I'd be the first to say Yes, please do it tomorrow.

IV

LANGUAGE IMPAIRMENT

One of the most distinct characteristics of humankind is language. Chomsky (1972) called language the "human essence" and Skinner (1996) said, "The uniqueness of language lies not in the mode of its expression or comprehension but in its ability to transmit symbolic meaning" (p. 111). Insights into the effect language impairments have on individuals affected can be found in Kapur (1997). One of these individuals is a clinical psychologist, Scott Moss, who sustained a debilitating stroke at the age of 43 years, within hours of passing a demanding physical medical examination for a new job. Moss writes, "When I awoke the next morning in hospital I was totally (globally) aphasic. I could understand vaguely what others said to me if it was spoken slowly and represented a very concrete form of action: otherwise it was a language deficit which crossed all language modalities. I had lost completely the ability to talk, to read, and to write. I even lost for the first 2 months the ability to use words internally, that is, in my thinking" (p. 76).

Moss was able to return to work, unlike Bill, one of the people described in this section. Bill remained globally dysphasic for the rest of his life, although he was able to learn a limited form of communication. Bill's alternative communication system almost certainly worked because he was capitalizing on his relatively intact right hemisphere skills. The right hemisphere is better at comprehension than expression, better at nouns than verbs and better at the affective components of language such as prosody and emotional expression. Bill showed all these characteristics. His communication system was far more useful for comprehension than for expression, he understood nouns better than verbs and his facial expressions and emotional gesturing appeared to be unimpaired.

Laurence, the second man described here, shows us the distress that can be caused by language difficulties. Laurence felt other people viewed him as crazy or stupid because he did not always understand them and they did not always understand him. His main therapeutic needs, I felt, were to be able to try to make sense of what had happened to him and to have people around him patient enough to ensure communication took place. Fulfilling these needs appeared to be more important than formal speech and language therapy, which Laurence had had for several years. Addressing the social and emotional needs of patients is as important as trying to remediate or compensate for the specific cognitive deficit. Most experienced speech and language therapists would probably agree that addressing the psychological needs of people with aphasia and their families is an integral part of language therapy.

Ron, the third person in this section has not shown similar emotional difficulties to Bill and Laurence. Not only is Ron's language problem primarily restricted to word finding difficulties and telegrammatic speech, he has more widespread brain damage and cognitive deficits. He has a deep dyslexia, problems with writing, visuospatial difficulties and an almost complete loss of autobiographical memory prior to his head injury. Nevertheless Ron was a rewarding person to work with and never stopped trying to improve himself.

All three of these men achieved a considerable amount yet because of the severity of their language difficulties all sustained significant disruption to their lives. This was recognized by Cot et al. (1993) when they wrote:

> Aphasia disrupts.
>
> _____
>
> Aphasia causes personal disruption because it impaired expression of thought, and it confines the person to a closed universe.
>
> _____
>
> Aphasia disrupts marriage when years, even decades of life as a couple are shattered due to the inability to share one's ideas and feelings.
>
> _____
>
> Aphasia disrupts the family as persons with aphasia quickly become strangers in their own homes, alienated from everyday life.
>
> _____
>
> Aphasia disrupts the social environment since, without dialogue, in a few short months the circle of friends and neighbours dwindles away. Aphasia also disrupts the person's relation with society. (p. 245)

10

BILL: LEARNING TO COMMUNICATE WITH SYMBOLS FIVE YEARS AFTER A STROKE

BACKGROUND

I first saw Bill in 1979 when he was 62 yr old. He had sustained a severe left hemisphere stroke 2 yr earlier. For the first few months after the stroke Bill had been an inpatient at the rehabilitation center but by the time I arrived he was attending as an outpatient 3 days a week. He spent part of his time there doing woodwork and part doing gardening. Although hemiplegic with no movement at all in his right hand and arm, Bill walked competently with a leg brace. He had no speech but acknowledged people with a raised hand and appeared to know all the staff and patients. He knew his way around and was an independent self-sufficient man. I saw Bill regularly but had no formal contact with him until 3 yr later by which time he was 65 yr old and 5 yr post stroke.

INITIAL ASSESSMENT

I started seeing Bill at the request of his social worker. She wondered if there was anything I could do to reduce the "terrible rows" at home. I began assessing Bill and found he had no words at all and only one sound "ba-ba-ba." When he wanted to communicate he pointed and said "ba-ba-ba." When he wanted to show his distress at not being able to talk he pointed to his mouth, said "ba-ba-ba," and made an expression of distress. On the British Picture Vocabulary Test (Dunn and Dunn, 1982) Bill's comprehension of single words was at a 2-yr-old level. He could copy letters and shapes accurately but could write nothing spontaneously, not even his own name. Anxious to show he had some skills, he took my pen, wrote some numbers on a page, and added them up. He was able to complete a few simple sums but had difficulty if these involved carrying from one column to another. He was unable to read anything aloud although he could distinguish real words from nonwords with 75% accuracy provided a two-choice format was used whereby one word was a real word and one was not. If the words on this lexical decision task were presented one at a time in the usual way, then Bill was at chance. He could select correctly his name from a choice of three stimuli (e.g., BLIL, BILL, BLLI) and could also put words showing days of the week in the correct order. He could also put in the correct order words showing months of the year, apart from June and July, which he frequently put the wrong way around. Apart from his name, months of the year, and days of the week, Bill appeared to be unable to read any other stimuli. He could not match printed common nouns such as BOOK with a picture or with the real object.

It may be surprising that the referral was made because of the arguments Bill was having with his wife at home. How can a man with no speech, one sound, very limited comprehension, and almost no reading or writing, manage to engage in an argument? I soon had the opportunity to observe one of these arguments for myself.

I telephoned Bill's wife to ask her to come to see me to discuss Bill's program. She agreed readily and we arranged a time for her to come with Bill. I did my best to explain the arrangement to Bill through the use of mime, a clock, and a calendar. I had recently changed rooms from one building in the rehabilitation center to another. Bill of course knew this, he was very aware of happenings in the rehabilitation center and had come to the new room for some of his assessment sessions. I had not met his wife before so did not tell her of the change. I assumed she would follow Bill. However, she had been to the center many times when Bill was an inpatient, prior to my arrival, and had seen the clinical psychology department in the old building.

The day of the appointment arrived and at the right time, I was in my room waiting for Bill and his wife when I heard shouting outside my door. I went to the door to find out what was happening. There was Bill, very red in the face and looking as if he were about to have another stroke yelling "ba-ba-ba" and pulling his wife towards my room. She had been trying to go to the old room. She saw me and said, "You see what he's like, you see what I have to put up with?" They came in and calmed down and we discussed the arguments and the means of communication between the two of them.

Soon after his stroke Bill had received speech and language therapy three times a week for several months. The speech therapist noted "no improvements" and Bill's sessions were stopped. A year later, the speech therapist saw Bill again and attempted to teach him Ameri-Ind (Skelly, 1979) a sign language based on Native American sign language. Amer-Ind is a one-handed system potentially useful for people with hemiplegia. Bill, however, became confused and distressed when attempts were made to teach him this method so the Ameri-Ind sessions ceased and no further attempts were made at speech and language therapy. Bill enjoyed his woodworking and gardening and was happy to come to the center 3 days a week for these activities.

The main problem at home was with communication. Married for 40 yr altogether, including 5 yr since the stroke, Bill and his wife had failed to develop an adequate method of communication since the onset of his language deficits. His wife said the arguments typically started when there was a change in routine. For example, if Bill needed his leg brace checked on a day he normally went to the rehabilitation center, his wife was unable to explain this to him. Consequently Bill yelled and pulled her arm to try to make her go to the rehabilitation center. As this often happened when they were in the car and his wife was driving, she was concerned about the danger of an accident occurring.

INITIAL REHABILITATION

I decided to talk to the speech therapist who had known Bill for the past 5 yr to see if she would collaborate with me in trying to teach him a simple system based on visual symbols adapted from work described by Gardner et al. (1976). Anne, the speech therapist, was willing to collaborate and we agreed to run the program jointly.

We asked Bill's wife to keep a record of the number of arguments they had and also to note any words and phrases she thought it would be useful for Bill to know. She started keeping records and made some suggestions about useful words, including spectacles, pills, and leg brace. In our first session with Bill, Anne and I made sure that he could match a drawing of an object with a real object. We drew a matchbox, a bottle of pills, a newspaper, a cup, a leg brace, spectacles, and other common objects on pieces of index cards and gestured to Bill to put the drawing in front of the appropriate object. This was easy for him. Like Gardner et al. we decided to use abstract as well as pictorial signs. Abstract signs were particularly useful for people's names and could be produced more quickly than obtaining photographs of the relevant people. The symbols for Barbara, Anne, and Bill were,

respectively, , and . We taught these within a few minutes by showing the symbol to Bill and then holding it against the appropriate person. Following three demonstrations we gave a name card to Bill and gestured for him to give it to the right person. He had no trouble with this task.

Following this session we added a verb card "give me," once again using an abstract symbol. We also adopted a modeling procedure to teach him the meaning of the symbols. One of us placed two cards such as "give me matchbox" on the table looking intently at the other therapist who would look closely at the cards and then give the matchbox. The second therapist would then use the cards to ask the first "give me matchbox." One of us would then use the cards to ask Bill "give me matchbox." Usually he understood what was required. If he hesitated or was incorrect we demonstrated again and physically prompted Bill to carry out the correct action by guiding his hand to the correct object and offering it to the person who had made the request. All went smoothly until we added other verbs "pick up" and "want." Bill failed to reliably distinguish between any two verbs. We abandoned "give-me," "pick-up," and "want" as these did not appear to be crucial in the communication process. "Matchbox" or "leg brace" was sufficient for Bill to understand what was required.

By the third session Bill had a dozen common nouns and five proper nouns he could understand. We purchased a small photograph album with clear plastic containers in which to keep the cards and he carried this in his jacket pocket. We knew from the earlier assessment that he could understand the days of the week and months of the year so these were written on two separate cards and placed in the album. We also confirmed he could tell the time. We suspected this because Bill was never late for his woodworking or gardening sessions. However, before making a card with a clock, we showed him a toy clock and "requested" that he make it the same as the clock on the wall. We did this through modeling and gesture. This caused Bill no problem. At noon—the end of the session—we observed where Bill went. He went straight to the canteen for lunch and not to woodworking from where we had collected him. We also used the cards to tell Bill the time and day of his next session. "Friday-11:00 o'clock." He appeared without a reminder on the correct day at the correct time. He could obviously understand and tell the time. A clock card was added to the album. We drew a clock face and added two cardboard hands with a paper clip that enabled the hands to be moved independently. Bill was able to manipulate the clock hands with his functioning left hand.

Would he understand a calendar we wondered? Using a printed calendar, a drawing of a birthday cake, and singing "happy birthday to you," I pointed to my birthday on the calendar. Anne did the same. We gestured to Bill to show us his birthday. He did so successfully. We showed the card with his wife's name on, pointed to the birthday cake drawing, and gestured to the calendar. Again Bill was correct so we stuck a calendar in the back of his album.

Towards the end of the second week, Bill's wife telephoned to say he was soon going to spend 3 days in the local cottage hospital for respite care so that his wife could have a break. She wanted us to inform Bill so he would be prepared. He had gone to this hospital several times before and each time an argument ensued.

Our goal for the 3rd wk was to ensure that Bill understood that he would be spending 3 nights at the local community hospital. We drew a card for his house and matched it to a photograph of the house. We drew a bed. We conveyed hospital by drawing a nurse and several beds. Again Bill appeared to understand as he raised his left index finger—his sign for understanding. With the calendar, the days of the week card, the card of his house, bed and hospital, we 'explained' that he would sleep (bed) at his house for the next 5 days and then go to the hospital for 3 days. We went though this procedure several times during each of the next three sessions, adjusting the days spent at home as appropriate. Bill gave his usual signal for understanding i.e., raising his left index finger. He seemed to grasp what we were saying. When we saw him after his return from the cottage hospital he pointed to the hospital card and held up three fingers. His wife confirmed that for the first time since his stroke he had gone to the hospital without making a fuss.

The following week Bill needed to have his leg brace checked at another hospital. Once again we were able to prepare him.

Bill was obviously enjoying his sessions. He often tried to tell us something through gesture and saying "ba-ba-ba." As soon as we worked out what he was trying to say we drew this on a card to go into his album. We met with his wife regularly to discuss the program with her. Initially skeptical she became enthusiastic about the system and soon began making her own drawings for the album. The first picture she drew was of a "button" and the second was of a "hammer." She explained that Bill had lost a button from his jacket and wanted her to replace it. He also did woodworking at home and on one occasion he could not find his hammer. It took her some time to work out what he wanted but as soon as she succeeded she made the card. We already had a card for woodworking with a picture of a hammer, saw, and woodworking apron. The hammer drawn by Bill's wife would not do for Bill. He recognized the drawing of the three tools as representing woodworking and did not accept them as three separate objects.

Most importantly, the arguments at home had all but ceased. They had been caused by frustration resulting from an inability to communicate. Once an adequate method had been established, Bill became frustrated far less often. Within 3 wk we had established an effective system for comprehension. Bill could understand his wife, Anne, and me without too much trouble. Other staff at the center could also use the system because a written word or phrase accompanied each symbol for those who did not understand what the symbols (particularly the abstract ones) represented.

Expressive language was a different matter. Bill used the cards to express his needs if prompted by us. We did this in our sessions. We began by pointing to the "How-are-you?" card and then using the "I am fine" card. Bill asked us, "How are you?" too. Sometimes we accompanied him to the canteen and prompted him to use the cards to ask for "a cup of tea, milk, sugar." He was happy enough to go along with our prompting but did not use the cards spontaneously until 9 mo after the onset of treatment. On this occasion he was in occupational therapy early in the morning waiting to go to woodworking. He jabbed his finger towards the wall and said "ba-ba-ba." Not surprisingly, the occupational therapist did not know what he meant. Pointing could mean 'over there,' or 'my house,' or 'my son's house,' or 'clinical psychology,' or any number of things. Realizing he was not understood, Bill reached in his pocket for his album, found the picture of the clock, pointed at the clock, and pointed to the wall again. The therapist realized the clock on the wall had stopped! Even after this, however, Bill rarely used the symbols for expressive language, preferring his pointing and his own sound, sometimes supplemented by rather hard to interpret drawings. Nevertheless as a comprehension system the method worked well.

LATER REHABILITATION

Three mo after Bill's program began, Anne moved to another part of the country and left the center. I continued seeing Bill once a week for the next 2 yr usually with a clinical psychology student. He remained enthusiastic about his sessions and enjoyed working with the students. He readily grasped new abstract symbols for proper nouns and had no difficulty learning people's names in this way. Sometimes when I gave him the name cards to distribute to the appropriate people I included the card for Anne. Bill always put this card on the floor and pointed to the distance. He knew she had left and gone away. When I went on holiday or to a conference I arranged the next appointment with Bill using the clock card, days of the week card and the calendar. Sometimes the next appointment would be 3 wk away. I would indicate with the cards "Bill," "Barbara," "Monday," "June 11th," "9:00 A.M." Never once did Bill miss an appointment yet he had no way of writing down or otherwise recording the information. His memory for appointments was phenomenal. I also sent him postcards when I was abroad using the symbols to communicate the message. I often wondered what the postmen thought about these unusual messages. Some of our cards were phrases to describe events that had happened. We made a card to say "Bill and Barbara made a videotape and Bob was the cameraman." The card looked like this
Another card said "Bill, Barbara + Phillipa" (a student) "did some singing." This

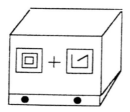

BOB

was depicted as + + . Bill often took these cards from his album to remind us about the past sessions. He could also refer to the future. For example we made one card that said, "I am going to stay with my son at Christmas." We thought it both unusual and helpful that someone with such a severe dysphasia could communicate about the past and the future.

It was now 5 mo since the beginning of the program and we summarized Bill's understanding and use of the symbols. We counted all those (1) we had introduced, (2) Bill "knew" i.e., he reliably matched the symbols with a photograph, drawing, or real object, and (3) he used spontaneously in our teaching sessions. These results can be seen in Table 10.1.

The apparent anomaly with verbs was due to the fact that he always made errors when tested with verbs yet sometimes used "give me" spontaneously.

At this time we decided to look more systematically at Bill's ability to understand pictorial and abstract symbols. Initially, we had been loosely following Gardner et al.'s (1976) approach, using abstract symbols for proper nouns and pictorial symbols for common nouns. Gardner et al., (ibid.) used abstract symbols for verbs like "pick up." We had included these at the beginning but Bill became confused. We also tried this system with two other very dysphasic men both of

Table 10.1. Words Introduced and Used by Bill for 5 Mo After the Program Began

CATEGORY	NUMBER OF SYMBOLS INTRODUCED	NUMBER OF SYMBOLS KNOWN, I.E., RELIABLY CORRECT ON TESTING	NUMBER OF SYMBOLS USED SPONTANEOUSLY
Names of People	19	18	15
Common nouns	37	34	6
Places	9	9	5
Feelings	5	5	1
Verbs	9	0	1
Phrases (How are you?, I am fine)	2	2	2
Questions (When, where)	2	1	1
Times	8	7	3
Sizes (Big, small, medium)	3	3	0
Others	3	0	0

whom were unable to learn "pick up," "want," and "give me." We thought these verbs were not particularly useful. If Bill or one of the other men wanted to request "spectacles" then showing the "spectacles" card was sufficient. "I want spectacles" or "Give me spectacles" was redundant. Verbs like "shave" or "get dressed" we considered more useful for someone like Bill. Furthermore, we thought that given the difficulty with verbs, it might be simpler to use pictorial symbols rather than abstract ones. After 6 mo on the program we decided to investigate systematically Bill's ability to learn nouns, verbs, and adjectives using both pictorial and abstract symbols.

We selected 36 common nouns, 36 verbs, and 36 adjectives previously unused in our sessions. Half were used for the pictorial condition and half for the abstract condition. There were equal numbers of high and low frequency words in each set. From within each category of words, one set was allocated to the pictorial condition and one to the abstract condition. We next drew pictorial or abstract symbols for each word.

As Bill was now seen once a week we taught 18 words in each session over a period of 6 wk. The 18 words were comprised of 6 nouns, 6 verbs, and 6 adjectives. Half of each set were pictorial and half were abstract. The teaching procedure was as follows:

1. Bill was shown a card with one symbol and this was placed below a photograph depicting the word. For nouns, the photographs were of objects. For verbs, the photographs were of a person carrying out the action. For adjectives, there were two photographs: one depicting the correct adjective (e.g., red) and the other depicting its opposite (e.g., green).
2. This procedure was repeated with the remaining five cards.
3. The six cards were then shuffled and presented again, one at a time.
4. This procedure was repeated four more times making six presentations.
5. Immediate testing was carried out by giving Bill the 18 cards one at a time and asking him to match each one with the appropriate picture.
6. Delayed testing. Step 5 was repeated at the beginning of the following session 1 wk later. These results were used to compute the effectiveness of abstract versus pictorial symbols.
7. The next step of 18 cards was presented following steps 1–6 above.
8. This procedure was followed until the 7th wk when only the delayed testing was carried out.
9. Correct responses at delayed testing were totaled.

The results can be seen in Table 10.2.

A Fisher's exact test showed there was a significant difference between the two conditions for nouns ($P = 0.045$), verbs ($P = 0.0027$), and adjectives ($P = 0.0001$). Bill learned 53 out of 54 pictorial symbols and only 28 of 54 abstract symbols. Furthermore, with the pictorial symbols he could learn nouns, verbs, and adjec-

Table 10.2. The Total Number of Words Bill Recalled with Abstract and Pictorial Symbols

	PICTORIAL SYMBOLS	ABSTRACT SYMBOLS	TOTAL LEARNING
Nouns	18	13	31
Verbs	17	8	25
Adjectives	18	7	25
Total	53	28	81

tives whereas with the abstract symbols he showed a tendency to learn nouns more easily. From these results we decided to stick with pictorial symbols and stopped employing abstract symbols apart from proper nouns.

The program itself was an undoubted success. Bill was able to understand changes in his routine. His wife and others could communicate with him. He enjoyed his sessions and always appeared on time and in good humor. His earlier frequent and often tearful bouts of frustration at his lack of speech ceased—he stopped jabbing at his mouth with a frantic expression on his face. His arguments at home were now very infrequent and working with him was a pleasure.

There were no scans of Bill's brain but he almost certainly had considerable left hemisphere damage to all the major language areas. In retrospect his response to the program was not surprising. Presumably, he was using his right hemisphere for most of his communication, and we know the right hemisphere is better at comprehension of language than it is at the expression of language. This is probably why the system was always more effective for comprehension than expression for Bill. We also know that the right hemisphere can comprehend nouns better than verbs. Once again this was true for Bill.

Perhaps the most surprising aspect was that it took 5 yr to develop a reasonably efficient system despite the fact that Bill was in a specialist brain injury rehabilitation center. I do not think it was lack of interest that caused the delay. The speech and language therapist had worked hard at the beginning trying to restore language functioning. Bill and his wife no doubt expected this and, if anything like other globally aphasic people, were very reluctant to take on visual symbol systems in the early days. Five years later, having now accepted that loss of speech (and other language skills) was permanent, they were ready to accept something new. The stress caused by the arguments also contributed, perhaps, to their motivation to learn an alternative means of communication.

FOLLOW-UP

One day in 1984, Bill failed to appear for his regular Monday morning session. Later that day his wife telephoned to say he had had another stroke over the weekend. He had lost consciousness and was in the hospital. Two weeks later, without regaining consciousness Bill died. He was 67 yr old and had taught me and several of my students a great deal. Whenever I hear skepticism about providing rehabilitation for people over 65 or for people more than 2 yr post insult, I think of Bill and his enthusiasm, not to mention success, at learning an alternative communication system.

11

LAURENCE: LISTENING TO THE MESSAGE AND NOT THE WORDS

BACKGROUND

Laurence developed epilepsy when he was approximately 11 yr old. He had about one seizure a year for a number of years but was otherwise well. He liked sports and was a good football player. One day early in 1982 at the age of 25 while playing football, he felt strange. There was a pressure in his head and he lost his balance and fell. A local doctor was called. Laurence was told he just had a headache. He said, "No, it's more than that." The doctor gave Laurence some tablets and sent him home to his wife and children. Later that day Laurence's mother called. She noticed that Laurence's eyes were crossed and told him to go to the local hospital. He was kept in and had some eye tests. The following day Laurence was sent to a university teaching hospital about 20 miles away. A tumor was discovered—an intraventricular giant cell astrocytoma in the left hemisphere. Surgery was carried out in January 1982. Laurence was said to have made a good recovery although he had both expressive and receptive dysphasia.

Laurence was unable to return to work. He had held a number of jobs before the operation, he had been a butcher, a fork-lift truck driver, and had worked for an electrical firm. After leaving the hospital, he was reluctant to meet people other than members of his family. He had been married since the age of 18 and had three children, the youngest was born in 1982, the year of Laurence's operation. His mother, brothers, and sister lived nearby, so he was not too isolated. He attended speech therapy on and off for the next few years.

In September 1987, over 5 yr since his operation, Laurence forgot to go to a hospital appointment at the rehabilitation department. As a result I was asked to see him to try to help with his memory problems. I made an appointment with him for October 1987. We were unable to meet for very long because of transport problems. Laurence had come from his home about 20 miles away by hospital transport. I was able to talk to Laurence and his wife about the nature of his memory difficulties and decided whether or not I was the appropriate person to see him.

Laurence had obvious problems understanding my questions and in expressing himself yet despite this he was a good communicator. He almost always found a way to make me understand what he was saying by pantomime or circumlocution or gesture. Furthermore, if he did not understand what I was saying he made this clear and I had to find another way to express my ideas. Laurence thought he had a "big problem" with dates, names, where he put things, and passing on messages. He felt he had no problem with faces and routes. I asked him about remembering things he saw on television and he replied, "That goes as well."

I realized that Laurence's main problems were with language and therefore a speech and language therapist would be in a much better position to help. Moreover, he was already having this help. I felt his memory problems were probably secondary to his language problems and I doubted he would benefit from the strategies and compensations I could teach. However, I was intrigued by Laurence. I had not worked closely with anyone quite like him. Ron (Chapter 12) had a multitude of problems and Bill (Chapter 10) was far more language impaired. I decided I would see Laurence for two additional sessions for a more detailed assessment before making a decision about treatment.

INITIAL ASSESSMENT

Laurence did surprisingly well on the National Adult Reading Test (NART) managing to read 20 words successfully. This suggested he was functioning premorbidly in at least the average range of ability, and possibly higher. On the Graded Naming Test he managed to name only one picture correctly (kangaroo) although he could describe many of the others. For example, when shown a picture of a "scarecrow" he said "put up to stop the birds." I also administered the old Wechsler Memory Scale (WMS) (Wechsler, 1945) and the Recognition Memory Test for Faces (Warrington, 1984). He did not do too badly on the WMS scoring 5/5 for orientation, 4/6 for personal and current information; and he successfully recalled 3 of the 4 visual reproduction cards (A, B, and C2). On the Paired Associate Learning Subtest he scored 9/18 on the easy pairs and 2/12 on the hard pairs. On the prose recall (Anna Thompson story) he managed 4 items in immediate recall and 3 in delayed recall. He was only able to recall 3 digits forward although he had a normal span on the Corsi blocks test. These results are not consistent with an amnesic syndrome and, although not good, suggest his memory problems were, at least in part, secondary to his language disorder. These results can be seen in Table 11.1

Laurence was interested to know as much as possible about the cause and nature of his problems, so we spent some time each session addressing these issues. Much of my explanation was in the form of drawings of the brain and the location of the language areas.

It became clear that the reason Laurence would not meet his old friends was because he thought they would think he was crazy. This seemed to bother him considerably. He also refused to go to a stroke club for people with dysphasia because the other dysphasic people were much older than he was and he felt out of place.

At the end of this brief assessment I felt Laurence should be seen by someone with more specialist knowledge about language disorders and decided to see if I could refer him to a more suitable person. In my report to the referring consultant I said:

> On the National Adult Reading Test Mr. _____ read 20 words correctly, suggesting that his premorbid intellectual level was at least in the average range and possibly higher. On the Graded Naming Test he was only able to name one picture, indicating considerable word finding problems. His immediate nonverbal memory span was normal and he showed normal performance on a nonverbal learning test. There is some evidence of memory problems, for example, his score on the Rivermead Behavioural Memory Test was 4 out of 12 which is in the moderately impaired range. This cannot be explained entirely by his language deficits as other dysphasic patients are able to achieve higher scores than this. To a large extent, however, I feel his memory problems seem secondary to the language problems. I spent some time explaining to Mr. _____ why he had difficulties with his memory and speech and also why he had visual field deficits. As you know, he is terrified that people will think him crazy and he himself feels very stupid when he comes out with the wrong word. I did my best to explain the difference between psychiatric and neurological problems.
>
> I feel that the best thing for Mr. _____ would be to have a psychologist see him at home to work on some specific memory and word finding strategies there. He is somewhat suspicious of this and wants to see the person first. Whether or not we can find anybody able and willing to take on this task is, of course, another matter. It is possible that somebody would agree to see him, at _____ as some of the people there have a great interest in language disorders and believe successful treatment can follow a very detailed analysis of the language deficits. I will ring a colleague there to see if she thinks this idea is worth pursuing.
>
> I told Mr. _____ that I will contact him in the New Year to keep him up-to-date with what is happening.

Table 11.1. Laurence's Results on the Initial Assessment (1987) and Following Further Surgery (1988)

TEST	1987 SCORE	1987 COMMENT	1988 SCORE	1988 COMMENT
National Adult Reading Test	20/50 correct	Predicted full scale IQ 106	5/50	Marked deterioration almost all words read phonetically
Graded Naming Test	1/30	Severely impaired	1/30	As before
Rivermead Behavioural Memory Test	Screening score = 4/12 (Passed pictures, faces, orientation, delayed route)	Moderately impaired	2/12 (Passed pictures and faces)	Severely impaired
Recognition Memory Test for Faces	35/50	Impaired	34/50	Essentially the same
Corsi Span	Age scaled score = 3	Normal	5	Normal
Corsi Span Plus 2 learning test	5 + 2 = 7 Learned in 3 trials	Normal	—	
Wechsler Memory Scale				
Personal and current info	4/6	Slightly impaired	4/6	As before
Orientation	5/5	Normal	4/5	Did not know date
Prose recall				
Immediate	4/24	Impaired	2/24	Slight deterioration
Delayed	3/24	Normal as percentage of copy	1/24	Slight deterioration
Digits forward	3	Impaired	2	Impaired
Digits backward	2	Impaired	2	As before
Visual reproduction	3/4	Normal	Not tested	
Paired associates				
Easy pairs	9/18	Impaired	Not tested	
Hard pairs	2/12	Impaired	Not tested	

Business Library - Issue Receipt

Customer name: Blower, Taylor-Jayne

Title: Case studies in neuropsychological
rehabilitation / Barbara A. Wilson.
ID: 1005204175
Due: 12/01/2015 23:59

Total items: 1
22/10/2014 15:12

All items must be returned before the due date
and time.
The Loan period may be shortened if the item is
requested.

WWW.nottingham.ac.uk/is

THE NEXT STAGE, JANUARY–AUGUST 1988

As I expected, it was not possible to find a clinical psychologist to see Laurence at home although I was able to arrange a referral to a specialist team in London. The team agreed to pay Laurence's traveling expenses if he could find his way there alone, and would also pay expenses for his wife or a friend if he traveled with a companion.

Laurence and his wife traveled to London by train in March 1988. Unfortunately, before arriving at the language department he had a seizure on the underground, fell, and sustained a minor head injury. This aggravated a cyst that had formed at the site of his tumor. He was taken home by ambulance and admitted for further surgery to drain a porencephalic cyst. This surgery was not successful and in May 1988 a repeat craniotomy and drainage were performed. Laurence returned to speech therapy and was found to have deteriorated in his language functioning.

A report from his speech therapist soon after this said, "Recent surgery has left him with a more marked comprehension problem than previously. Reading comprehension is limited to single simple words and auditory comprehension to two element phrases." She noted that situational context and nonverbal information facilitated his comprehension and she also felt that his poor memory affected his ability to comprehend written and spoken information. Laurence's expressive abilities were felt to be better than his comprehension. He had difficulty with finding words and sequencing information. Again, it was agreed that his poor memory hindered his communication. The speech therapy department agreed to continue seeing Laurence weekly to work on his auditory and written comprehension, word finding, and sentence construction. It was suggested that Laurence should be re-referred to me. Consequently, in August 1988 the consultant asked me to see Laurence for treatment as he was unable to travel to London. I agreed, although I felt rather out of my depth. Because of his speech and language difficulties I would have preferred to work jointly with a speech and language therapist. The current situation, however, meant this was not possible. Laurence went to one hospital for speech therapy and to another, 20 miles away, for psychology.

FURTHER ASSESSMENT AND REHABILITATION, SEPTEMBER 1988–SEPTEMBER 1990

I saw Laurence approximately once every 2 or 3 wk over the next 2 yr. The first question I wanted to know when I saw him again was whether or not he had changed on the tests I had administered almost a year earlier. These results can be seen in Table 11.1. There would appear to have been some decline in Laurence's memory functioning and a marked decline in his ability to read the nonphonetic words on the NART.

I administered further tests at this time including the Raven's Standard Progressive Matrices on which he scored 35/60, i.e., in the lower end of the average range.

Over the next 2 mo I gave Laurence numerous object naming and reading tests. He was asked to name various sets of cards from the Winslow Press Photograph Library (ref) and the Renfrew Picture Cards (Renfrew, 1975). He usually recognized a picture and could tell me something about it but he could not find the correct name. In February 1989 he was given the Test for Reception of Grammar (TROG; Bishop, 1982) which he found very difficult. Four pictures at a time are presented, together with a spoken word or sentence. The subject is required to point to the correct picture. Laurence's overall score was equivalent to that of a 5-yr-old, although his pattern of performance was inconsistent and did not follow the normal age pattern. He managed some fairly complex structures such as, "Not only the girl but also the cat is sitting," while failing some relatively easy ones such as, "The boy is chasing the sheep." This may have been due, at least in part, to his problems with some of the vocabulary. Laurence took a very long time to decide on the correct picture and frequently requested several repetitions of the sentence. He benefited to some extent from seeing the sentence written, while in oral presentation he appeared to forget the beginning of the sentence. Even so, he made many errors in both the auditory and written modalities.

I investigated Laurence's reading in more detail at this time. He made errors on an easy lexical decision task, i.e., deciding whether a printed letter string was a real word or a nonsense word. He showed a slight but inconsistent effect of word length, reading GAS and "PIN" in 4 sec each and "NEWSPAPER" and "LIGHTNING" in 22 sec each. He made numerous errors, however, reading NEIGHBOUR as, "NAILBOROUGH" in 47 sec, and giving up on VEGETABLE after 71 sec saying, "VEG-VEG-ET . . . . . . I give up." He had no parts of speech effect but a definite effect of regularity of spelling. These results, shown in Table 11.2, suggest that Laurence has some characteristics of a person with surface dyslexia. This was more marked with his spelling. He made numerous phonetic errors, such as HUNNY for HONEY and SENNSIBL for SENSIBLE. On a homophone confusion test he read all words correctly but identified only 7/22. With the remaining words, he described the homophone, for example he read, "HOARSE" and mimed riding a horse.

I also looked again at his digit span. His recall of spoken digits was fairly consistent and he almost always recalled two digits. Occasionally, he managed three digits. Next I tested him with visually presented digits. The digits were written individually on cards and presented to him one at a time, before Laurence was shown a card with all nine digits on and asked to point to the ones he had just seen in the same order as he had seem them. Again, he almost always managed to recall two digits successfully and occasionally recalled three. I then repeated the

Table 11.2. Results of Laurence's Reading Assessment November 1988–January 1989

TASK	SCORE	COMMENTS
Lexical decision	31/39	2 False positives (bant, rost) 6 False negatives (burn, shawl, germ, pity, groan, pest)
Parts of speech	32/32	No effect of parts of speech
Reading words of different lengths	32/49	Regular word errors = 5 Irregular word errors = 12 Effect of irregularity
Word length effect	36/57	Slight word length effect on the words he read correctly, but not clear cut
Homophone confusions	7/22	Identified the homophone for the remaining words, e.g., for "hoarse" he mimed riding a horse

Corsi Block test. He successfully recalled all lengths up to and including five and one out of three strings of a sequence of six taps.

By January 1989 it was time to try some strategies to improve Laurence's word retrieval problems. When searching for a word Laurence could often say how many syllables or how many letters the word contained. If he could find the initial letter he was much more likely to retrieve the word he was looking for. He often said, "If I can see the first one I can get it." I considered forward chaining as a treatment method, i.e., give him the first letter of a word and if this did not help give him an additional letter and so forth.

First letter cueing, of course, is not new in language therapy. Nickels (1992) and Best et al., (1997) are among others who have successfully used this method to enhance word retrieval. I drew up a list of common words, which seemed to cause Laurence particular difficulty, and asked his wife to do the same. When the preliminary list of words was ready I wanted to see if Laurence could repeat after me and read aloud the words he could not retrieve. These results can be seen in Table 11.3.

I took these 40 words and put them into 4 groups, trying to ensure a balance of one-, two- and three-syllable words in each group. One group was for a no treatment condition, one for forward chaining, one for verbal rehearsal, and one for reading rehearsal. Each session for the next 4 meetings we practiced three of the sets. First I showed him a picture of an object and asked what it was. He was then prompted using one of the three treatment methods.

Forward chaining involved writing down the first letter of the word when Laurence gave an incorrect response or a nonresponse. If he still failed an additional letter was written down by the first, then a third letter, and so forth until he retrieved the word correctly. For *verbal rehearsal* he repeated the correct name

Table 11.3. Naming, Repetition, and Reading of Some Common Everyday Objects

PICTURE	NAMING	ABLE TO REPEAT	ABLE TO READ
Bath	"Path (No first word is wrong.)"	Yes	Yes
Belt	"I have one."	Yes	Yes
Bread	"Eat it."	Yes	Yes
Bucket	"For water."	No	Yes
Cards	D.K.*	Yes	Yes
Clock	"Quarter past 9."	Yes	Yes
Coat Hanger	D.K.	1) Hanger 2) Coat 3) Coat hanger	Yes
Coach	D.K.	Yes	Yes
Corn cobs	"My son likes them."	Corn cops	Yes
Crutches	"If they broke."	No	No
Draughts	D.K.	Yes	Yes
Elephant	D.K.	Yes	Yes
Fireplace	D.K.	Fire Place (as two words)	Yes
Fork	"Eating."	Yes	Yes
Frying Pan	(Mimed)	After 4 goes and with some hesitancy	Yes
Globe	"America."	Yes	Yes
Grass Hopper	"Fly."	At 3rd go	Yes
Helicopter	"Not a plane."	1) No response 2) Heli 3) No response	Yes
Ice Skates	"Ice . . . ice."	Yes	Yes
Iron	"What I fixed last week."	Yes	Yes
Jewelry	D.K.	Yes	Yes
Keys	(Mimed)	Yes	Yes
Lawn Mower	"Grass."	1) Something mower 2) Yes	Yes
Lorry	"Driving."	No	Yes
Mouth Organ	D.K.	Yes	Yes
Nails	(Mimed)	No	Yes
Paddling Pool	"Swimming—kiddies."	Yes	1) Ing pool 2) Yes
Pillow	(Mimed sleeping)	No	Yes
Rose	"I gave one to my wife."	Yes	Yes
Ruler	"At school—12 inch."	Yes	Yes
Saw	(Mimed)	Yes	Yes
Scales	"Weight reading."	Yes	Yes
Skipping Rope	"Boxers use them a lot."	Yes	Yes
Spade	(Mimed)	Yes	Yes
Stapler	"Nails."	Yes	Yes
Sunbed	"When its Sunday—during the—its hot."	1) Sun 2) Bed 3) Sunbed	Yes

(*continued*)

Table 11.3. Naming, Repetition, and Reading of Some Common Everyday Objects
(continued)

PICTURE	NAMING	ABLE TO REPEAT	ABLE TO READ
Swan	D.K.	Yes	Yes
Table	"Where people eat—no bits to go with it."	Yes	Yes
Television	(Mimed)	Yes	Yes
Toaster	"Bread."	Yes	Yes
Tooth Brush	"Brush."	Yes	Yes
Torch	"Use it."	Yes	Yes
Trumpet	(Mimed)	No	Yes
Violin	(Mimed)	Yes	Yes
Whisk	D.K.	Yes	Yes
Yacht	D.K.	Yes	Yes

*D.K., Don't Know.

after me three times. *Reading rehearsal* required Laurence to read the correct word three times. We went through the three different treatments in random order several times each session. Following the four treatment sessions, I tested Laurence on all 40 words in random order. He retrieved none of the words in the no treatment group, two words in the reading rehearsal group, four in the verbal rehearsal group, and five in the forward chaining group. Again these were not brilliant results but forward chaining seemed to be a reasonable strategy to try. These results can be seen in Table 11.4.

I thought I should combine forward chaining with expanding rehearsal, i.e., once he correctly retrieved the word, I should test him after 5 sec, 10 sec, 20 sec, and so on in an attempt to establish more permanent learning. However, before we were able to implement the next stage of treatment, Laurence once again developed a severe headache and double vision. He wrote me a note that he brought to one session saying,

HEADACHE (TIRED), DOUBLE-VISION
TINGLES ALL DOWN
RIGHT SIDE!
(ELECTRICAL FEELING)
——
BALANCE ?

He was referred again to the neurosurgeon and was readmitted to the hospital for further drainage of the cyst that had enlarged over the past few months. Another stormy few weeks passed. In July 1989, a peritoneal shunt was placed directly into the cyst and Laurence returned home 2 wk later still complaining of bad headaches and double vision.

In September 1989 Laurence returned to clinical psychology. The TROG was

Table 11.4. Pictures Shown in Each Condition

FORWARD CHAINING	VERBAL REHEARSAL	READING REHEARSAL	NO TREATMENT
Paddling pool	Mouth organ	Skipping rope	Draught board
Table	Bucket	Iron	Ruler
Lawn mower	Toothbrush	Coat hanger	Fireplace
Nails	Belt	Cards	Clock
Coach	Torch	Yacht	Scales
Helicopter	Frying pan	Grasshopper	Ice skates
Whisk	Rose	Spade	Fork
Pillow	Sunbed	Crutches	Lorry
Stapler	Violin	Trumpet	Globe
Jewelery	Corn cobs	Elephant	Toaster

Total correct on final test

5	4	2	0

Total correct at follow-up

4	1	1	1

readministered. Laurence passed a fewer number of blocks (7 as opposed to 9 earlier) but the same number of actual sentences correct (55 on both occasions). Thus there would not appear to have been a significant change. Laurence's visual digit span was a little better. He could now manage four digits after visual presentation both when the response was visual and when it was oral. With orally presented digits, however, he still only managed two reliably with very occasionally a string of three digits correctly reproduced.

In October 1989, we decided to revisit the word retrieval issue. His wife said there were not any particular words Laurence had difficulty with at home except people's names. He always had problems there even with his family. She wrote down a few examples of his problems at home. She said she told Laurence he had dirt on his finger and he looked at his foot. On another occasion she asked if he wanted rhubarb crumble and had to show him what it was, even though he had it every week and usually understood the words. On this occasion, however, he did not know what she meant. His wife also said that if Laurence asked what time he had to be somewhere she had to keep repeating the time until in the end she replied with the nearest hour or half hour which caused him less trouble. The final example involved using the telephone. If someone he knew well telephoned, Laurence talked quickly and without hesitating but if it was someone he did not know he panicked and called his wife.

We administered the picture–word task we had tried with Laurence in January.

He recalled four of the forward chaining words and one each in each of the other conditions.

Once again Laurence became ill. He had three seizures during the second week of October yet kept his appointment on the 16th as he really looked forward to his sessions. He said he had tight feelings down his right side and felt numb all over. When he walked he experienced double vision and felt he had more problems with reading and understanding words than he had a week earlier.

Soon after this Laurence was readmitted to the hospital for further tests and adjustments to his anticonvulsant medication. He began his weekly sessions again in November. Observations and discussions with Laurence confirmed our earlier findings. When shown a picture of an object he had frequent problems with the name, yet could usually say how many syllables and could often reproduce the "rhythm" of the word. He could say with a fair degree of accuracy how many letters there were. If he could access the first letter of the word through writing or going through the alphabet he could often retrieve the word itself. This did not always work though, e.g., when shown a picture of a glass and given three letters, G–L–A, he still sometimes failed. When given the correct word Laurence would often say, "Yeah, I know it's a word, I can hear it but it doesn't mean anything." It seemed Laurence found it easier to remember words if he saw them written. He could not "hold on to" the name of a student who saw him until he saw it written, after which he reliably recalled the student's name whenever he saw the student.

Before implementing an expanding rehearsal treatment, Laurence was given a few more tests in order to test his visuospatial sketchpad functioning. Laurence was asked how many windows there were in his house. We asked his wife the same question to confirm the answer. Laurence had no difficulty in producing the correct response. A further test of the visuospatial sketchpad functioning (described by Phillips [1983]) was also given. In this test the subject is shown a matrix of squares ranging from 2×2 to 4×5. Some of the squares were filled in and some were empty. Laurence was asked to look at one grid for 2 sec, this grid was immediately replaced by a second grid in which one square was different. The task is to identify the square that was different. Laurence was able to manage a grid of 12 squares giving him a span of 6, which is just below the range for normal control subjects (Wilson, 1993). On the Block Design Subtest of the British Ability Scales Laurence successfully completed all 16 designs although he was outside the allotted time limit on 8 of them. His visuospatial functioning then appeared to be relatively normal.

He also succeeded on a simple auditory recognition test, in which a series of environmental sounds were presented on a tape recorder. These included a train, a dentist's drill, a siren, and animal noises. Laurence was required to identify the sounds by pointing to the appropriate picture on a card in front of him.

The expanding rehearsal treatment was implemented in November and December 1989. Although the original plan had been to combine forward chaining and expanding rehearsal, this was accidentally overlooked and expanding rehearsal was used alone.

The plan was to teach one word each week. The procedure for each word was:

1. Show picture of the object, together with the written word;
2. Ask Laurence to read the word and look at the object;
3. Remove the word and ask Laurence to name the object immediately;
4. Ask for the name again after 10 sec, then 20 sec, then 40 sec, 60 sec, 90 sec, 120 sec, 180 sec, 5 min, and 10 min—use nonverbal tasks, e.g., Raven's Matrices for filler tasks for test intervals over 1 min;
5. A successful response was defined as production of the correct word/name within 10 sec.

There was a slight problem in obtaining a stable baseline because Laurence sometimes could not find a particular word at all and sometimes he found it easily within 10 sec. Nevertheless, we found seven everyday words with which Laurence had particular difficulty. He learned each of these words within the sessions and could successfully recall the word even after a 10-min interval. The problem was demonstrating carry-over to the following week. Obviously, this method needed the expanding rehearsal to continue over a much longer period of time than we could offer in the sessions. We considered asking his wife to test him at home but felt this would not be fair to her and might distress Laurence. If we follow the principle of "normalization" (Gunzburg, 1976) and try to let people live as normal a life as possible within the limits of their disability, then it is not normal for family members to regularly act as therapists or experimenters at home.

We felt our findings on expanding rehearsal were inconclusive and more work needed to be done. Others, however, have been more successful. Moffat (1989), used expanding rehearsal to reteach words to a woman with dysphasia associated with dementia. Camp (1989) and Camp and Stevens (1990) used expanding rehearsal to teach new information to people with Alzheimer's disease.

Another question posed at this time was whether or not Laurence's problem in retaining even short amounts of orally presented verbal information was due to an echoic memory deficit, i.e., to a failure in the auditory sensory memory system that holds information for less than a quarter of a second, or whether he had a more straightforward short-term memory deficit. In January 1990, we decided to explore this further by presenting him with a series of digit span tasks beyond his span of 2 to 3 digits to see if there were position effects. We also repeated this procedure with two modifications: (1) the digits were followed by an auditory tap on the table as the signal to recall and (2) the digits were followed by an orally presented suffix—"now"—as the signal to recall.

We predicted that if Laurence had an echoic memory deficit there would be:
(1) no recency effect [as this reflects short-term memory (STM)] and (2) no difference in recall between the tap on the table condition and the command "now"
condition. If, however, Laurence had a short-term/immediate memory deficit
then there would be both a recency effect (he should get the last one or two digits
correct) and poorer performance with "now" than with the tap on the table (as
"now" would interfere with STM).

The results seemed to support the STM hypothesis. With digit strings presented orally for immediate spoken recall in the correct order, Laurence almost
always recalled the first and last digits of each string, i.e., there was both a pri-
macy and a recency effect. When the signal to recall was a tap he correctly recalled 6/6 strings of three digits, 4/6 strings of four digits, and 2/5 strings of five
digits. On all strings where he made errors he recalled the final digit correctly.
However when "now" was the signal to recall, he correctly recalled only 2/6
strings of three digits, 1/6 strings of four digits, and 0/6 strings of five digits. Furthermore, on only three of the incorrect strings was Laurence correct on the final
digit. This would appear to be fairly conclusive evidence for an immediate or
short-term memory deficit and not a problem with echoic memory.

Further work on expanding rehearsal for the seven words was carried out between January and April 1990. Laurence learned to recall reliably five of the
seven words within 10 sec. The two verbs in the list, "carrying" and "pouring"
continued to cause trouble. He sometimes retrieved these but typically took between 23–39 sec to retrieve each of these words.

In May 1990 when he was discharged from speech therapy it was felt that little
progress had been made. Laurence also had a break from clinical psychology. He
developed yet more problems with his shunt and his cyst, which required another
operation. For several weeks he was in and out of the hospital. He recovered sufficiently to return to his sessions in June 1990. I continued to see him every 2 or 3
wk until September when I made my good-byes before leaving to take up my
present post in Cambridge. Most of the sessions over the last 3 mo were spent in
conversations and explanations about the nature of his problems (Laurence never
ceased asking about this and requesting information over the 3 yr since he first
came to see me) and discussions regarding his feelings about his life.

"Tell me how it began," I said one day. He said he had his first epilepsy "turn"
when he was 11 or 12 yr old. He went on to say "then another turn a year later
and then one turn each year until about 17, and then every few months but sometimes more." His wife, who was present during this conversation, said she saw
the first seizure when Laurence was 17. After that he had one more before they
were married (at 18 yr old) and no more until he was 20. He had one or two after
that until the tumor was diagnosed.

I asked Laurence to write his story, tell me what happened and how he felt
about it. I shall reproduce the first 8 pages of Laurence's account in the hope that

it shows, despite his spelling mistakes and problems with grammar, what a good communicator he is. A well-known American speech and language pathologist, Audrey Holland, said to me many years ago, "Don't listen to the words, listen to the message." Laurence conveys his message very well.

(Dr)

    BARBARA WILSON
—8 YEARS AGO I SLOWLY GOT
MORE OF A, HEADACHE/A/BALLAN-
-CE ETC, I WENT TO MY LOCAL D^{RS}
TO SEE WHAT SORT OF PROBLEMI
~~D~~ HAD—THE DR SAID HE COULD NO—
—T THINK OF WHAT, WRONG. SO HE
SAID—I WILL SEE ANOTHER D^R ? LATER.
    AT THIS TIME MY VISION WAS
GETTING LESS SO I ~~ME~~ WENT TO
HOSPITAL (EYES)—AND I HAD TO DO
SOME TESTS EX ? EG (6 pm)
    WEN I HAD SOME EYES SCANES
I HAD TO SEE DR B____. AND SAID
THAT I WILL HAVE TO STAY IN —
    IN EARLY IN THE MORNING I
WAS TOLD—THAT I HAD TO GO TO—
(—S _____ HOSPITAL, NEUROLOGY)
—(HEADACHE/
I DID HAD A PROBLEM BEFORE
THAT ___ EPILEPSY/(CONVULSIONS)
    AFTER THAT THEY
DOWNE SOME TESTS, DOWN
STAIRS (X-RAYS). I WENT BACK
TO THE WARD. ~~IT WAS~~
    LATER/ON?—(ME & J _____)
        SENT
WE WERE IT ~~CALLED~~ FOR ?
    AFTER THAT THEY
DOWNE SOME TESTS, DOWN
STAIRS (X-RAYS). I WENT BACK
TO THE WARD.
    LATER/ON?—(ME AND J_____)
WE WERE IT SENT FOR?
    IT WAS A TUMOUR THAT
THAY FOUND I HAD—? TUMOUR!
    I COULD NOT THINK
    ————————————

    WOT A SHOCK
    THE NEXT DAY, THERE WAS
ANOTHER THING? THERE WHOSE
SOME—GROIN/TUBE—BRAIN/
SCANS/PICTURES? I DID NOT
LIKE <u>THAT</u>

WHEN I WOKE UP I WAS
IN A AGONY—
—(HEADACHE/FOR AGES
        AFTER THE OP, I COULD
NOT REMEMBER.
        I WAS MILES AWAY.
BUT SLOWLY I CAME BACK.
        ALL THE HOSPITAL
STAFF, THERE REALY
LOOKED AFTER ME
—DRS, SISTERS, NERSES, ETC, ETC
(THANK CHRIST FOR THAT)

        MY SPEECH. DID NOT MAKE
SENCE. TO ME?
        ANY MY THINKING—GONE
        I STAYED THERE FOR A
MONTH.
        IT WAS ONE THING. WHAT
I REALLY WANTED—
_____, LONG GHAIR.
(AND DON'T LAUGH)
ON THE FIRST OF JAN. 87
        I HAD TO GO TO THE
HOSPITAL/   I HAD
BEEN GETTING SORE—
—THROAT. A DR SAID—IT
WOULD BE A BETTER IDEA
        TO REMOVE THE TONSELS.
        FOR THE FIVE DAYS
THAT I KEPT/STAYED THERE
        I FELT VERY SORE.
MOST OF THE PEAPLE
THAY WERE ONLY KID'S
HOW ENBARISING!
BUT I DID NOT CARE
        MY EPILEPS HAD STILL CONTI-
NUD—(GRAND MAL/PETIT MAL)
AND A CHANGE OF
TABLETS. ETC. IF THAY ~~WAS~~ WERE
LIKE SWEATS - IT WOUD HAVE BEEN OK!
        I HAD BE~~EN~~EN SEEING DIVE-
-RENT PEAPL~~Y~~E / DRS—
SPEECH THERAPY/ EYE DEPT /
PSYCHOLOGY / PROF M_____,
        ~~ALO~~ ALSO
DR BARBARA WILSON/PSYCHALOQIST)
        STILL
ON - 88 I WAS HAVING MORE
FITS, SO I HAD TO GO BACK

TO THE NEURO. AND WEANT
FOR A BRAKE - CYSTS (OP)
            ON MAY 88, AT A FOLLOWING
MONTH, I HAD TO COME BACK,
AND, ANOTHER OP WAS FOR
THE SAME BIT
            MY EPILEPSY DID G~~ED~~ NOT
CONPLEPLY STOP ANY FITS.
            IT HAS ALWAS BEEN A
HOPE. ~~AT~~ THAT IT COU7D
BE A DREAM.
            ON JULY 89 FOR A 2
WEEK, I HAD TO HAVE AN O.P
WHICH WAS CALLED A
~~SHU~~ SHUNT?
AT THIS TIME. I DID NOT HAVE
A O.P. AUG 21ST-SEPT 6ST
                  OK!
MY EYES WERE X, BALLENCE
ETC.
NO CHANGE. THE FITS
~~DID~~ WERE MORE X 2/3 (ETC),
SO ON MARCH 12TH, I HAD
TO GO BACK, AND STADED
FOR A MONTH. ALL ~~THE~~
WARKERS WERE DOING SOM
JOBS SO I HAD TO
GO TO ANOTHER LEVEL.
            IT WAS THREE WEEKS. BE-
-FOR I WAS TOLD THAT I
HAD TO HAVE A O.P.—
CYSTS.
            (STILL AT THE ~~NUE~~ NEURO)
ON THE 8TH OF APRIL.
I HAD 3 PETIT MAL
FITS—. WHEN I SAW
MR _____ HE SAID—IT MAY
BE COUSED—DUE TO THE
PREVIES 4 DAYS WHEN I
HAD A O.P. THEN HE
SAID—LAURENCE. YOU CAN
GO HOME.
            (DR WILSON/BARBARA)
I DONT NOW IF I MAY - NOT SAY THIS
BIT?—BUT WHEN I STAYED THERE
/ THEIR THE MAN ~~HOW~~ THAT
I HAD NEXT TO ME HE JUST DIED—
            THE ~~NEXT DAY~~ SAME TIME—
LATER ON. A MAN/MIDDLE AGED.

NAVY ELECTRISON H DIED !
WE HE SAID THAT HE DID
NOT FILL BAD/OK !
     I CAN STILL SEE HIS FACE
NOW—THINKING ABOUT NEURO
I HAVE NOT BEEN OUT
FROM HOME, PERHAPS THE SHOP
OR NEXT DOOR TO SEE OLD FRED
WHO JUST PAST AWAY AGED
65. ISE HE WAS SUCH A
FREANDLY MAN ..
     HE USE TO MUCK ABOUT
         BUT
WITH ARE KIDS BUT HE SLOWLY
GOT WERSE.
     BEFORE I HAD A
ANY IDIERS ABOUT CONVOULSION
—IT WHOSE SOME-THING A WHEN
             NOT
A PERSON PAST OUT. I DID NOT
THINK THAT IT COULDNT
HAPPEN TO BE. THERE IS
CLUBS AND HELPERS FOR
PEAPLE WAON HELP
AND I NEEDED,
     AT SCHOOL I WAS A
FOOTBALL PL;AYER, RUNNER,
CRICKET, AND BOXING IN
THE NAVY CADETS AND I
REALY LIKED THAT

Before I left to go to Cambridge I tried again to find another psychologist to see Laurence but I was unsuccessful.

The following year I learned that Laurence was receiving speech therapy again as the speech therapist wrote to me asking for copies of my reports.

SINCE 1990

Apart from one brief meeting with Laurence while visiting my former place of work, I did not see him again until July 1997. I heard about him every now and again from a medical colleague who saw him every few months.

I went back to the old hospital to see him for 2 hr one hot Friday afternoon. Laurence looked well, and was enthusiastic about the meeting.

We repeated a few tests—the TROG, Digit Span, and the Phillips (1983) visual spatial sketch pad task. Despite several demonstrations of the sketch pad task, Laurence was unable to understand the instructions and could not complete any of the matrices. His digit span was 2 forwards (during the period of investigation in 1990, he had sometimes managed to recall 4 digits). His Corsi Block span was 4 (previously it had been 5). He also showed slight deterioration on the TROG. He passed a total of 6 blocks and 50 actual sentences.

I also readministered the seven pictures used in the expanding rehearsal experiment interspersed with seven untaught pictures. He recalled three in each condition so there was no apparent long-term effect of the treatment.

Laurence still tried to find the first letter. He said, "If I can't think what it's called I go through it in my head." I asked him if he meant he goes through the alphabet and he agreed.

I learned that Laurence's wife had left him and he was living alone. He seemed very sad. He said he had been in the hospital four times for operations. He thought he had had the present shunt for about 3 yr and it was fine. He said,

> "This one—I can't think what it's called now—a tube. I went in—something tumor, cyst, cyst, shunt. Later after a year it didn't work so they did it again and put another one inside and then it started again. It's OK now but my hand is zizzy," (I think he meant tingley) "and I can't see out of this eye." (his right eye).

He said he had had no more seizures since the last shunt.

"What do you like doing?" I said. "Do you still like football?" "Not really," said Laurence, "I never see it." "Do you watch it on television?" "Not really," he said. "So how do you spend your day?" I asked. "Walk, I walk all over," replied Laurence. "Do you have any friends." "No," said Laurence. "I got a brother and my mum lives round the back—not far from there. I got a sister and I see my oldest one." (He meant his oldest child.)

So Laurence seems to lead an empty life for a man in his 40's who is physically fairly able and who would, given the right support and structure, be able to cope with some sheltered employment.

12

RON: PICKING UP THE PIECES

BACKGROUND

Ron was almost 31 yr old at the time of his head injury. He was married with a daughter of 20 mo and was working for the gas board where he lectured apprentices. On the 2nd of September 1978 Ron was at his next door neighbor's, helping to paint the house. He was working on the garage roof when the accident occurred. His wife Lesley described what happened.

> I heard the ladder go and I knew it would be Ron. I just ran out and he was on the floor. The garage roof had rotted and it collapsed under the weight of the ladder. Ron was just footing the ladder and the chap was painting up at the top, but luckily he was OK. He just came down with the force of the ladder but Ron's head was in the ladder and as he came through the gap he crashed his head on the concrete floor. We phoned an ambulance and he was admitted to hospital.
>
> He was unconscious and there was blood coming from his ear—and we knew that was a bad sign. I kept saying to the young doctor there, 'Has he got brain damage, has he got brain damage?' That was in my mind straight away, but the doctor said, 'No.' But they couldn't get him to open his eyes and I don't know if that's a normal thing. I stayed the night and there was no change. My mum arranged for Dad to come and pick me up at 6 in the morning. I'd just left the hospital because they'd said 'No change,' and I was going back to change and then come back. As soon as I got home I had a telephone call to say he'd been transferred

to a specialist unit. The next day he had the first operation to remove a blood clot.

Then the following day they had to do another operation to remove part of the brain because his brain had swollen so much. Then he was in a coma for 2 months. When Ron came out of the coma—well you wouldn't have known he was out of the coma. He couldn't walk, talk, speak, see, do anything really. He was just propped up in the chair. All he could say was 'juice.' 'Juice' or 'Joyce' we couldn't make out what he was saying, it was all gobbledygook.

Then to feed Ron you had to say, 'Swallow it.' When you said 'swallow' he would swallow so that's how he first started to eat. He was understanding *that,* as he knew what to do, but he couldn't make you understand anything he wanted. We were just feeding him. If he said 'juice' or 'Joyce' we would give him something to eat or drink, or take him to the toilet. We didn't know what he wanted. We don't really know if Ron knew what he wanted. Later on he definitely knew when he wanted to go to the toilet.

At first he didn't know who we were. He didn't know who I was, who anybody was. He had no memory at all. It had all been wiped out . The nurses said to me that I was the only one . . . he was very difficult behavior-wise because he couldn't understand anything. If you were washing him or dressing him, he just couldn't understand anything. So he was very difficult and the nurses used to say that it was only me who could go in and bathe him and they couldn't handle him. They seemed to think I could handle him the most. He didn't like the bath. It was very difficult.

When our friends came, Ron nearly killed Dan, which is quite opposite to how Ron was or how he is now. It was explained that it was scar tissue and that it would subside, which it did but not for another couple of months.

The next step after that was—because he was unmanageable and they wanted his bed—they said to transfer him to the cottage hospital. The sister called me in and said it would be the worst thing for Ron because they would drug him because he was so unmanageable. They'd give him drugs to keep him quiet. I got appointments at two rehab. centers but they wouldn't take him because he was too bad. He had to be able to look after himself. I was getting no joy, I went somewhere else, but no joy. Then Rivermead accepted him. I don't know if it was anything to do with the fact that I'd written to the M.P. [Member of Parliament] saying I'd applied to these places and no one would accept him. Then the place at Rivermead came up. I just put it to the M.P. that here's a 31-yr-old man. If you're going to spend all this money operating on him, there's no point if he's not going to have any rehab. after. The next minute I heard from Rivermead but I don't really know if he (the M.P.) had anything to do with it. It may have just been the timing and that Rivermead had a place available.

One of the other centers said to come back in a year or so's time. They'd done tests on the eyes and they said one of the optic nerves hadn't actually broken. There was something there. At this time he didn't have any sight at all, so they said he could get something but they weren't prepared to take him then because he was too bad. There was nothing for him. He couldn't be left. He literally had to learn to walk again, to walk upstairs, and to walk downstairs. And he had to learn to see again.

He had another scan before Rivermead and they said when the results came back that he couldn't possibly see because one side of his brain was like an 80-yr-old and the other side has got the damage to the optic nerve. I told them that when I took him home he pointed to the floor. There was a pattern on the carpet and I thought perhaps he could see it. But they said 'No.' At Rivermead they verified that he could see but his brain wasn't telling him what he was seeing. It was when he went to Rivermead that something was showing—that he was seeing something, not that he understood what he was seeing.

I can tell you the first time he strung words together. It was New Year's Day 1979. He said, 'Have you got one?' Mum had lit a cigarette. He could smell it. He couldn't see it but he could smell it. 'Have you got one?' was what he said. We said it was the best New Year's present we could have. We didn't know he wanted a cigarette, we tried him with an orange, a banana, we didn't think of a cigarette. Mum was sitting quietly smoking and we tried to give him everything except the thing he wanted.

He didn't get any therapy because he wasn't able to respond to anything. He couldn't function at all, not really. The only thing is the doctor, the surgeon came and did tests with smells and things. He said there was no response at all, nothing. Then he suggested the cottage hospital but Rivermead, they obviously did tests and the first thing they did was teach him to use a toothbrush. They taught him the basics.

THE INITIAL ASSESSMENT

Ron was admitted to Rivermead in March 1979. In May he was assessed by a clinical psychology student. I first met Ron during his second admission in June 1980. The student who saw Ron in May said he was too impaired to administer any of the standardized tests due to dysphasia and visual problems. (He had tunnel vision by now.) Consequently, she devised a number of simple tests to estimate Ron's intellectual abilities. She reported that Ron knew his name and could copy it but could not write it spontaneously. He could also copy a circle and a triangle, although he made distortions when attempting to copy a star, a daisy, and a cube. She assessed color matching by giving him colored circles that he had to match to colored rectangles. He matched the colors accurately by holding one circle against each rectangle in turn until he found the correct match. When asked to name colors, he was only reliable with red. Shape matching was assessed in the same way, just using circles and rectangles. Ron could do this task accurately. He was then asked to construct a tactile block design using up to four blocks with either a smooth or sandpaper surface. He was given the sample design to feel and had to replicate the design with either one, two, or four blocks. Although successful with one and two blocks, he failed on three- and four-block designs, apparently because of difficulty with spatial arrangements in addition to visual problems.

Ron's visual memory was assessed by showing him some shape drawings such as a circle, a diamond, and a cross. He was required to look at each shape for 10 sec after which the shape was removed and Ron was required to reproduce the drawing. He was able to reproduce the simplest shapes accurately, although he was only partially successful with the more complex shapes.

To summarize, Ron, although still unable to say more than a few words, could perform simple matching tasks of shape or color and could reproduce simple drawings after a brief delay. The results were intended to provide a baseline against which to assess future improvement.

In June 1980, during Ron's second admission to Rivermead, I was asked to reassess him to see if he had improved. I readministered all tests from May 1979 plus some of the standardized psychological tests Ron had been unable to complete the previous year. It was, by now, 21 mo since his head injury. Ron had improved on all tests given to him previously. He could almost write his name without copying, making only one mistake in his surname. He was however very slow. His copying was accurate and he could complete the tactile block designs provided he could build his design on top of the original ones.

Despite his severe language problems, I gave him the Wechsler Adult Intelligence Scale (WAIS) because I wanted to establish a baseline. He failed all the performance items largely due, no doubt, to his severely restricted vision and to spatial difficulties. He was able to do some of the verbal subtests although his verbal IQ was only 55 at this stage. The results can be seen in Table 12.1. It was also clear that Ron's understanding of the questions was greater than his score would indicate and his expressive dysphasia was responsible for the poor result.

The Raven's Coloured Matrices were also administered and here Ron's raw score was 23, that is, an IQ equivalent of 70–80. On the Benton Visual Retention Test his total correct score was 3 (the average score is 8). His immediate recall of a prose passage was 3 (average being 9) with a delayed recall of 1.5. Ron was also asked to identify photographs of objects. Because of his severe word finding problems, however, the procedure was modified. Three words were presented to Ron and he had to select the correct word. For example, he was shown a photograph of swimming goggles and given the words "snorkel," "goggles," "glasses." He correctly recognized 13 out of 20 objects. A normal score would be 18 out of 20. It is hard to know to what extent Ron's failures were due to naming (word finding) difficulties or to visuoperceptual difficulties.

The most interesting result for me at this assessment was connected with Ron's reading. Having been unable to read in May 1979, this was the first time, as far as I knew, that his reading had been tested. He was given the prepublication version of the National Adult Reading Test (NART; Nelson, 1982), which contains irregularly spelled words. Ron was able to spell out the letters of the first word, ACHE, but not to say the whole word. He named most letters by going through the alphabet out loud until he reached the correct letter. With the second word DEBT he said the letters and then added, "Something to do with money." With the word PSALM he pointed to the second letter and said, "That's Stevie" (his brother); and with the fourth letter he said, "That's Lee" (his daughter).

We abandoned the NART and looked at some simpler words. "BUS" and "CAT" he read immediately. I then wrote BUSY and he thought it might be

"BUSSING." He thought JUMP was "something to wear," and chose JERSEY when given a choice of JUMPER, JUMP, or JERSEY. Finally, BOAT was read as "TRAIN." These results made me question whether Ron had deep dyslexia. This condition was first described by Marshall and Newcombe (1966) and is an acquired dyslexic syndrome whereby people are typically able to read some words reasonably well, particularly if the words are concrete and of high imageability. Consequently people with deep dyslexia are better at reading nouns than verbs, and find prepositions particularly difficult. Nonwords such as PLAG are usually impossible for them to read. The most characteristic errors are semantic so that a stimulus word will be read as a word with a similar meaning. Visual errors are also common, as are morphological errors such as inflectional or derivational ones. Sometimes a combination of visual and semantic errors may be observed. As noted above, Ron showed several of these characteristics when he read, for example "TRAIN" for BOAT (semantic); "BUSSING" for BUSY (visual); and "JERSEY" for JUMP (derivational).

I decided to refer Ron to Max Coltheart who, at the time, was working in London. Max had a great interest in acquired disorders of reading and had asked colleagues to keep a look out for people with reading problems following brain injury. Max sent me a copy of his lexical decision test in which subjects are required to decide if a printed word is a real word or a nonsense word. Ron was 68% correct on this test, that is, above chance but not good.

In my report of July 1980 I noted that Ron was cheerful and cooperative at all times during the assessment although he needed lots of reassuring, and beamed with pleasure at any compliment. The really striking thing about his behavior, though, was the tremendous effort he made when trying to cope with any task he was asked to do. No matter how difficult, he attempted it bravely, using anything and everything at his disposal. If he could not find the word he needed he gestured or pantomimed with an eloquence reminiscent of Marcel Marceau. If he could not follow an instruction, he questioned and rephrased until he comprehended.

There was no doubt that Ron had made significant improvements over the past year although still remaining severely brain damaged. In my report I commented upon Ron's efforts to understand what was said to him and to solve his everyday problems, although I could make no forecast as to how much further improvement would follow.

REHABILITATION

The two areas of Ron's rehabilitation program in which psychologists were involved were (1) reading remediation and (2) lessening inappropriate speech.

Table 12.1. Main Psychological Test Results for Ron

	MAY 1979	JUN. 1980	SEP. 1981	NOV. 1983	APR. 1989	OCT. 1992	SEP. 1994
Matching shape	Can match circles and rectangles	Not administered as copying, so much better					
Matching color	Can match red, green, yellow, blue	Not administered as copying, so much better					
Copying	Can copy own name, circle, triangle	Can copy own name, circle, triangle, star, daisy	Can copy own name, circle, triangle, star, daisy				
Memory for shapes	Can reproduce simple shapes after 10 sec delay	Can reproduce simple shapes after 10 sec delay					
Prose recall	Cannot do	Immediate recall = 3 Delayed recall = 1.5	Immediate recall = 3 Delayed recall = 1.5	Immediate recall = 7.5 Delayed recall = 5			Immediate recall = 7 Delayed recall = 6
Tactile block design	Can copy 1 + 2 block designs failed 4 blocks	Can do 4 block designs	N.A. as now doing WAIS block design				
Writing name to dictation	Cannot do	Cannot do	Cannot do	Can write first name correctly and surname (with one error)	Can write name correctly	Can write name correctly	Can write name correctly
WAIS Verbal subtests raw score and			Cannot do	Information 1 (1) Comprehension 0(0) Arithmetic 6(6)	Information 7(5) Comprehension 10(5) Arithmetic 7(7)	Information 12(8) Comprehension 14(8) Arithmetic 8(7)	

(scaled score)		Similarities 4(5) Digit span 5(1) Vocabulary 9(2) Verbal IQ = 55	Similarities 9(8) Digit span 6(2) Vocabulary 19(5) Verbal IQ = 75	Similarities 7(7) Digit span 6(3) Vocabulary 29(8) Verbal IQ = 80	
Raven's Matrices	Cannot do	Raw score 23 IQ equivalent 70–80 (Colored matrices)	Raw score 32 IQ equivalent 90 (Standard matrices)	Raw score 35 IQ equivalent 90 (Standard matrices)	Raw score 28 IQ equivalent 93 (Colored matrices)
Benton Visual Rentention Test	Cannot do	Total correct = 3			Total correct = 3
National Adult Reading Test	Correct = 1 (ACHE) Spelled out letters for A–C–H–E	Correct = 1 (HEIR)	Correct = 2 (ACHE, HEIR)	Correct = 1 (ACHE)	
Lexical Decision	68% Correct 7 False negatives 9 False positives		77.5% Correct 3 False negatives 6 False positives		
Schonell Graded Word Reading Test	24 Correct Reading age = 7 yr 5 mo	32 Correct Reading age = 8 yr 2 mo	38 Correct Reading age = 8 yr 10 mo		
Rey-Osterreith Complex Figure	Copy = 10/36 Recall = 4.5/36	Copy 15/36 Recall = 6/36			
British Ability Word Reading List		52 Correct Reading age = 7.5/8 yr	60 Correct Reading age = 8.0–8.5 yr		
Rivermead Behavioural Memory Test		Screening score = 4/12			Screening score = 2/12
Graded Naming Test			2 Correct (kangaroo, handcuffs)		

N. A.. not applicable.

(1) Reading

Max Coltheart and his assistants Sally Byng and Susan Rickard came to Rivermead to see Ron in September 1980 and confirmed he had deep dyslexia. Ron
was discharged in October 1980 so Max and his colleagues continued seeing him
at his home. In May 1981, they began seeing him regularly in efforts to reduce
his reading difficulties, the therapy being carried out by Sally Byng and Susan
Rickard. They began with single letters. Ron could neither name letters nor write
them to dictation but in reading aloud and in spontaneous speech, it was evident
that, despite his considerable word finding difficulty, he had knowledge of some
characteristics of the word he was seeking. For example, he often knew how
many letters a word had and sometimes the approximate meaning of a word,
hence the semantic errors. Sally and Susan decided to teach Ron individual letters so that he could perhaps eventually identify the initial letter of a word and
use this as a self-cuing device.

When therapy began Ron could reliably name letters "A" to "G." He was
given two new letters each week and within 6 wk he could reliably name and
write to dictation all 26 letters of the alphabet. Sally and Susan noted that Ron
was usually able to access the letter directly without having to say the alphabet
under his breath until he reached the correct letter. Occasionally however he still
used the alphabet sequencing cue.

The next step was to give Ron three-letter words to learn and by September
1981 he could write 25 words to dictation from memory. Prior to the treatment,
Ron could only write his name. Sally and Susan planned to continue with a
phonological approach to reading whereby Ron would be taught the sounds of
the letters. This was influenced by some work done in France by de Partz (1986).
Before this, however, Ron was readmitted to Rivermead for a further 3 mo period
of rehabilitation.

Ron's reading was reassessed during this admission along with a reassessment
of his other cognitive abilities. On the NART his semantic errors were even more
in evidence. For ACHE he said "HEADACHE, HEAD, WHEN YOU'RE NOT
WELL." DEBT he read as "MONEY," and PSALM as "SERMON." He also
made derivational errors such as "JEANS" for DENY (denims?), and "BARBE-
CUE" for BOUQUET (banquet?). On the Schonell Graded Word Reading Test
(Schonell and Schonell, 1963) he scored 24 correct, giving him a reading age of
7 yr 4 mo, and once again showed errors characteristic of someone with deep
dyslexia. These included errors such as "MERMAID" for ANGEL, and "IDEA"
for IDIOSYNCRASY; visual errors such as "GENERAL" for GENEROUS, and
"POST" for POSTAGE; as well as derivational errors such as "REALLY OLD"
for GENEROSITY (geriatrics?), and "DONKEY" for SHEPHERD (sheep?).

At this stage Ron was reading correctly some 39% of all nouns presented, 28%
of adjectives, and 20% of verbs. Prepositions were not administered.

Ron also continued to improve generally on other psychological tests (see Table 12.1). In particular, his WAIS results showed a significant improvement to a verbal IQ of 75 and a performance IQ (which he could not manage at all previously) of 69. He was given the Standard Raven's Matrices this time (Raven, 1960), which is harder than the colored version given before, and his predicted IQ on this nonverbal reasoning test was 90, that is, just within the average range. This was despite continuing visual problems that not only caused him to have a very restricted circle of vision but also caused him to be very slow both in positioning material so that it fell within his narrow circle of vision and in comparing one stimulus with another.

As before, Ron was enthusiastic and cheerful, putting enormous efforts into all tests. He never seemed frustrated by setbacks and failures but instead looked more carefully or searched for different words until he could understand or make himself understood. All the staff who knew him commented on his good humor, persistence, and cooperation.

The continuing visuospatial problems are illustrated by Ron's copy of the Rey-Osterreith Complex Figure, as can be seen in Figure 12.1.

In November 1981, Ron saw John Marshall and Christine Temple of the Radcliffe Infirmary in Oxford. They administered a reading test and wrote, in a letter to me,

> He (Ron) read 14/60 words correctly (7 nouns, 6 adjectives, and 1 verb). There was no length effect over 4 to 7 letters, but there was a fairly substantial word-frequency effect. Letter spellings and phonetic try-outs were common. Frank semantic errors were very rare (PINK—'orange . . . it's a color . . . the color is P . . . pink.' although circumlocutions and gestures that indicated that the word's meaning was known (at least approximately) were quite common (APRON—'A,P,R,O,N, . . . not a man's job, a woman's job . . . they hold it when they're doing something . . . something to wear.'
>
> Our impression was that there was considerable 'dissolution' of meaning within the semantic system. Ron was sometimes unsure of the correct response even when given (auditorally) a set of items to choose from.
>
> Many thanks again. It was fascinating to see a 'remediated' deep dyslexic.

(2) Inappropriate Talking

Although it may seem strange to discuss inappropriate talking in someone with a severe nominal dysphasia, Ron sometimes irritated people with his loquaciousness and circumlocutions. He took a very long time to say what he wanted to say, he repeated himself, and he came across as rather childish in his desire to please. In September 1980, I was asked by the nurses at Rivermead to devise a behavior program to reduce the amount of Ron's talking. Following a meeting with the ward sister, Ron's social worker, and myself, we devised the following plan:

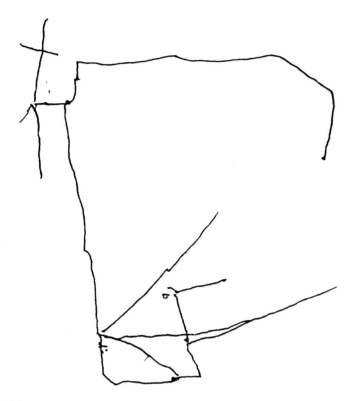

Figure 12.1. Ron's copy of the Rey Osterreith complex figure.

1. Nurses will be asked to record over the coming weekend the number of times Ron talks to the staff and the approximate length of each conversation.
2. The ward sister, social worker, occupational therapist, and clinical psychologist will meet together with Ron next week to explain to him that people find his overtalking stressful. In addition, they will write down the information in his notebook.
3. We will use a signal (a tap on Ron's shoulder) to indicate to him that he should stop talking.
4. We will discuss the program with Sally Byng who sees Ron at home.
5. We will ask the new clinical psychology student, Louise Russell, to work on conversational skills with Ron.

Over the weekend the nurses recorded Ron's conversations. Between Friday evening and Sunday evening he engaged in conversation with the nurses for a total of 47 min during 20 separate interactions. Virtually every interaction was described as "appropriate" or "polite." On only two occasions did they say otherwise. On one of these a nurse reported "childish conversation" and on another, "slightly giggly." Thus it appeared that the problem was not quite so serious as perceived.

Nevertheless, we discussed the matter with Ron who appeared to be only too pleased to have a signal to tell him when he was 'going on' too much. As always, he wanted to succeed and do things the right way. Meanwhile Louise Russell, who had recently started a 3 mo placement with me, saw Ron to help with his conversational skills. In particular, Louise decided to try to reduce the number of times Ron said, "Nice to see you," and to provide acceptable alternatives.

Ron, because of his language problems together with his friendliness and sociability, had difficulty finding opening conversational gambits. Instead, he used one phrase, "Nice to see you," very frequently—to the extent that other people found it irritating. Louise commented that "Ron has been irritating staff, patients, and his wife by his repeated use of the phrase. He is, in general, somewhat overtalkative, a tendency exaggerated by the circumlocutory style he is forced to use as a result of his dysphasia. He also tends to talk about himself too much. However, his good humor and determination led us to overcome our initial reluctance to embark on this program." Louise knew about the shoulder tapping and used this technique in conjunction with his program.

She began collecting a baseline by recording the greetings Ron used when he was fetched from occupational therapy to psychology and when he was returned to the ward after his session with Louise. Each journey took about 4 min. On four of the five baseline sessions Ron only used the phrase, "Nice to see you" and no other phrases. He said it three times on the 1st day, five times on the 2nd, four times the 3rd, and seven times on the 4th day. On the 5th day he said, "Hello," when collected from occupational therapy, and "Nice to see you," when being returned to the ward.

The baseline stage was immediately followed by the intervention stage. Ron's previous discussion with the staff had clearly sensitized him to some extent. He was initially embarrassed and cross with himself when the purpose of the sessions was explained gently to him. However, in his typically determined way, Ron said he was grateful to be told about his difficulties so he could do something about them. Ron and Louise decided on the following phrases that Ron could use as alternatives to "Nice to see you." "Hello," "Have you had a nice weekend?" "Goodbye," "See you soon/tomorrow/next week," and "How are you?"

It became apparent that when Ron concentrated consciously on what he was saying he had more difficulty saying it. This, together with a problem Ron had of initiating the phrase, was solved by giving Ron a piece of paper with the phrases on. He practiced these and in his sessions with Louise he graphed his greetings using colored squares. "Nice to see you," was colored yellow, "Hello," was red and so on. Ron did the recording himself at the beginning of each session. Because of his memory problems he needed frequent reminding of the purpose of the program. Once he had recorded the greetings used each day when coming from occupational therapy and returning to the ward, Ron practiced using the phrases in imaginary situations. Over the next 9 days Ron used "Nice to see you," on eight occasions, that is, on average less than once a day. He used, "Hello," nine times, "Goodbye/See you," eight times, "Have you had a nice weekend?" once and "How are you?" twice.

A video was made of one of the sessions and Ron enjoyed watching this on a small monitor. He was able to recognize his mistakes and seemed to benefit from the feedback he was receiving.

After the "Nice to see you" program, Louise's sessions were more concerned with helping Ron practice how to cope in social situations demanding a variety of responses. She hoped to enable Ron to talk less about himself, respond more appropriately to the social situation in which he found himself, and adapt to the needs of the particular people involved. These situations would include meetings with the occupational therapist, talking to various people on the telephone, and meeting the other psychologist. Appropriate modeling of the alternative response was a constant feature of the program. The shoulder tapping was also employed when Ron talked too much.

Ron and Louise met on 14 occasions over a period of 6 weeks. Although he stopped saying, "Nice to see you," so frequently, he did not appear to recognize when he had used this phrase and expressed surprise when told he had said it. Despite preparing to use another phrase, such as, "How are you?" he sometimes said, "Nice to see you," thinking he had said, "How are you?"

Ron also frequently asked questions such as, "When you say 'Hello' should you put the person's name in? If you do put it in should you say the name before or after 'Hello'? How often can you say, 'How are you?' Is it the same as, 'Have you had a nice weekend?' Can you only say it on certain days?" (Ron had worked out for himself that you could say, "Have you had a nice weekend?" only on Mondays.

Ron also said that sometimes he refrained from talking altogether because he was not sure how to say things. Sometimes at the end of a session he would say, "Lovely to see you," or, "Nice to see you," because he was so pleased at the help he was receiving. He said these things in such a sincere and genuine manner that Louise felt she could not draw attention to Ron's mistakes. Furthermore, in the role-play situations Ron behaved very naturally and was particularly inventive at producing amusing and appropriate pieces of conversation.

Members of the staff reported that Ron appeared more sensitive in conversation than he had previously, and was also more aware of his tendency to monopolize conversation. He asked people to stop his saying "Nice to see you," and to stop his rambling in conversation. It was unnecessary to tap him on the shoulder as he responded to normal conversation cues. For example, he paused and allowed the other person to enter the conversation. Although he made more mistakes when pressured to use the "right" phrase, he was skilled at thinking up appropriate conversational gambits when in role play.

SINCE 1981

Ron came back to Rivermead for a further reassessment in November 1983. Once again his scores had improved and the results of the tests can be seen in Table 12.1. As before, he was keen to complete the tests, he concentrated well and attempted everything asked of him. It was noticeable that he was now better able to find his way around the unit, his conversation was more appropriate for a man of his age, and his word finding problems were less severe. Nevertheless, he continued to experience severe cognitive problems and these together with his poor vision meant he could not lead anything like a normal life. His motivation appeared to be as fierce as ever and it was considered by those who saw him at the time that he would continue to improve although at a slower rate now that 5 yr had passed since the head injury.

I did not see Ron for the next 5 yr but in 1989 I decided to follow up a group of patients with acquired dyslexia and Ron was among this group (Wilson, 1994). I went to see him and his wife at their home. In my letter to Ron and Lesley, in which I summarized the results obtained during this visit, I wrote:

> There is no doubt that Ron's reading has improved. He still shows signs of 'deep dyslexia' in which typical mistakes are those to do with meaning. For example, Ron read the word BIG as 'LARGE,' and he read NORTH as 'SOUTH.' Another kind of error made by people with deep dyslexia is connected with the visual appearance of a word. For example, Ron read HAMMER as 'HAMMOCK,' and LEADER as 'LADDER.' Yet another characteristic of deep dyslexia is that nouns are usually easier to read than verbs, adjectives, or prepositions. Ron read, for example, the word WITH as 'WHICH,' and THE as 'THEN.' Some of his mistakes were very sophisticated, such as, 'JEALOUSY' for JEOPARDY and 'BARRISTER' for JUDICATURE. This implies that Ron must have had a good vocabulary before his accident. As I said to you last week, deep dyslexia is a rare and interesting condition which helps researchers understand how people learn to read and how the brain is organised for reading. So Ron still appears to have deep dyslexia but nevertheless his reading is considerably better than when I last saw him.
>
> Another area which seems to have improved is Ron's memory. He recalled more of a short story I read to him this time compared with last time. Furthermore, he forgot very little of the story after a delay.
>
> In some areas Ron does not seem to have changed. Mental arithmetic, for example, is still difficult for him. This is partly because he does not understand all the

parts of each question and partly because he forgets where he is up to when he is working out the answers.

As always, Ron showed patience, determination and cooperation when doing the tests and gets top marks for his persistence.

In 1992, Ron took part in another follow-up study that was looking at people who were too impaired to be assessed on standardized tests when first seen in rehabilitation (Wilson and Cockburn, 1997). By now Ron had moved to a home for people with physical disabilities. While his own physical disabilities were limited to the fact that he had poor vision, his main problems continued to be cognitive. He had moved to the home in 1989, soon after my previous visit. I asked him how he now spent his day and he replied:

> Wake up early in morning. Have shower. Sort breakfast out. Eat breakfast. Sit down and have coffee. Do dishwasher—1 hour and 20 minutes. Then I get all clean stuff in cupboards. I hoover room. Then in kitchen I do surfaces. Might do chess sets. People buy them. They drive here and buy them. I read the paper and have dinner. Might see TV for half an hour and the weather and the news. Afternoon, I might be in the work-shop. In here I read the paper, do all the tea, have a coffee with friend. When I've finished—dishwasher—say 7.30—put in cupboard. See my friends. I read the paper—I love it—it's hard. Might be in the bar. My dad phones Tuesday. Lesley's going to phone today. I see her every 2 weeks.

Thus, although Ron still had some telegrammatic speech and could not always find the word he wanted, he communicated well and could give a good account of how he spent his day.

I wrote a "thank you" letter to Ron, who had also asked for a report on his problems. In the letter I wrote:

> You have continued to improve but still have 'deep dyslexia,' 'nominal aphasia' (i.e., problems finding the right name or word for something), and verbal memory diffi-culties. You are good at solving non-verbal problems like the block design test we did the other day, although your tunnel vision means you can only see part of the de-sign at any one time, not the whole of it. This means you keep 'losing' the pattern from your narrow range of vision. You are also good at communicating despite your language impairments, and you can make people understand what you mean quite easily. One of your main strengths, Ron, is your perseverance. You don't give up easily and keep trying to find a solution to any problem you are faced with.

I saw Ron once in 1993 and six times in 1994. He made fewer mistakes in reading and on a test looking at content versus function words, administered in 1993 (loaned by Karalyn Patterson), most of Ron's errors were visual. On Colt-heart's high and low imagery test, Ron scored 23/28 correct on the high imagery and 12/28 correct on the low imagery words, and once again the majority of er-rors were visual.

Ron was given a test of naming in 1994 (Hodges et al., 1992) and managed to name 20/48 items correctly. Once again Ron clearly demonstrated that he recognized many of the objects he could not name. For the TOASTER he said, "I want toast so I turn on the—COOKER." For ELEPHANT he said, "It's an E . . . I can't get it." Ron was also asked to name from description using the Hodges et al. (1992) items. He scored 5/24 without help but often found solutions for the ones he could not name: for example, when asked, "What is the name of a small green animal which leaps around ponds?" Ron answered, "Give me one," (meaning "give me the first letter") I replied, "F," to which he responded (using the subvocal alphabetic sequencing to access R, O, and G): "There's four of them F–R–O–G—FROG." The definition for FOX was, "A cunning animal which has reddish fur and a bushy tail and is often hunted for sport." Ron responded, "Three letters or four letters?" I informed him there were three. Ron answered, "Three? I think it's four. The people who are going to kill him—they wear red things and a hat—three letters." "Do you want the first letter?" I asked him. "Go on then," said Ron. To the letter "F" Ron thought for a moment and then said, "F–O and the last one you want is X—FOX." Even when Ron answered correctly he frequently needed to cue himself. Thus, for the naming to description for MOTORCYCLE he said, "Bike, Bike, no not a bike, an engine bike . . . . M . . . MOTORBIKE."

In 1994, Linda Clare, a trainee working with me for 6 mo as part of her training, saw Ron to find out whether he learned better using a trial-and-error or error-free learning method. The latter method does not allow people to guess or make errors during learning trials, and it has been established that people with severe memory problems learn better when they are prevented from making mistakes during learning (Baddeley and Wilson, 1994; Wilson, Baddeley, Evans and Shiel, 1994). We wondered whether Ron would also benefit from errorless learning. A summary of Linda's report on this study follows.

RON, A COMPARISON OF ERRORLESS AND ERRORFUL METHODS OF LEARNING IN NOMINAL APHASIA

Aim

To investigate whether errorless and errorful learning methods of learning to name pictures of objects and living creatures are differentially effective for a person with nominal aphasia.

Method

The picture-naming section of John Hodge's Semantic Battery was administered on two occasions (4 May and 2 June). Pictures which were not identified correctly on either trial were presented again (2 June). Twenty-one items were not named correctly on any of the three trials.

The twenty-one pictures were matched on three dimensions: high or low frequency, living or nonliving, and whether Ron had made an incorrect guess or given no answer. They were then randomly allocated into three matched sets of six words each. The three sets were each assigned to one of three learning conditions:

1. Errorless: written stem completion after being told the correct name.
2. Errorful: guessing the correct word and attempting to write it down.
3. Forced choice recognition: selecting the name from a set of four (with correction if necessary); sets included visually and semantically related words.

In a pilot trial (2 June), three words from each condition were taught in an alternative sequence. Five learning trials were given followed by an immediate and delayed test (15 min delay).

On July 14, errorless and errorful conditions were taught separately using the full set of words in each case. Teaching involved five learning trials, followed by an immediate and delayed test (20 min delay). A further test was conducted after a 1 mo delay (16 August).

Results

In the pilot trial, results were similar for each condition:

	IMMEDIATE (MAX 3)	15 MIN DELAY (MAX 3)
Errorless	1	1
Errorful	0	1
Forced choice	1	1

The main trial showed equivalent results under each condition when tested immediately and with a 20 min delay. However, after a 1 mo delay there was a clear advantage for names learned under the errorful condition:

	IMMEDIATE (MAX 6)	20 MIN DELAY (MAX 6)	1 MO DELAY (MAX 6)
Errorless	5	5	1
Errorful	5	5	4

The errorful method appeared more effective in that gains were maintained over a longer period. This may have been due to the greater amount of effort involved in the learning process under this condition.

Linda Clare
19 August 1994

In June 1994, I gave Ron the *Autobiographical Memory Interview* for the first time. He had virtually no memories at all of life before his accident scoring 0.5/21 on recall of factual information for his childhood, and 0 for recall of autobiographical incidents. For his early adult years, he scored 6.5/21 for factual information and 0 for recall of autobiographical incidents. He did better on recall of recent information, that is, within the past year, scoring 13/21 for recall of factual information and 7/9 for recall of autobiographical incidents. These results support the view that Ron has a dense retrograde amnesia. When asked to remember an incident from his childhood, he said, "Thirty years—no—all I know is I've seen you the other years—I know—Oxford."

The next time I saw Ron was in August 1996 when I administered more reading tests the results of which showed that Ron continued to have difficulty with some words, he still made visual and semantic errors although he read 160/254 words from a list of regular and irregular words.

After the testing I told Ron I wanted to write a chapter about him for this book. He agreed and I then said, "What can you tell me about your accident?" Ron replied:

> My house—the wife—I was in the Gas Board—I was a lecturer—my friend—my house with Les—his house was where my house was. He said, 'Can you come and help?' I went to his house and I fell. Two months and a little bit—coma. When I was home I see the Gas Board and all my friends. It was nice.

My next question was: "Tell me about Rivermead?"

Ron said, "That was my friend there who you don't see him any more. He was nice he was. That's it really." (The friend was another head injured man who Ron liked very much. Ron had previously asked me if I still saw this man and I explained that I tried to see him for one of the follow-up studies but he had moved and I could not trace him.)

I said, "What about your therapy?

Ron answered, "Exercises—arms and feet and everything. Not long ago I see one—not long ago she was here. 'Oh, hello,' she says, 'Hello Ron, how are you?' 'It's me, I'm here.' I said, 'Hello, how are you?' She was here because someone she works with might be coming here."

"Can you remember any of the other therapy?"

"Not a lot—it's a long time—I can't remember."

"Can you remember going home from Rivermead?"

"It was weekends—weekends going home—then Sunday here again. After—I do 2 days a week in Black Notley—go in a workshop where I was working. We made thousands and thousands of money. It's not there now. The building—all gone now."

"When did you come here?" (the home for people with physical disabilities)

"About 7 years I reckon."

"How do you spend your week now?"

"I read my paper and in summer I do my garden. It's lovely that is. All my plants. It's lovely."

"Anything else?"

"I might be in the workshop if they want a chess set. They're lovely. Some of the staff get one. I'm doing some tomorrow. All my plants—they gone—when they did my room. The home gave me £100.00 for the plants I haven't got. It's lovely."

"How do you feel about being here?"

"It's alright. We tried—or my wife and her dad did, tried. They were terrible— nothing to do. Here—I've got the workshop and the bar's open in the evening— and they're friendly here—we all sit down of an evening and it's nice."

"How often do you see Lesley now?"

"Three weeks because she works—we phone every week. She's got a 2 hour drive. She brings all my cakes. She says, 'We'll do all your stuff. She cuts my (Ron mimed cutting his moustache). She does my clothes and says, 'Right, we're going into a restaurant.' We have steak. She buys all my apples. She's here 5 hours and then she has a 2 hour drive home. She's got her life. I've got my friends here, and the bar."

"When I write this chapter is there anything you want me to say about you and your head injury?"

"It's up to you."

V

REMEDIATION OF ACQUIRED
DISORDERS OF READING

We have already encountered three people in the previous part with severe reading problems caused by brain damage. In this part three others who received treatment for acquired dyslexia are described.

McCarthy and Warrington (1990) claim that ". . . the analysis of the reading process has possibly received more attention from psychologists than any other cognitive skill" (p. 228). A number of different acquired dyslexic syndromes have been described since Marshall and Newcombe (1966, 1973) suggested that the complex ability to read could be subdivided into several interlocking skills that could break down independently, causing different forms of dyslexia.

One of these forms, deep dyslexia, was described in Chapter 12. Ron showed the typical characteristics of deep dyslexia in that he (1) made semantic errors in reading aloud (e.g., he read CANARY as "BUDGERI-GAR"), (2) also made visual and derivational errors (such as "GRAVEL" for GRAVE and "LISTENING" for LISTEN), (3) found nouns easier to read than verbs, (4) made more errors when reading difficult to image, abstract words than when reading highly imageable concrete words, and (5) found nonwords such as ROST virtually impossible to read.

The other main syndromes of acquired dyslexia are surface dyslexia (described in Chapter 9 on Jason), phonological dyslexia, and letter-by-letter reading. The three people in this section are Ted who showed a positional dyslexia (he could not read the initial letters of words), Derek who completely lost the ability to read after a gunshot wound to the head, and Jenny who also became totally alexic after a severe head injury sustained in a horseback riding accident.

Given the extent of interest in the acquired dyslexias there are surprisingly few published papers that address the subject of treatment of these conditions although there has been an increase in the number of such papers in recent years.

Benson and Geschwind (1969) in their chapter entitled, "The Alexias," devote only 1 of 30 pages to the subject of treatment. In contrast, Walsh and Lamberts (1979) describe the use of errorless discrimination learning and picture-fading techniques to improve the reading of moderately mentally handicapped children. In the former method the children respond initially to one word only. Other words are introduced gradually and, at first, these words are dissimilar from one another in size, typeface, color, and so forth. Later the words become more alike. This method was tried with Derek (Chapter 14) unfortunately with little success. In the picture-fading method each word is accompanied initially by a picture that is gradually faded out until the child is eventually reading the word alone.

Albert (1979) reported that some neurologically impaired patients with letter-by-letter reading (or alexia without agraphia) could "read" if they traced the letters with their fingers. This method certainly helped Ted (Chapter 13) although he did not like the method. It also helped Derek (Chapter 14) when he first started to read again after his accident. Derek only needed to trace the letters for a short time, however, as soon after this he was able to read by the visual rather than the kinesthetic or tactile route.

One of the earlier papers describing treatment of a patient with acquired dyslexia appeared in 1979 when Moyer reported on the treatment given to a 30-yr-old man following embolic stroke. Previous treatment included improving the subject's discrimination by encouraging him to trace sandpaper letters (the tactile method again). He was also required to respond as quickly as possible to words printed on individual cards. In addition he was given paragraphs to read for homework. The principle teaching technique here was practice and the main outcome measure was the time taken to read. Moyer's patient increased his score from a mean of 66 syllables per min to 94 per min some 3 mo later. At the end of treatment he said he was able to enjoy reading the newspaper for the first time since his stroke.

Moody (1988) used Moyer's technique with a letter-by-letter reader who also improved his speed of reading over a 15 wk treatment period. His reading, however, was still far behind that of a normal reader.

An interesting treatment program for a French dyslexic patient is reported by de Partz (1986) who set out to reteach the ability to translate directly from orthography to phonology, that is from print to sound. This method was used with some success with Ron (Chapter 12). Patterson (1994) describes a number of treatment strategies in some detail.

Of the three people described in this section, two (Derek, Chapter 14 and Jenny, Chapter 15) learned to read again after severe head injuries left them virtually totally alexic. Both, however, were far from normal readers showing characteristics of surface dyslexia and letter-by-letter reading.

13

TED: THE MAN WHO COULD READ "ASTROCYTOMA" BUT NOT "DOG"

BACKGROUND

In 1986, talking to a speech therapist over a cup of coffee, I heard about Ted, a 71-yr-old man who had suffered a left hemisphere stroke the year before. Apparently he had difficulty identifying the initial letters of words. I pricked up my ears for, although this problem was often seen after right hemisphere lesions causing neglect of the left side of space (see Chapter 19), Ted had a left hemisphere lesion so, if his problem was due to neglect, he should be neglecting the right side of space or showing a nonlateralized neglect, i.e., omitting or neglecting letters across the page and not just initial letters. The speech therapist wanted to refer Ted to me for rehabilitation and I was happy to see him.

Ted was a bright man who had worked as a courier for the Royal Air Force before his retirement. In 1978, he sustained ischemic macular damage to the left eye and remained with only light–dark vision in that eye. For several years after this Ted was treated for hypertension. He also had a myocardial infarction in 1984. Then in 1985 came the stroke. A CT scan showed an infarct in the territory of the left posterior cerebral artery, plus infarcts in the left thalamus and putamen. On neurological examination Ted had a right homonymous hemianopia but no facial or motor weakness or sensory loss.

In the formal referral letter to me, the speech therapist said, "He is a recovered

Broca's aphasic." She reported that Ted had good verbal comprehension even of complex tasks, fluent expressive language with a wide range of grammatical constructions, and only occasional word-finding difficulty.

Ted lived nearby, he could walk to the hospital and was happy to come along for 2 to 3 h once a week.

INITIAL ASSESSMENT

I began with the WAIS and Ted obtained a verbal IQ of 112 (above average), a performance IQ of 90, and a full scale IQ of 103. The only subtest yielding a substantially subnormal age scaled score of 5 (with 10 being average) was digit symbol where Ted was slow for his age. Both his short- and long-term memory appeared normal. His digit span was 7 forwards and 4 backwards. His everyday memory as assessed by the Rivermead Behavioural Memory Test (Wilson et al., 1985) was in the normal range. He was slow but showed no signs of neglect on the Behavioural Inattention Test (BIT; Wilson et al., 1987). He showed some very mild word-finding difficulties, 12/15 on an object naming test, but managed 14/15 correct on naming to description (both tests by Coughlan and Warrington, 1978). Nothing really remarkable so far.

When I began to look at Ted's reading ability, however, I became really intrigued. He read "ASTROCYTOMA" immediately yet struggled over DOG. He tried "LOG," "BOG," and finally settled for "FOG." Sometimes he tried a letter-by-letter approach. For example with YACHT he said "E–A–C–H–T—no that's not right—YACHT." He spent some time looking at BURY and finally said "FURY." He showed fewer problems reading text no doubt because the context helped him. Anxious to try some rehabilitation strategies I also realized Ted had a very unusual and highly specific disorder that needed some detailed and specialized neuropsychological assessment. Consequently I contacted Karalyn Patterson to talk about Ted and to ask if she would be interested in seeing him. Karalyn and I saw Ted together on numerous occasions and later published a paper based on our findings (Patterson and Wilson, 1990). Attempts at rehabilitation (reported later) took place concurrently with our investigations to establish the characteristics of his reading deficit. The results of these investigations are now summarized.

DETAILED ASSESSMENT

Vision and Visual–Spatial Functioning

We needed first to establish that Ted's reading impairment was not due to a failure to see the stimuli adequately. The combination of the right homonymous hemianopia and macular damage to his left eye meant that Ted relied on the nasal field of his right eye to see. Acuity in that field however was good, and certainly sufficient to support letter recognition and identification. He could trace letters with his finger and once again given his lesions should, if anything, be neglecting stimuli on the right not the left. He rarely misidentified the last letters in a word and when shown words such as KICK, EYES, and LILT and asked to point to the two letters which were the same, his performance was faultless. We felt confident then that poor acuity was not responsible for Ted's problem with initial letters.

Support for rejection of unilateral neglect as an explanation also came from his performance on the BIT mentioned above and from Ted's ability to copy drawings. He was always slow but accurate. His scanning was systematic unlike many patients with unilateral neglect and when asked to read a passage omitted no words at all although he made two initial letter errors consistent with his usual reading errors. He could also name geometric shapes arranged in a horizontal array. With four shapes presented in all possible combinations over 24 trials, Ted made no errors or omissions. Of course this is probably an easier task than reading but it did demonstrate that Ted did not have a general deficit with initial stimuli.

Word Reading

Perhaps the two most striking findings—because unexpected in reading impaired patients—were that Ted was better at reading (1) long words than short ones and (2) irregular rather than regular ones. Thus, he could read IDIOSYNCRASY but not MAT and he could read YACHT but not LAND. As we pointed out in the 1990 paper, this can be explained by the likelihood of guessing the word if the initial letter is obscured. No other word would fit (A)STROCYTOMA or (I)DIO-SYNCRACY while many would fit (M)AT or (L)AND.

In order to further explore this hypothesis, we presented Ted with words that had and did not have orthographic neighbors identical in everything but the initial letter. Consider, for example, the words BATCH and BIRCH. Of similar length and fairly close in orthographic structure, they differ in that BATCH has several orthographic neighbors identical apart from the initial letter (catch, match, patch, watch) whereas BIRCH has none. When tested in this way Ted read correctly 85% of "one" body words (e.g., soap), 68% of "few" body words (e.g., deaf) and 60% of "many" body words (e.g., real). The relative closeness of his performance on "few" and "many" body words suggests it is not the number of "neighbors" that is crucial but whether there are neighbors at all.

As a rule, Ted did not omit a letter but made substitutions thus preserving the length of the target word. With many words like MAT and LAND an omission of the initial letter would produce a legitimate word. To test whether Ted would make omission errors when words of this type were presented, we asked him to read 50 such words (e.g., BLIGHT, FRAIL, and STRAIN). He did not make a single response of the LIGHT or RAIL variety. His errors were of two types, substitutions such as BRIGHT for FRIGHT and additions such as SPOUT for POUT. Very occasionally however, Ted did make an initial deletion error. We gave him 400 monosyllabic words 3–6 letters in length. Many, although not all of these words became other legitimate words without their initial letters. On 4 (1%) of these words Ted omitted the initial letter. A summary of the results on these 400 words can be seen in Table 13.1.

We next looked at all the four-letter words from this set of 400. There were 199 of them. We examined Ted's responses to these words and asked what proportion of responses in each position were correct. We counted from right to left so that a response like SPOUT for POUT would be correct in positions 4, 3, and 2. We also did a similar analysis for four-letter nonwords such as NEEN, TINK, and PLEN. These results can be seen in Table 13.2.

The deficit identified was restricted to visually presented words. A set of 70 words (whose main characteristic is that each could be made into a variety of

Table 13.1. A Description of Ted's 126 Errors in Oral Reading of 400 Monosyllabic Words, 3–6 Letters in Length

ERROR TYPE	EXAMPLES			NUMBER	(%)
Substitution on initial letter	frail	→	"trail"	84	67
	safe	→	"cafe"		
Addition before/after initial letter	pout	→	"spout"	10	8
	boom	→	"broom"		
Substitution of + addition to initial letter	fall	→	"shall"	4	3
	cove	→	"above"		
Deletion of or deletion of + substitution of initial letter	pear	→	"ear"	14	11
	shear	→	"rear"		
Other (typically errors of initial letter and also elsewhere in word)	haste	→	"vast"	14	11
	purse	→	"horse"		
	yearn	→	"earth"		
Total				126	100

Table 13.2. Proportion of Ted's Reading Responses Reflecting Correct Letter in Correct Position in Four-letter Words and Nonwords (Counting from Right to Left)

		POSITION IN STRING			
	NO.	1	2	3	4
Words	199	0.68	0.98	0.97	0.98
Nonwords	19	0.47	1.00	1.00	0.94

other words by a letter substitution on the initial letter, e.g., BROWN has the orthographic neighbors CROWN, DROWN, FROWN, and GROWN) was presented to Ted on two different occasions, once printed in lower-case letters and once spelled aloud. He identified only 44/70 (63%) of the words correctly from their written form, but 68/70 (97%) of the words from their spoken letter names. Goodglass and Kaplan (1983) pointed out that identifying orally spelled words is exceptionally difficult for most people with Broca's dysphasia and is certainly harder for the majority of normal readers than identifying printed words. The fact that Ted was better at the harder of these two tasks provides an indication of both the extent to which he had recovered from his reported Broca's dysphasia and the specificity of his deficit in identifying the initial letters of visually presented words.

Letter Reading

We tested this by presenting Ted with the stimuli used for Jenny (see Chapter 15). Thus Ted was presented on two separate occasions with 26 letters of the alphabet in four different sizes and in both upper and lower case. We did this to determine whether or not size affected Ted's ability to recognize letters. Although size had no effect at all, Ted found upper case (77% correct) easier to identify than lower case (58% correct). In this he was similar to letter-by-letter readers (Patterson and Kay, 1982). Were certain letters particularly difficult or easy for him? Only one lower case letter "a" was correctly identified on all eight occasions. No letter was always wrong, although "b" was only correct on one occasion and four letters (l, n, p, and y) were only correct on two occasions.

We knew that when presented with real words Ted was influenced by the number of orthographic neighbors but what would happen when he was presented with letter strings where no lexical constraints existed?

Ted was given 43 strings of lower case letters to read. Each letter of the alphabet occurred once in each position and the string ranged in length from three to five letters. Once again the initial letter deficit was marked. Indeed he was even worse with the first letter position (26% correct) than when reading the first letter of four-letter words (68%) or nonwords (47%), or single letters (58%).

Could Ted's problem be due to attentional dyslexia? Patients with this kind of dyslexia are able to identify single letters but make mistakes when strings of letters are shown (Shallice and Warrington, 1977). Perhaps Ted, like patients with unilateral neglect, could simply not attend to the first letter? Well, we saw earlier that Ted was not like patients with neglect and, if anything, was the opposite of people with attentional dyslexia in that he was *worse* with single letters than with strings of letters. He did, nevertheless, have a position-specific disorder. When asked to name each letter in a meaningless string of four letters, and naming from left to right, Ted was 27% correct on the first of the four and 96% correct on the final, fourth letter. Asking him to name from right to left significantly improved his performance on the first letter, i.e., the last of the four to be named (42% correct), but it was still much poorer than his performance on the fourth letter, i.e., the first to be read (88% correct).

Spelling

Most of our assessment focused on Ted's reading but we did on occasion look at his spelling. On a list of 100 irregular and regular words he correctly spelled 94 of them. He could also recognize, virtually without error, words spelled aloud to him. On one occasion he was given 45 written word bodies (like _IGHT and _AIN) and asked to fill in the blank to make a word. On eight of these items Ted said one word and wrote another. (He had not been asked to name the resulting word but always did so.) This, no doubt was simply a reflection of Ted's initial letter reading problem.

REHABILITATION

Ted always insisted his problem was due to poor vision and that he needed new glasses. People with perceptual problems frequently argue their eyes are at fault (see, for example, Jenny in Chapter 15). Ted was a bright man but we were unable to make him understand that poor vision could not explain the very specific problem with initial letters. Throughout the several months of the assessment and treatment he requested new glasses. He saw a neurologist regularly and an optician occasionally. Both of them confirmed new glasses would not solve the problem.

Because of the superficial similarity to patients with neglect dyslexia, our first rehabilitation attempts were influenced by strategies used to remediate scanning and attentional deficits in patients with unilateral visual inattention (e.g., Diller and Weinberg, 1977; Riddoch and Humphries, 1994). Diller and Weinburg (1977) recommended drawing a thick red line to the left of a prose passage. Patients were requested to find the line before starting to read. The rationale was to disengage attention from the right and draw attention to the left. Neglect patients appear to have problems attending to the left but can be helped to do so if a dominant stimulus is present on the left side only.

Fifty one- and two-syllable words which Ted had misread earlier were selected. He was asked to read these words again on two separate occasions, one week apart. This was the baseline. Ted's performance was much as before. He made a total of 32 errors, i.e., 68% correct over the two occasions. Following this, a thick red line was drawn to the left of each word. Ted was asked to find the line first before trying to read the word. He was given the 50 words to read on two separate occasions a week apart and the total number of errors recorded. This time he made 35 errors, i.e., 65% correct—marginally worse than in the baseline. The problem was that Ted knew the line was not part of the word. Unlike neglect patients, Ted had no difficulty drawing his attention to the left side of space, so he saw the line, moved to the word and, not surprisingly, had difficulty with the first letter. Ted himself confirmed his problem was not in seeing or attending to the word but in identifying it. He said, "I can see them (the initial letters) as well as you can, I just can't tell you what they are."

The second attempt to help Ted was a modification of the red line procedure. He knew the red line was not part of a word but what if we repeated the initial letter, would that help? The procedure was as before. A new set of 50 words was drawn up and two baselines taken. Once again the error rate was in the 32% range. In stage two the initial letter was repeated (e.g., SSOCK). Once again this made no appreciable difference. Ted appeared to realize that the first letter was irrelevant so ignored it and began reading the word at the second letter, which had now become the initial letter. He continued to request new glasses while we had one final attempt at providing an additional stimulus in front of the word to be read. This time we tried putting an X in front (e.g., XMAD) but this too failed to help. Once again he realized the X was irrelevant, moved on to the M and typically read it as BAD or SAD. Maybe if another letter had been used Ted would have done better given that a patient with positional dyslexia reported by Katz and Sevush (1989) benefited from an extraneous Q to the left of words but not from an extraneous X. We feel this is unlikely to have happened with Ted, however, given that he was different from other positional dyslexics in several ways (Patterson and Wilson, 1990).

At this point a colleague, Arnold Wilkins was visiting during one of Ted's sessions. Arnold persuaded Ted to look at the words through a narrow tube with a magnifying lens at one end. This had the effect of isolating letters or syllables from their surroundings. Ted disliked this tube intensely and we were unable to obtain sufficient data to evaluate its efficacy. Although Ted enjoyed his reading sessions particularly the assessment, he was quite resistant to the rehabilitation strategies as he wanted to read again in the same way he had read prior to his stroke. He clung to the belief that somewhere a certain pair of glasses could be prescribed that would do the trick.

Looking at some of the literature for helping children with developmental dyslexia to read, I came across the *Hairy Hat Man* (Tomkins, 1978) and wondered if this might help Ted. Following this principle, we tried to teach letters by drawing an identifying feature. Thus the letter S was drawn as a snake, the letter Y was formed into a yacht and the letter N was illustrated as the "north" on a compass. Ted showed very poor learning on this. He took three 2 h sessions to learn the above three letters, he made numerous mistakes, he was very slow, and showed no generalization from the above letters to printed letters. Once again he did not like this method.

The method of expanding rehearsal (otherwise known as spaced retrieval) was considered next. This approach is based on work by Landauer and Bjork (1978). Expanding rehearsal is a useful teaching method for amnesic patients (e.g., Moffat, 1989; Wilson, 1995c). The information to be remembered is presented, tested immediately, tested again after a brief delay, then after a slightly longer delay, and so forth. Ted was shown one letter, say "b," told "This is a b," asked to repeat the name immediately, then asked for the name again after 1 sec, 2 sec, 3 sec, and so on. Although he could retain one letter at a time if no other tasks were introduced, it proved impossible for him to retain the name of the letter once we introduced a second letter or prevented him from rehearsing by, for example, engaging him in conversation.

Finally and almost in desperation I resorted to one of our earlier assessment techniques and asked Ted to trace the initial letter with his finger before reading the word. We knew he could usually identify letters traced by us on either of his hands. He could also trace any letter accurately himself including initial letters. Sometimes such tracing appeared to help him. I decided to monitor this more formally by using the first set of 50 one- and two-syllable words employed in the red line therapy described above. It will be remembered that Ted made 32 errors on two baseline occasions. This time I asked Ted to trace the first letter of each word before saying the word. He was told this would help him to discover or to cue himself as to the true identify of this initial letter. This strategy led to a significant improvement in Ted's performance and he only made 8 of a possible 100 errors. A comparison of four of the treatment strategies can be seen in Figure 13.1.

Despite our enthusiasm at having found a reasonably successful method, Ted was not happy with the tracing method. He found it too slow and said, "It's not normal reading." Nevertheless when reading text—and he continued throughout these months to read his daily newspaper—he resorted to the tracing method (or tactile reading) when really challenged by a particular word. As long ago as 1979 Albert reported that some neurological patients with acquired dyslexia can "read" if they trace the letters with their fingers. Indeed, Derek (Chapter 14) used this method quite extensively when he first relearned to read.

Soon after the tracing method was completed, our detailed assessment was also nearing its end, and one of the last investigations was concerned with numbers. We had observed much earlier that Ted had similar difficulty identifying the initial number in a string as he did with letters. Thus 601, would be read as 501 or 201. The later assessment, however, looked at combined strings of letters and numbers. The questions were (1) Does Ted always know that a letter is a letter?, (2) Is it the first *position* in an array that causes difficulty or the first *letter*? It was clear from the results (Patterson and Wilson, 1990) that (1) sometimes Ted confused letters and numbers, reporting letters as numbers and vice versa and (2) numbers were vulnerable in precisely the same way as letters. However, and this

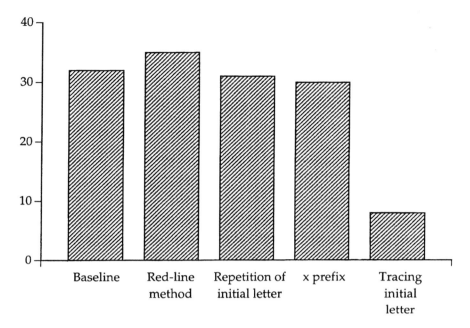

Figure 13.1. Percentage errors in four different treatment methods for Ted's initial-letter-reading deficit.

is the point of introducing this matter here in the rehabilitation section, if Ted muddled numbers and letters then preceding a word with a digit instead of a red line, an X or repetition of the first letter might have reduced his initial letter errors. In fact Karalyn Patterson tried this manipulation. She gave Ted 40 "many body" (i.e., words identical in all but the initial letter) words to read with (1) no stimulus before the word, (2) a digit before the word, (3) an X before the word, (4) a letter that would also make a real word (e.g., (F)RAIL), (5) the initial letter printed in red, and (6) another four-letter word (e.g., CASH) preceding the stimulus word (e.g., LAND). Unfortunately the digit preceding the word did not lead to significant improvement, neither did the other conditions apart from condition (6) putting another four-letter word in front of the stimulus word (χ^2 1 d.f. = 9.60, $P = 0.002$). These results can be seen in Table 13.3.

It is hard to see however, how this additional word solution would be of much practical help in Ted's daily life. Newspapers and books are not written in this way and it would be hard to persuade any friends and relatives who might write letters to do this. If they did it would no doubt confuse Ted as to the real meaning of the communication. At least with the tracing method, Ted had a ready-made, portable solution at hand.

In retrospect I would like to have tried combining two approaches, for example

Table 13.3. Ted's Performance in Reading "Many Body" Words (e.g., Land) in Six Different Conditions

CONDITION		NO. CORRECT (OUT OF 40)	PROPORTION CORRECT
(1)	land	24	0.60
(2) 2	land	26	0.65
(3) x	land	31	0.78
(4) b	land	30	0.75
(5) (red 1)	land	31	0.78
(6) cash	land	36	0.90

See text for description of conditions.

printing the initial letter in red. I often recommend using two or more strategies to amnesic patients for learning new information and it is possible this would have reduced Ted's error rate even more.

FOLLOW-UP

The following year, 1987, I had moved to another job and Ted's sessions had almost come to an end. We went to see him every now and again to complete the assessments for the 1990 paper. In February 1990, in an attempt to answer some of the referee's points following submission of our paper, Ted was seen once more. We found his vision had deteriorated significantly. He was unable to see most of the test materials and this performance on all visual tasks was poor. His ability to identify upper case single letters had dropped from 77% on previous testing to 27% in 1990. He showed perseveration in his responses calling 10 of the 26 upper case letters R. Although his attempts at reading words suggested he still had major problems with initial letters, he was now producing errors and omissions unlike any we had seen before. For example he read LIMP as "SLAP" and TAG as "RAW." Ted was also very slow and halting in his responses. Sadly for him and for us the sessions, which he had so enjoyed, came to an end.

14

DEREK: RELEARNING TO READ AFTER
A GUNSHOT WOUND

BACKGROUND AND HISTORY

Derek was born in 1954. At the age of 18 he joined the Royal Air Force but was discharged because of tuberculosis. He spent 2 yr as a slaughter man before joining the Special Airborne Services (SAS) Regiment of the Rhodesian Army. In October 1977, during a battle in Mozambique, Derek was shot in the head. At first he was left for dead in the bush but a friend went to reclaim the body 3 days later. Derek was found to be alive although his brain was visible through his shattered skull. Taken to Salisbury (now Harare) in Rhodesia (now Zimbabwe), Derek underwent surgery to clean the wound and repair a leak of the cerebrospinal fluid (CSF). For 3 mo he hovered between life and death. Derek's father in England learned of his son's plight and scraped together enough money to go to Rhodesia and bring his son back to England where he was admitted to a neurosurgical department. Derek was very agitated and disturbed. He had meningitis and a communicating hydrocephalus.

The bullet which struck Derek had entered the left occipital area and lay in the left temporal area. In total four operations were carried out, two in Rhodesia and two in England. During the first operation the wound was cleared and the dura (one of the linings around the brain) was closed. The second operation was for repair of a sinus causing the CSF leak. The third operation, after Derek's return

209

home, was for insertion of a right frontal ammaya reservoir to remove the CSF and for further toileting of the left occipital wound. During this operation a swab was found to be present in Derek's brain. This appeared to have been left behind during one of the operations in Rhodesia and presumably was the cause of the meningitis. Fragments of shrapnel and bone were also found to be present in the left frontal area, so a fourth operation was carried out to remove these fragments.

The following 3 mo were rather stormy for Derek, he developed epilepsy and caught an infection requiring treatment with anticonvulsants and antibiotics. However, the scar healed well and by the end of June 1978 he was ready to be admitted to a rehabilitation center. The discharge summary described Derek as "fully conscious and speaking fluently but still with visual agnosia, receptive aphasia, apraxia, and difficulty in reading, writing and calculation." He was also reported to have marked memory problems and a right homonymous hemianopia. Motor power was normal in the upper limbs with a mild diffuse weakness in the lower limbs. The sensory system appeared normal.

I first met Derek 16 mo later when I started working at the rehabilitation center. Derek was by now an outpatient attending the rehabilitation center 3 days a week. He was referred to me by his physiotherapist for help in reducing his weight problem. I put him on a program to help reduce his weight and became aware of his inability to read and write. I wanted Derek to keep a 2 wk baseline of everything he ate or drank. Of course he was unable to do this, nor was he able to record the baseline on a tape recorder because of his severe memory problems. After some discussion his father agreed to keep the baselines. We found a powerful reinforcer (namely an extra day at the center) if Derek was able to lose two pounds over the week. Several months later Derek had achieved his target of 30 pounds weight reduction.

Meanwhile, I became aware of Derek's desperate desire to read and write again. He had, as far as we knew, been a normal reader before his injury and had indeed passed examinations to enter the Royal Air Force. Reading his rehabilitation center folder of notes it was clear that in his first months at the center Derek had numerous problems. His behavior caused concern to the staff who believed Derek was suffering from hallucinations as he often tried to climb walls to escape from "creatures which were chasing him." He had been unable to recognize objects or to judge depth and distance. When taken through the parking lot, for example, he was frightened of the large strange objects, which were, of course, cars. He also became very frightened when he saw a change in coloring in the paving stones underfoot. One stone was a darker color than its neighbor and Derek thought this signified a change in depth and that he was about to fall through a hole. The behavior problems and difficulties with judging depth had resolved by the time I saw him, his speech was fluent and grammatical, although he had word-finding problems and perseveration with naming to confrontation.

THE ASSESSMENT

In October and November 1980 Derek was given a neuropsychological assessment. This showed his vocabulary was in the low-average range; his reasoning skills were borderline between low-average and impaired; and he had severe difficulty with tasks involving arithmetic, perception, construction, memory, and reading. These results can be seen in Table 14.1

The reading difficulties caused Derek most distress, however, so prior to a treatment program carried out with Peter McGill (a trainee with me at the time), we began on a detailed assessment of Derek's reading ability. These results can be seen in Table 14.2. Max Coltheart, then working in London, also came to see Derek on two occasions. We also reassessed Derek's visual fields and confirmed the previous finding of a right homonymous hemianopia with intact left visual fields.

REMEDIATION ATTEMPTS

The first serious attempt to teach Derek to read again began 3 yr after the gunshot wound had left him with a profound reading disability in the context of widespread cognitive deficits following brain damage. At that time little had been published on the remediation of dyslexia acquired in adulthood. Benson and Geschwind (1969) devoted 1 page of a 30-page article on "The Alexias" to the topic of rehabilitation. They described some of the techniques that had been used including kinesthetic aids, sight reading, and alphabet drilling but were not optimistic. The only paper we could find was one by Moyer (1979) describing a very different patient from Derek. Moyer's patient, a 30-yr-old man had sustained an embolic stroke. The main teaching technique was practice in reading paragraphs on which the patient was timed. He increased the speed with which he read new material from an average of 66 syllables per minute to 94 syllables per minute some 3 mo later. This method was obviously not appropriate for Derek at that stage.

At the same time Albert (1979) reported that some neurologically impaired patients who demonstrated alexia without agraphia could "read" if they traced letters with their fingers. We could have tried this method with Derek although, once again, his pattern of difficulties was different as he had agraphia as well as alexia, and he was not a letter-by-letter reader as are patients with alexia without agraphia. Instead we turned to the literature on teaching children with developmental learning difficulties.

Walsh and Lamberts (1979) described the use of errorless discrimination learning and picture fading techniques to improve the reading of moderately mentally handicapped children. In the former method the child has to respond initially to

Table 14.1. Derek's Main Neuropsychological Test Results

Wechsler Adult Intelligence Scale-Revised

VERBAL SUBTESTS	AGE SCALED SCORES	PERFORMANCE SUBTESTS	AGE SCALED SCORES
Information	5	Digit symbol	0
Comprehension	5	Picture completion	3
Arithmetic	1	Block design	0
Similarities	5	Picture arrangement	6
Digit Span	1	Object assembly	2
Vocabulary	8		
Verbal IQ	65	(Impaired)	
Performance IQ	50	(Severely impaired)	
Full scale IQ	56		

Color Naming (Woollen skeins from the Gelb-Goldstein color sorting test were used)

1. Derek was unable to name colors
2. He was unable to point to the correct color named by the examiner
3. He was unable to match to sample
4. He was unable to group shades of colors appropriately

Object Naming (10 objects in the room, e.g., door, sink, window, telephone, etc. were selected)

1. With only 1–2 sec between each object 2/10 correct (many perseverations)
2. With 10–15 sec between each object 6/10 correct

Peabody Picture Vocabulary Test

1. Asked, "What is this?" or "What is__doing?"
   4/20 correct (many perseverations)
2. "Point to the__." (normal administration)
   19/20 correct

Usual and Unusual Views

Unusual	2/20	(many perseverations and circumlocutions)
Usual	4/20	

Gestural Apraxia Test

19/20 (First attempt)
20/20 (Second attempt)

Table 14.2. Derek's Reading, Writing, and Spelling Assessment

Initial Assessment

1. Derek was able to select his own name from a choice of three alternatives.
2. He was able to match to sample printed words.
3. He was unable to read common first names.
4. He was shown 44 words and short phrases from the social sight vocabulary (Gunzburg, 1973) plus his own first, middle, and last names (total = 47). He failed to respond to 33 of these, gave two correct answers, "Gentlemen" and his own middle name, together with the following incorrect answers:

Stimulus	Response
Keep left	"Q"
Stop	"X"
Derek	"It's my own Christian name . . . Campbell."
Men	"X"
Open	"YZ"
In	"X"
Women	"Ladies"
Open here	"Ladies" (immediately after correctly naming Gentlemen)
Danger	"Part of my Christian name . . . Campbell." ("Is that your Christian name?" "Yes." "What's your surname?" "Derek.")
Coffee	"Surname" ("What's your surname?") "Campbell—part of that."
Campbell	"P---" (produced middle name). "It's part of me."
Sugar	"Campbell."

These errors can be classified as:

1. 5 random errors (keep left, stop, men, open, in)
2. 3 semantic errors (women, Derek, Campbell)
3. 2 perseverative errors (open here, sugar)
4. 1 visual/semantic error (danger)
5. 1 visual error (coffee)

Reading Single Digits

0/10 correct

Reciting Alphabet

Unable to do whole alphabet
A–F without error

Reading-Related Tests (carried out by Max Coltheart)

1. Derek was unable to read single letters.
2. He could tell whether a letter was upside down or not (so he knew something about letters and was able to perceive them adequately).

(continued)

213

Table 14.2. Derek's Reading, Writing, and Spelling Assessment (*continued*)

3. He performed at chance on a lexical decision task (i.e., deciding if a printed letter string was a real word or a nonword).
4. He was unable to read any words presented.
5. He could repeat single spoken words or nonwords (so his problem could not be due to articulatory difficulties).
6. He performed above chance, although in the impaired range on deciding whether single letter pairs of mixed upper and lower case were the same letter or not (e.g., Aa, Bp). Derek's score was 71% correct, which is significant on a Chi-Square Test ($P < 0.05$).

Writing and Copying

1. Derek was able to write his own name to request with both his right and his left hand.
2. He was unable to write words to dictation.
3. He was able to copy single letters.
4. He was able to copy three-letter printed words.
5. He was unable to write to dictation words he had copied although sometimes approximated the correct response (e.g., BT for BAT).
6. He was only able to copy the first letter of words presented in script.

Spelling

1. Of five three-letter words presented orally Derek was correct with three and made one error with each of the other two.
2. When asked to spell four- or five-letter words Derek was usually able to give the first two or three letters. He made one semantic error saying S–A–T when asked to spell chair.
3 When three-letter words were orally spelled to him, Derek correctly named 2/5 and made single letter errors for the other three.
4. With four- and five-letter words Derek again named 2/5 correctly, gave one perseverative error, one nonresponse, and one partially correct response (BARK for B–O–O–K).

one word only. Other words are introduced gradually and, at first, these words are dissimilar from each other in size, typeface, color and so forth. Later the words become more alike. In the picture fading method each word is accompanied by a picture that is gradually faded out until the child is eventually reading the word alone. For Derek we decided to adopt the former, errorless discrimination method. Walsh and Lamberts (1979) was only one example of a range of recent (at that time) studies showing the efficacy of errorless learning with people with developmental learning difficulties. Gunzburg (1973) argued for teaching a social sight vocabulary (i.e., socially useful words likely to be encountered in everyday environments) rather than more advanced reading. We took this as our starting point.

STAGE 1: WORD IDENTIFICATION

We selected six words we considered to be useful for Derek in his everyday life. These were his first name, middle name, and surname, together with LADIES, GENTLEMEN, and EXIT. Testing with all six words was carried out at the beginning and end of each session. We followed Cullen's (1976) suggestions for teaching reading aloud when using an errorless learning approach. This involves showing the first word (e.g., EXIT) and saying, "What does this word say? It says EXIT." Thus the answer was provided before Derek responded. Derek was then asked to repeat the answer. Errors were thus avoided by providing him with the answer before his response. After five correct responses, a second word was added. After five correct responses of the second word the two words were interspersed. Then a third word was introduced and so forth. This procedure continued for 3 wk before being abandoned. Derek was above chance when tested on the six words but was nevertheless failing to reliably read aloud the six words. In retrospect, we would have made two changes. First, we would not have tested so frequently. By testing at the beginning and end of each session we were encouraging Derek to make errors, so were not really following an errorless learning approach. Second, we would have combined errorless learning with expanding rehearsal (also known as spaced retrieval) whereby we gradually increased the interval between Derek being given the correct answer and being asked to retrieve that answer. As work using errorless learning with amnesic subjects was to show several years later (Wilson et al., 1994), we need to avoid passive learning as far as possible. However, as always, it is easy to be wise after the event.

STAGE 2: WORD RECOGNITION

We decided to change emphasis and work on word recognition rather than word production as we knew from our assessment that Derek was better at this. Walsh and Lamberts (1979) had worked on discrimination, i.e., recognition with their learning disabled children. Furthermore, Hendrickson et al. (1978) found their reading-disabled children responded better to modeling, whereby the teacher identified the word first, than they did to error correction by the teacher. The procedure we followed was this:

1. We used the same six words as previously.
2. One word was presented and identified by the psychologist.
3. This word was presented first with one, and later with two other words to Derek in a random order.
4. Derek was asked to point to the target word.
5. Errors were corrected by telling Derek to "try another."

Testing was carried out six times over the 15 sessions of treatment by asking Derek to "Point to (EXIT)." Of 180 trials where there were two words to choose from, he was correct 156 times (88.6%). He was also tested 60 times on pairs of untaught words (Barbara, Peter, Danger, Out, Men, and Women). He was correct on 54 trials (90%). When tested with combinations of three taught words, Derek correctly pointed to the target word on 48/60 trials (80%). His performance was the same with three-choice recognition on untaught words.

On three occasions all six words were presented and he was asked to point to one word. He was correct on 17/18 trials (94.4%). However when all six un-taught words were presented he scored 100% correct. Thus, although he did well at recognition, there was no effect of treatment and he was still unable to read any of the words aloud with any degree of consistency. We abandoned treatment and tried to persuade Derek and his father that the relearning of reading skills was an unachievable goal.

A few months later, Derek was discharged from the rehabilitation center and began attending a day center for adults with developmental learning difficulties. Here he met Sam White, an untrained helper interested in adult literacy.

STAGE 3: THE PHONETIC APPROACH

Derek called in to the rehabilitation center regularly to tell us how he was getting on. One day in 1982, 5 yr after the gunshot wound, Derek told me that Sam White was going to try to teach him to read, so I decided to do another baseline before Sam began his teaching. Over a period of 4 days I retested Derek on his ability to read aloud the six social sight words selected for treatment and on all letters of the alphabet both upper and lower case. He performed very poorly, reading none of the words on any occasion and very few of the letters. Q was read correctly once, X once, T once, and L once.

Sam began his teaching program using the phonetic approach. He started by going through the alphabet teaching Derek the sounds of the letters. On the first day, Sam presented the first three letters, A, B, and C in the upper case and Derek was taught the corresponding sounds. He was asked to practice these and make sure he learned them by the following session, 2 days later. Derek retained the knowledge of the sounds of these letters and in the second session he learned the sounds for D, E, and F, one at a time. His homework was to practice all six sounds. Teaching proceeded in this way for 3 days a week. By the end of the 3rd week Derek had learned all 26 sounds when upper case letters were presented. He came to see me half way through this stage to demonstrate his knowledge. He came again at the end of the 3rd week. Not only did he score 100% on letter–sound correspondences, he was able to read the six social sight vocabulary words from the original program without error, even though Sam White had not used these words at all. Lower case letters were tackled next in the same way with even faster learning. On his next visit to me I administered the Schonell word reading test, Derek scored at a 9-yr-old level. This test had not been administered before because Derek could not read any words. These results can be seen in Figure 14.1.

Sam continued his program by teaching Derek to recognize the vowels from an array of words. They proceeded to work on short regularly spelled words and finally practiced irregularly spelled words. At this point formal teaching sessions were abandoned and Derek worked alone at his reading. His motivation was extremely high and he practiced as often as possible. He persuaded everyone he saw to listen to him read and came to see me weekly to demonstrate his newly acquired skill and to allow me to monitor his progress.

At this stage he was reading almost every word phonetically, remembering very few words as whole units. In an interview with Derek in February 1983, he told me he had been an excellent reader prior to his injury. He said that when he was learning the alphabet with Sam, he confused *m* and *n* and *d* and *b* for a long time but the hardest letter to learn was "f" until he associated this with a four-letter word. He went on to say that his memory was appalling and when he was learning words he learned rapidly, but if he learned a second one the first one disappeared, but, he said, "I'm a tenacious and motivated chap and I never get fed up with it [reading]."

By now Derek was reading slowly but with good understanding, using context to help him. His reading age increased within a year to over 12 yr. He had changed from a person with alexia to a person with surface dyslexia and letter-by-letter reading. He could read 35% of nonwords making regularizations with other words, e.g., to BADY he said, "It's baddy, but its spelled wrong." He read regular words well but was impaired on irregular words. He sounded out words letter-by-letter and showed a word-length effect. When Derek first started reading again, he always traced the letter with his finger and if prevented from doing this became alexic again. Thus, once he had become a letter-by-letter reader he showed the behavior described by Albert (1979) who said some patients with alexia without agraphia are able to "read" if they trace the letter first. Derek, however, learned to read without this compensatory strategy. His tracing of the letters ceased within a few months. He read for pleasure and sometimes sent audiotapes of his reading. He particularly enjoyed military books both pictorial and factual. Why had Derek learned to read so rapidly with the phonetic method, 5 yr postinjury when the whole-word method had failed so dismally? His motivation was a factor, no doubt, but he was highly motivated 2 yr earlier when we began the first program. Coltheart's (1985) dual-route model of reading can explain this. A simplified version of the model can be seen in Figure 14.2.

We know that Derek was able to do some visual feature analysis, as in the original assessment he could tell if a letter was upside down or not. He was unable to

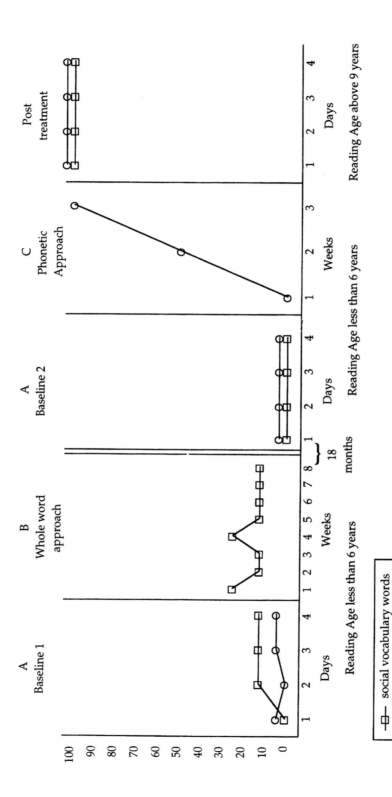

Figure 14.1. Percentage of stimuli Derek read correctly.

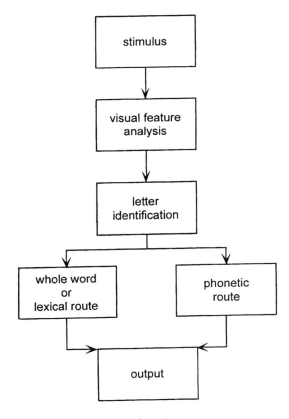

Figure 14.2. Coltheart's dual-route model of reading.

identify letters, however, so this prevented him from reading. Furthermore, as it turned out, his whole word/lexical route appeared to be permanently damaged because even after he had learned to read the letters, he was still unable to use this route, and had to depend on the nonlexical or phonetic route. Had we known about Coltheart's model in 1980 when we began Derek's reading program, then we might have referred to this in our analysis and decided to address the letter identification deficit, which occurred at an earlier stage in the reading process than the whole word route. However, not only was the model unpublished at the time, but we had no way of knowing the whole word route was damaged while the phonetic route remained intact. It was unfortunate that we used the route resistant to treatment. Had the phonetic route been the resistant one, our treatment could well have worked despite Derek's lack of letter identification. After all, young children can read whole words as visual units or icons before they have knowledge of individual letter sounds.

Furthermore, if the whole-word route seemed resistant to treatment we could have predicted that the letter identification system might have been resistant to treatment too. Without trying, one does not know whether something will respond to treatment or not. The dual-route model is good at identifying what is wrong in Derek's case and also for explaining why one treatment worked and another did not. Identifying what is wrong, however, does not inform us as to *how* to remediate or reduce the deficit. Wilson and Patterson (1990) also address this argument and use Derek as an example. The most important message from Derek's dramatic success is that it is sometimes possible to reteach alexic patients to read even several years postinsult, and solutions to problems should always be sought.

Although Derek was never given any formal teaching for his writing deficits, his writing improved in parallel with his reading and he often wrote letters to me and his social worker. His spelling was surface dysgraphic but quite understandable.

FOLLOW-UP

In 1983, Derek moved back to the town where he had spent his childhood, which was a long way from the rehabilitation center. He still wrote occasionally and kept in touch with several of the rehabilitation center staff. In a letter written in 1985, Derek said, "It gives me a grait feling of prid to think that I have realy acheved something well."

He managed to join the volunteer service of the regiment he belonged to before going to Zimbabwe (then Rhodesia) and is now a Lance Corporal. He has even made some parachute jumps despite some opposition from Army doctors, and, despite epilepsy, hemianopia, and persistent cognitive difficulties. Derek described this in a letter:

> There was a parachute jump from an aircraft planed . . . I went to see the instructor and it was the man who I know quite well so he asked me a cople of questions and I told a fuw white lies and then he said if enything goes wrong tell them you have not seen me. . . . Well I landed OK but the 4th man to jump broke his leg and when every one sore the umbulance go out thay all thought that it was me so there were quite a lot of releved faces when thay sore me come stroling in whith my used parachute over my sholder.

In 1988, Derek married and now works part time as a slaughterman for his battalion. Despite very frequent epilepsy he appears to be happy and seems to lead a fairly normal life.

A recent assessment of Derek's reading showed that his reading age on the Schonell Graded Word Reading Test was at a 13-yr-old level. He remains a surface dyslexic and a letter-by-letter reader. Examples of surface dyslexic errors include, OUNT for AUNT, BOWEL for BOWL, and "DOAG" for DOUGH. His spelling is surface dysgraphic, for example he wrote, WRESAN for REASON and CUD for COULD. On a lexical decision task he made 6/40 errors comprised of five false positives and one false negative. He made a number of homophone confusions, for example, TOWED was defined as, "a little animal revolting to most people," (toad) and GROAN was defined as, "I've grown something in the garden." He also shows a marked word-length effect supporting the conclusion that he remains a letter-by-letter reader, reading OIL in 1 sec, FELLOW in 4 sec, and NEWSPAPER in 10 sec. No parts of speech effect was found.

Despite dramatic improvement and the fact that Derek still reads for pleasure, it is clear that restoration of reading skills was far from complete. It is true that on tests assessing reading age he scores like an average 13-yr-old. However, 13-yr-olds do not show a surface dyslexia and they do not read in a letter-by-letter fashion. Returning to the approaches to rehabilitation described in Chapter 2, what mechanism can explain Derek's improvement? Restoration of function was, at best, partial. Anatomical reorganization may have played a role but in the absence of detailed pre- and postbrain imaging, it is impossible to prove or disprove this suggestion. Derek certainly did not attempt to by-pass or avoid his problems. Quite the contrary, he strove to learn to read again. Finding an alternative solution is, perhaps, the best way from explain his success given that he now reads in a very different way to how he read prior to his gunshot wound. Instead he now appears to be dependent exclusively on the nonlexical route. Furthermore, because of an inability to see words as whole units, he has to resort to a letter-by-letter strategy.

Derek has been an example to me: he was one of the first brain damaged patients I worked with; he forced me to problem solve; he educated me about the nature of brain injury; and most importantly he was a fighter who refused to give up on his goal of relearning to read. When asked what he thought about his reading now Derek said, "It's a bloody miracle."

15

JENNY: REGAINING QUALITY OF LIFE FOLLOWING A HORSEBACK RIDING ACCIDENT

BACKGROUND

Jenny was 17-yr-old when she had a devastating accident in May 1981. An excellent horsewoman, who had won many prizes, she had just returned from a 20 mile ride with her prize-winning horse. Jenny followed the same routine as she did every evening. She untacked and fed the horse. After that she mounted the horse in order to jump the hedge into the field before dismounting and leaving the horse for the night. Jenny always jumped the hedge without a bridle or saddle. This was something she could accomplish with ease. On this particular night, however, something happened. Jenny mounted the mare bareback but instead of jumping the hedge, the horse went in the opposite direction down into the lane for about 400 yards with Jenny clinging on, straight into the road. A car was coming, the driver braked but at that moment there was a failure in the brake pipe system (discovered later when the spilled brake fluid covered the roadway for several yards). The car hit Jenny and the horse. Jenny was thrown 30 feet. The horse was badly mutilated and had to be destroyed immediately.

Jenny's parents do not know the full story of the accident. They do not know what caused the horse to bolt that Thursday evening, causing its death and Jenny's severe head injury. They only knew she was an excellent rider ". . . brilliant, top-notch, 100%."

Jenny was taken to the local general hospital in a coma. She was not expected to live. Her parents were very angry at the way they and Jenny were treated. Obviously, there are at least two sides to any story but Jenny's parents' perception of their treatment is repeated in various forms by other relatives. They felt they did not receive appropriate attention, sensitivity, or compassion. Furthermore, Jenny's elder brother, a fit young man, had died a year earlier after he had contracted influenza from a rare virus that affected his heart. Whatever the true circumstances surrounding the early care of their daughter, Jenny's parents felt the medical and paramedical professionals had failed them.

Jenny was sent to a regional center for a brain scan. Her parents were told there was nothing to be done and she was unlikely to live. Her father believed the hospital wanted parts of Jenny's body for transplant. As he put it, "I knew what was coming. I knew it was spare parts they were after. I said, 'Don't you touch any spare parts. NO SPARE PARTS.'"

Returned to the local hospital Jenny's parents kept vigil at her bedside. They remembered that they had to keep calling the nurse to come and suction fluid from Jenny's lungs because she was not breathing easily. She was lying in a coma with tubes in for drip feeding and tubes to clear the fluid from her lungs. It appears that Jenny was not having physiotherapy at the time. Many early head injured patients do have chest physiotherapy to help clear their lungs and also have their limbs moved to help prevent contractures, which are fairly common after a severe head injury. Jenny's physiotherapy did not start until several weeks later.

Her father tried to stimulate Jenny during her coma by playing pop songs on a tape recorder. Coma stimulation is a controversial area and proper evaluative studies have yet to be done. It is possible that stimulation encourages faster or better recovery if provided for a few minutes several times a day. It is also possible that such stimulation can irritate a damaged brain and for some people this could be dangerous (for example, if there is swelling and pressure on the brain).

When describing Jenny's behavior during the playing of pop songs, her father said she would become very red and flushed and appeared to be straining and fighting to come round. Her mother, however, interpreted the flushes as Jenny's reaction to pain. Perhaps both interpretations were correct.

A stormy 3 mo followed with Jenny's parents fighting to get the best care for their daughter. Jenny gradually emerged from the coma after 3 mo. It was an extremely long coma considering that a 6 h coma is usually indicative of a severe head injury and a 24 h coma indicative of a very severe head injury.

When Jenny first came around her father took her outside in a wheelchair. She was taken to the pub and to places she knew before the accident. She just sat slumped in the chair. She could move her lips as if she were talking but no sounds emerged. She would sit in the chair, leaning on the tray placed across the front, and if someone talked to her she moved her lips in silent reply. After about 3 wk,

Jenny slowly began to speak again always in the same monotonous tone, no ups and downs, or rhythms to her speech.

At this time, the hospital decided to refer Jenny to Rivermead. Her father did not want her to go as it was too far away (about a $2^1/_2$–3 h drive). He agreed to let her go for 2 wk. Meanwhile Jenny was sent to a smaller hospital while the referral to Rivermead was made and Jenny was placed on the waiting list.

In January 1982, Jenny's father visited Rivermead and although extremely cautious about committing his daughter to another institution, he was persuaded when he heard the staff discuss "quality of life," a phrase that struck a chord with him. Jenny came to Rivermead in February 1982. She was to spend the next 13 mo there, apart from some weekends and short visits home.

A medical examination revealed a tremor and ataxia, caused by damage to the cerebellum, a squint, some right-sided weakness, and a poor memory. Her sense of touch was normal and so were her heart and lungs. One of Jenny's problems, which became apparent later, was the difficulty she had in regulating her temperature. She sweated easily and frequently complained of being too hot. It was not unusual to see Jenny outside on a cold winter's day without a sweater or jacket. This, presumably, was due to damage to the hypothalamus.

For the next 2 wk, Jenny spent much of her day in physiotherapy and occupational therapy. She was in a wheelchair, needing help for most activities. Not only was Jenny very ataxic, she had a shortened right leg as a result of two fractures sustained at the time of the accident. Her balance was poor, her movements were ungainly, and she was very slow. In occupational therapy she was noted to have perceptual problems and slurred speech (also a result of the cerebellar damage).

After 2 wk, Jenny was assessed by the speech therapist who found that Jenny's understanding of language was good and that she could express herself fluently and grammatically. There were two areas of major difficulty. First Jenny was no longer able to read and second she was unable to identify visual material. Jenny was referred to clinical psychology for further clarification of these problems.

THE NEUROPSYCHOLOGICAL ASSESSMENT

I first saw Jenny in March 1982 when she was 18 yr old. It was 10 mo after her accident. I began with the Wechsler Adult Intelligence Scale (WAIS). We came to the picture completion subtest and as I showed her each picture and asked, "What is missing?" I became aware that Jenny might be failing to recognize objects. The first picture was of a door without a handle. When asked what was missing she said, "The beginning." The second picture was of a pig without a tail. "What's missing here, Jenny?" I asked. "The front leg," she replied. "What is actually in the picture, Jenny?" "A hippopotamus," said Jenny. In the picture arrangement subtest when asked to put three pictures in order to make the most sensible story, not only did she fail, she said the story was about a dog looking for rabbits. It was actually a story about a bird building a nest.

I knew Jenny could hold a sensible conversation, she did not have obvious word finding difficulties, and she could define words on the vocabulary subtest without much difficulty. Her definition of REPAIR was "fix something that's broken," and for OBSTRUCT she said, "Get in the way of." She could also repeat back six digits in the correct order indicating her immediate memory span was adequate. She appeared to be able to "see" the pictures although her father kept insisting she needed new glasses. I thought she might have a visual object agnosia, i.e., a problem recognizing objects that was not simply due to poor vision or a naming disorder.

Over the next 2 wk I investigated Jenny's object recognition skills in more detail. With everyday objects she made some bizarre errors. For example, she said an ONION was "A BALL" and a BUTTON was "A COIN." Her exact words, when shown the button, were, "It's got two dots in it, it must be a coin, a two pence or five pence coin." A THREE-PIN PLUG was identified as "A PEN HOLDER" and a CLOTHES PEG was called a "HAIR COMB." She correctly identified a pen, a ruler, and a watch.

People with agnosia are sometimes helped if they see the object rotated in front of them. To see if this would help Jenny I slowly moved each object around and around in Jenny's vision. This rotation failed to promote correct identification although Jenny frequently provided other incorrect names. For example, she no longer thought the clothes peg was a comb but now identified it, on rotation, as a pair of scissors. In the same way the three-pin plug became a playing card box rather than a pen holder.

I also tested Jenny's ability to recognize objects by touch. In fact, some people with agnosia can recognize objects through touch even though they fail to recognize them visually. Jenny, however, was equally poor at recognizing by touch: the ONION became "AN APPLE" instead of "A BALL;" a PENCIL SHARPENER, which Jenny had previously identified as money when she first saw it, became "A KEY" when she felt it.

We could demonstrate that Jenny's inability to recognize through her sense of touch was not the result of poor sensation in her hands by getting her to say whether two objects she touched were the same or not. A screen was placed in front of Jenny with her hands out of sight on the other side of the screen. When she was given one object to hold in one hand and asked to find a similar object with the other hand, she made no mistakes.

We also had to make sure, of course, that Jenny could see adequately. If she was simply unable to identify the objects because she could not see them then we could not diagnose visual object agnosia. First, she was tested on a perimeter (a machine for measuring visual fields) to find out whether she could see all around.

In fact she had a full visual field in her left eye but, in comparison with the general population, she had a slightly reduced field in her right eye.

This slight reduction in the visual field of her right eye could not explain Jenny's failure to name objects. After all, people with one eye can recognize objects quite adequately. Even people with tunnel vision, such as Ron in Chapter 12, do not have major difficulties recognizing objects.

Dr. Jules Davidoff from the Radcliffe Infirmary in Oxford also tested Jenny's ability to detect patterns and her ability to match one item with another in an attempt to assess her ability to see. The standard visual tests using letters were unsuitable for Jenny as she was no longer able to identify or recognize letters. Instead, she was shown patterns containing vertical lines. In the first set of these there were wide spaces between the lines. The spaces then became narrower and narrower until the lines were no longer visible and the design appeared to be one solid block.

Jenny performed normally on this test. Dr. Davidoff commented, "Her performance on detecting patterns was very good as was her visual matching, except for small details." I then asked Jenny to copy items and to count dots on a card. Both of these she could do well although she usually did not recognize the items she had copied." Thus Jenny could obviously see well enough to count dots, match one pattern with another, copy drawings, and copy real objects. We were confident then in excluding poor eyesight as an explanation for Jenny's difficulty in recognizing objects.

Jenny was also asked to identify photographs and line drawings, as opposed to real objects. She had great difficulty in naming most of the pictures we gave her. When shown a drawing of a KANGAROO, for example, she said, "[it was] A DOG OR A CAT," a picture of a PERISCOPE was described as "A BOY FISHING" and a photograph of an IRON was called "A SHOE."

When Jenny gave an incorrect answer her response was usually the name of something that was similar in general appearance to the object, picture, or photograph. The smoothness and roundness of an onion is captured in Jenny's "ball" or "apple;" the approximate shape of an iron becomes a "shoe." These kinds of errors are not typically found in patients with naming problems due to damage in the language areas of the brain. More typical responses to an onion would be something like, "It's a . . . a . . . a . . . thingummy . . ." or "A carrot—no—a turnip . . . no, I can't tell you the name," or "It's a . . . I can't tell you . . . but you can peel it . . . you use it in stews."

So Jenny confused the object with something *visually* similar whereas patients with naming problems tend to confuse the object with something that has a similar *meaning;* or else they cannot find the word at all despite the fact that they may be able to describe the object in a way that shows they have recognized it.

In fact, Jenny was able to describe the visual appearance of objects and she could draw them. Her problem was that she could not *recognize* them in order to give them their names. When shown a KEY, for example, she named it "A PEN

LID" yet she described it in the following words: "At the top it's round, with a little hole in it. At the bottom it's straight with two pieces like a handle."

Even though Jenny's responses were unlike those of someone with a typical naming disorder, it was necessary to make sure that her problems were not due to a difficulty finding the right word for the object she was trying to name. I did this by asking her to name an object we described ourselves. For example, I asked her, "What is the name of something we chop up and use in stews and it makes your eyes water?" Immediately Jenny said, "An onion." Similarly, when asked, "What is the name of something that is on the flex leading from the television and when you want the television switched on you must first of all put this thing into the wall?" She replied, "a plug." Jenny was in fact correct on over 95% of the "naming to description" tasks.

Jenny's language abilities could be summarized as follows: (1) her spoken language was normal, (2) errors she made in recognizing objects and pictures were unlike those commonly seen in somebody with word-finding difficulties, and (3) she could name to description well. We could safely conclude therefore that Jenny did indeed have visual object agnosia owing to the fact that she was unable to recognize objects although she could see them, describe them, copy them, and provide their correct name if provided with a description of their function.

Further investigations of Jenny's object recognition difficulties revealed that she had particular problems recognizing animals. Her father had once commented that when he had taken Jenny out in her wheelchair before she came to Rivermead he showed her a houseboat on the river and, pointing to some dogs he could see on the houseboat, said, "Look at those animals." Jenny answered, "Are they ducks?" "Ducks," said her father, "they're guarding the houseboat." "Oh," said Jenny, "they must be Alsatians." They were indeed Alsatians, or German Shepherd dogs as they are now known, and the interesting thing to note here is that Jenny was able to work this out only after her father had said they were guarding the boat.

On another occasion Jenny saw a picture of a Concorde airplane and asked if it was a flying horse. I tested Jenny with a set of toy farm and zoo animals and she managed to correctly identify only 3 out of 20 (a kangaroo, a camel, and a horse). She called the GIRAFFE "AN ELEPHANT," a RABBIT was called "A PUPPY," a SHEEP was called "A LION," and a TIGER was "A BEAR." Once again, however, Jenny was able to supply a correct name once a description was provided. If I said, "This animal has wool and says 'baa,'" she would supply the name, "sheep." In fact she scored 100% in animal identification through description. All descriptions included function or information that was not solely visual.

Another feature to emerge was the inconsistency of Jenny's errors. Although she called a PLUG a "PEN HOLDER" on one occasion, she called it a "MATCH-BOX CASE," a "TORCH," and a "PAIR OF SCISSORS" on other occasions. She also had great difficulty drawing from memory as can be seen from the examples in Figures 15.1 and 15.2.

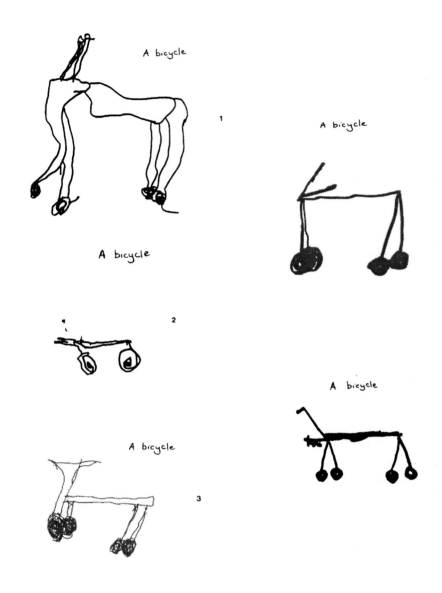

Figure 15.1. Examples of Jenny's drawing from memory.

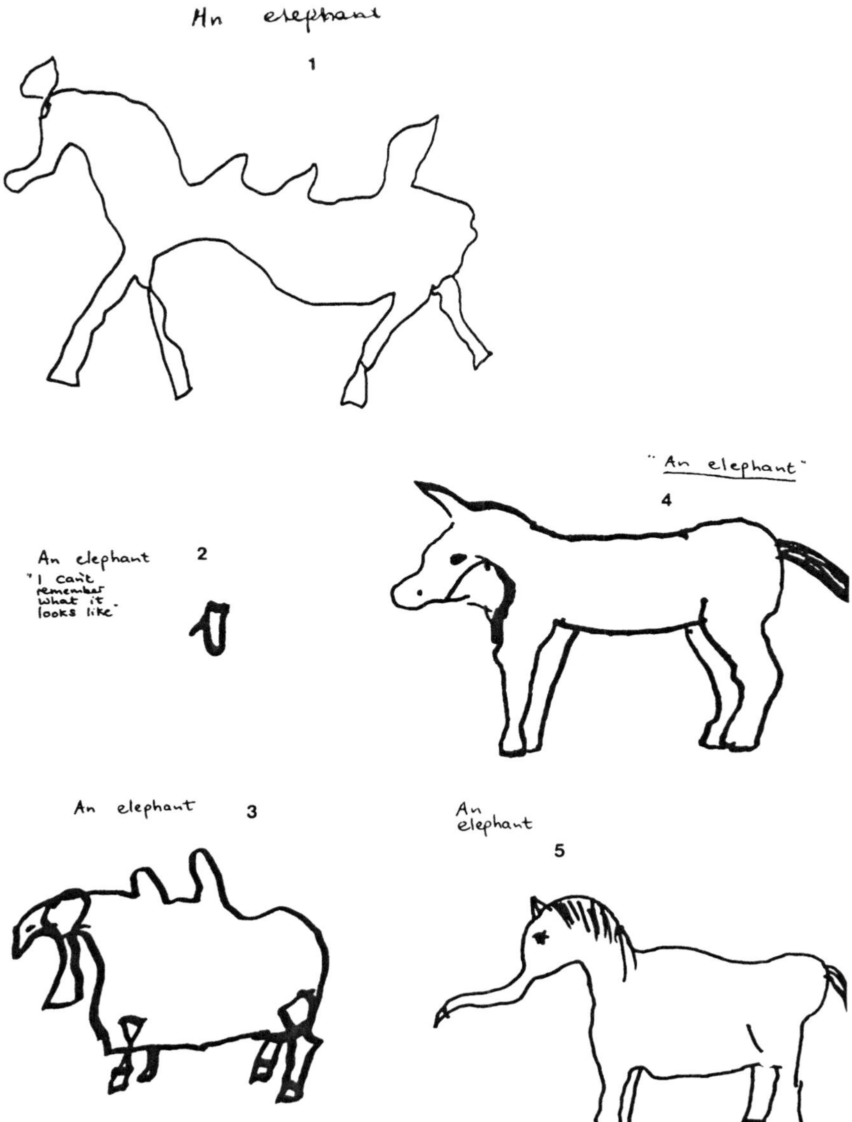
An elephant
1
An elephant
"I can't remember what it looks like"
2
An elephant
3
"An elephant"
4
An elephant
5

Figure 15.2. Examples of Jenny's drawing from memory.

Not only was she unable to draw from memory, she could not describe the physical appearance of many things. On one occasion Dr. Davidoff and I asked her, "What is an eagle?" Jenny replied, "a carnivorous bird." We then asked, "What does it look like?" She said, "It's got lots of teeth, four legs, and a long tail." Similarly she described a camel as "A ship of the desert . . . with four humps and eight legs." When shown a picture of a SWAN she said it was a "DUCK." When asked how many legs it had, she replied, "there are none in the picture, but under the water I think there are four."

Jenny had little trouble recognizing people's faces. She always recognized the people treating her at Rivermead and on some (but not all) tests of face perception she scored normally and was able to recognize different facial expressions. A report on the early investigations with Jenny can be found in Davidoff and Wilson (1985).

Another area of difficulty for Jenny was her reading. She was virtually unable to read—or to write or spell. Prior to her accident Jenny was studying for her "O" levels and had no major problems with reading, writing, and spelling. The neuropsychological assessment revealed that she could not read any words in normal size print from any of the reading tests I gave her, although she could read a few individual letters such as O and S. I wrote out some words in large print, which she read successfully. These were LITTLE, TREE, HORSE, JENNY, PETER, and SADDLE. She failed to read BARBARA (read as "WATER"), BRIDLE (read as "BROKE"), FETLOCK (she did not know this word), WATER (read as "HORSES"), EYE (read as "ARE"), PAPER (read as "POOR"), BOOK (read as "BOX"), and PONY (read as "FUNNY").

Next I spelled words out to her. She was correct on four: debt, pony, tree, and little. With many others, however, she was wrong, "M–I–L–K" was identified as "MIKE;" "C–L–O–C–K" as "CLOSET;" and, "S–A–N–D" as "SAD."

Her own oral spelling was also poor. She could spell up, bit, pencil, and fire. She spelled IS as "I–S–E;" RED as "R–E–D–D–E;" CHAIR as "C–H–E–R–E," and PAINT as "P–E–N–T–E". She did not have a deep dyslexia like Ron in Chapter 12, nor a surface dyslexia like Jason in Chapter 9, but was more like Derek in Chapter 14.

She showed some characteristics of letter-by-letter reading whereby the reader is unable to read a word as a whole unit although the word can be read if the individual letters are read or identified either overtly or covertly. There is no "parts of speech" effect as there is in deep dyslexia or little "regularity" effect as in surface dyslexia, but nevertheless letter-by-letter reading is slow and effortful. The longer the word the longer it takes to read. Patterson (1982) pointed out that in letter-by-letter reading a letter identification deficit is usually, but not invariably, present leading to the misidentification of some letters. Jenny certainly showed this to a marked degree so when shown UNCLE, for example, she said, "C–N–C–I–E." Her writing of individual letters was much better but not perfect.

She made three mistakes when writing the alphabet: N was written as H, Q as G, and Y as T.

When writing words Jenny could write her own name although she frequently left out one letter of her surname. She also managed tree, horse, little, and bun. With most other words she made errors including BOORK (for book), SITTE (for sit), PLAINE (for playing), SCOORLL (for school), and DAREBRRA (for Barbara). Numbers also caused difficulty. Although able to read single and double digits such as 5 and 42, she read 301 as 31. With writing she made mistakes with double digits too, so 21 was written as 201, 536 as 5036, and 301 as 3001. We were able to obtain copies of school reports from 1976–78 that described Jenny as "an excellent pupil, intelligent, and able" (1976); "she produces excellent creative writing and vivid poetry" (1976); "Jenny has a mature attitude to her studies and with her determination to succeed deserves to do well," (1977); and "Her determination stands her in good stead for the future" (1978).

REHABILITATION

A typical day for Jenny at Rivermead would be to get up at 7:00 A.M., be helped to wash, dress, and have breakfast on the ward. At 9:00 A.M. she left the ward for physiotherapy. Her physiotherapist would be responsible for Jenny and two other patients.

At 10:30 A.M. Jenny went to the canteen for a short break before going to occupational therapy from 10:45 A.M. to 12 noon. At 12 she returned to the ward for lunch. The afternoon sessions ran from 1:30 P.M. to 4:30 P.M. with a 15-min break in the middle. Three times a week Jenny would have a session with the psychologist for an hour during the afternoon. Sometimes this was increased to two sessions if there was a memory group running. Jenny attended the memory group for 9 wk (5 days a week) in total. Twice a week she went to the hydrotherapy pool. The rest of the afternoons were split between physiotherapy and occupational therapy.

Treatment in physiotherapy included balancing exercises, practicing transfer from wheelchair to bench and back, sitting to standing exercises, arm exercises whilst standing, walking practice using a rollator (a walking frame with wheels), and later walking without this aid, hydrotherapy, and attending a weekly horse riding class organized by the local Riding for the Disabled group.

By the time Jenny first left the unit 13 mo later she was physically independent. With a shoe raise on her right shoe to correct her shortened leg, she was able to walk unaided indoors but still required a three-wheeled frame for anything other than short distances outside. She could safely both stand while using her hands and manage stairs.

The occupational therapy sessions covered, to some extent, similar ground.

Here Jenny practiced walking with her three-wheeled frame and also continued transferring from her wheelchair to a chair or bed. She relearned the skills required for dressing, washing, and certain household tasks. She also practiced perception and memory tasks in occupational therapy.

As well as therapy Jenny received support and counselling from the unit's social worker who liaised with Jenny's previous social worker from her home town who, in turn, kept in touch with Jenny's family. The social worker helped to sort out any emotional, economic, and practical crises arising during Jenny's stay. The social worker investigated sources of financial aid for Jenny's family and spent time each week with Jenny giving her advice and counselling: Jenny's feelings, her fears and anxieties, her attitudes toward personal relationships, and her future expectations—all of these were discussed at length, with the social worker who tried to help Jenny to build up her confidence. Jenny was introduced to the local Physically Handicapped and Able Bodied (PHAB) Club and she attended several of their weekly meetings. Jenny's attitude toward this club was ambivalent, she did not like going to a club that was so up front about handicap. She was unwilling to consider herself physically handicapped, and once said to me, "I'm me, I'm Jenny, I'm not physically handicapped."

Sometimes Jenny became depressed and said she wanted to die, to go to heaven, and see her brother and her horse but for the most part she was cheerful, optimistic, and energetic.

TREATMENT FOR OBJECT RECOGNITION DIFFICULTIES

Jenny's object recognition difficulties resolved to a large extent over the next few years (Wilson and Davidoff, 1993). It is difficult to know to what extent this was due to natural recovery and to what extent it was due to the rehabilitation program. She spent some time each day in occupational therapy engaged in perceptual tasks but also spent part of her thrice weekly psychology sessions in object recognition retraining. Jenny's program was very similar to that devised for Paula (Chapter 16) in which three different methods for improving object recognition were compared. The first method simply involved telling Jenny the names of objects she could not identify so, for example, she was shown a key (which she had previously identified as a pencil) and told, "It's not a pencil, it's a key." The second method required Jenny to copy the object in the hope that once she had done so she would be able to recognize it better. This idea was based on the observation that Jenny had once read the word LITTLE as "TELLY," although when asked to copy the word she did so accurately and once copied she also read it correctly. The third method was to ask Jenny to concentrate on the prominent or important visual features of the drawings and to come to a conclusion about the object's name once she had done this.

The most effective method appeared to be telling Jenny what each drawing was. Despite a poor memory she was able to retain this information well and was able to generalize to other objects or drawings provided these were similar to the ones whose names had been given. Generalization was also built into the program by giving Jenny different examples of each object and providing the names as before.

With real objects, photographs, and line drawings, Jenny improved over the next few months. This improvement will be discussed further in the follow-up section.

READING REMEDIATION

Having recently found a successful treatment for Derek (Chapter 14), it was decided that Jenny's major problem was an inability to read individual letters correctly and that the first important goal would be to teach her to recognize letters of the alphabet in both lower and upper case. Before beginning treatment however, some further assessments were necessary. Jenny was able to read large print better than small print and yet she did not appear to be short-sighted as we saw earlier. We decided to investigate more systematically the importance of print size. Alan Baddeley from Cambridge had visited Rivermead soon after Jenny's admission. He saw part of her assessment and became interested in her reading difficulties. He sent a set of alphabetic letters he had used in an earlier study and a set was made up for Jenny. For each upper and lower case letter four cards were prepared. There was one letter on each card in one of four sizes. The largest was 7 mm high and the smallest 2 mm. We ended up with 208 cards (four sets of upper case letters and four sets of lower case letters). These were mixed randomly and presented to Jenny, one at a time, over the course of a week. We noted that Jenny usually found the larger sizes easier to read although there were some letters that were always read out correctly irrespective of size (such as S), and others that were never identified (such as Y). We also found that, of the letters Jenny could read, she could usually identify them when presented in both lower and upper case.

We began a teaching program which we operated for 15 to 20 min during each of the 3 h long psychology sessions Jenny attended weekly. Although Jenny was interested, motivated, and cooperative, she continued to experience great difficulty in relearning to read letters of the alphabet. We decided to select the 10 letters with which she experienced the most difficulty and teach these one at a time. We wanted to make sure Jenny had one letter "under her belt" before proceeding to the next. The first letter we chose was Y. Before the session I made 16 cards each with the letter Y on them. Each one was different in terms of color, shape, and size. Jenny was shown a card several times and each time she was informed that the letter on it was a Y. This particular Y card was then jumbled up with a number of other cards, some of which showed different Ys and some showed different letters, and Jenny had to identify these.

At the end of the session Jenny was given a test in which she was shown 10 different letters to identify. We needed to test Jenny in this way in order to find out (1) if she was making any progress, and (2) if there was progress, was this due to spontaneous recovery, general improvement over time, or learning specifically related to progress in identifying the Ys we taught her.

During these sessions we also gave Jenny lots of feedback. We told her when she correctly identified a Y. We also gave verbal prompts whenever necessary. We would chant, "Why can't I remember Y" and "Y-y-yes it's a Y." Jenny also received a red check mark every time she managed to identify the letter Y correctly. We also agreed that Jenny would be rewarded with a visit to the field to see the horses or that I would buy her a book about horses once she had obtained 20 red check marks. The checks served two purposes: they acted as a reward and also provided feedback to Jenny, indicating progress that was much desired, and—as it turned out—eventually achieved.

Jenny took 6 wk to learn to reliably identify the letter Y. In the meantime she managed to collect sufficient check marks prior to this to be taken for a few visits to the horses and to be given one book about horses. We worked through the remaining letters of the alphabet in similar fashion although none of them took quite so long as Y. The letters K, Q, and Z proved very difficult. We got around the problem of Q one day when I asked Jenny to tell me what the letter looked like. She said, "It looks like an O with a tail." "Right," I replied, "an O with a tail is a Q." Jenny repeated this regularly. For K we thought about kicking Ks and drew pictures of a K. This helped for a while but for years afterwards Jenny confused X and K. She usually addressed her letters to Okford rather than Oxford.

Jenny was remarkably good tempered throughout the period of 9 mo it took her to learn 10 letters of the alphabet. I am glad to say that after the painstaking slog of those initial months, progress with other letters was a little quicker. Her ultimate triumph over difficulties with letter identification can be measured best by the fact that by March 1983 she could read virtually all of the 208 original letter cards despite the fact that she had not seen them for 10 mo. She still made the occasional error, particularly with lower case letters when K, X, and Z were presented. Her reading of printed words had improved a little although she was very slow, and her spelling showed only some very slight improvement.

Jenny was now ready to move on to letter–sound combinations or "rules." We selected 10 rules that Jenny found particularly difficult to read, write, or spell: for example, IGH, WR, and AW. She had retained knowledge about other combinations: she knew, for example, that the K was silent in the KN combination and that PH made the sound of F. Having spent some time establishing which combinations of letters Jenny knew we started with OA words such as BOAT, OATS,

STOAT, etc. Unexpectedly however, Jenny went home for 3 mo just as this program started. She returned in July for 3 wk for a "top-up" before she was due to start a course in September 1983 at a college for people with physical disability.

On her return to us in July we found that she had retained her ability to read, write, and spell many OA words but had not improved on the other letter–sound combinations. This time we worked through all of these at each session because of the short time we had left. By this time Jenny was learning much more quickly. After 3 wk she was reading, writing, and spelling correctly between 80% and 90% of all the letter–sound combinations we had been teaching her.

Before we began our letter–sound program, examples of Jenny's spelling included the following:

dlew	(for blew)
toiy	(for toy)
soyil	(for soil)
cherche	(for church)

All of these were spelled correctly within 3 wk of our program.

On a formal spelling test however, Jenny still spelled IS as IZ, AM as AME, and GRASS as GRAS. The interesting thing to note is that her writing was decipherable because for the most part it was phonetically correct. Jenny now demonstrated a tendency to find regular words easier to read than irregular. It will be remembered that this is a characteristic of people with surface dyslexia. Besides spelling phonetically, like Jenny, people with surface dyslexia make homophone confusions. Homophones are words that sound alike but are spelled differently (for example, see and sea). These words present particular difficulties for those with surface dyslexia who might be able to read them correctly but define them incorrectly. Jenny made exactly this kind of error: she read the word POUR then defined it as meaning, "when you haven't got any money." She read the word USE and said, "The farmer worries about the ewes at lambing time."

It would appear then, that Jenny had changed from being unable to read at all to becoming a letter-by-letter reader who also had surface dyslexia.

SINCE RIVERMEAD

Jenny left Rivermead in July 1983 ready to take up a course at a college for people with physical disabilities in September. At discharge the physiotherapist reported that Jenny was able to walk outside without a frame, although if she did not concentrate she lost her balance. She also showed a tendency to stiffen up. The physiotherapist recommended that Jenny use the frame at home when walking outside. Her father, however, would have none of this and refused to take the frame home.

Jenny's occupational therapist reported an improvement in Jenny's perceptual abilities and observed she was much more competent in recognizing and handling money. She could plan menus, prepare food, and carry out some simple cooking.

Soon after starting at the college Jenny began horseback riding again. She had been going to Riding for the Disabled once a week at Rivermead but wanted to do proper horseback riding once more. She soon had a fall and broke her leg which required extra physiotherapy.

At the end of the first term Jenny's report stated that her memory problems caused her to have considerable learning difficulties and obvious frustration. The report went on to say that Jenny's spoken English was excellent with a good choice of words, a sophisticated structure, and an ability to make puns. Several teachers commented on her sense of humor.

In February 1984 Jenny returned to Rivermead for a 3 day follow-up assessment. Staff were still concerned about her flushing and sweating attacks, which remained problematic. However her tremor had improved, so too had her walking.

I reassessed Jenny's object recognition together with her reading, writing, and spelling skills. I continued to see her occasionally over the next few years. She had another 2 wk spell at Rivermead in August 1985 after which I saw her occasionally at home or she visited another hospital where I worked after leaving Rivermead.

IMPROVEMENT IN OBJECT RECOGNITION

Whether due to natural recovery or rehabilitation (or more likely to a combination of the two), there is no doubt that Jenny improved and continued to improve for some time as can be seen in Table 15.1.

With a set of 28 real objects she improved from 25% correct in March 1982 to 100% correct by April 1988. On the Graded Naming Test (McKenna and Warrington, 1983), she improved from 3% correct in 1982 to 53% in May 1992. The nature of her errors also changed. For example the YASHMAK from the Graded Naming Test was originally described as "a rather elderly gentleman wearing a hard headed hat." The LEOTARD was described as "a bandy legged woman wearing a riding jacket." In 1992 Jenny correctly identified the leotard and said the yashmak was "a head-dress worn by a person in the desert." Some of the failures on the Graded Naming Test were almost certainly due to the fact that Jenny had never known the name of the object. Other errors appeared to be due to a word finding deficit (e.g., the ANVIL on the Oldfield-Wingfield, 1965 test was "like a workbench"). Of the remaining errors, both visual and semantic errors were in evidence. Visual errors included a description of a TUNING FORK as "tongs for putting the washing in hot water," and a TASSEL was called

Table 15.1. Improvements in Object Recognition 1982–1992

	MAR./APR. 1982 (%)	NOV./DEC. 1982 (%)	FEB. 1984 (%)	JUL. 1985 (%)	APR. 1988 (%)	MAY 1992 (%)	CHANGE FROM FIRST TO LAST ASSESSMENT (%)
Real objects	25	38	71	95	100	100	75
Photographs							
Unconventional views	5	10	35	35	42	53	48
Conventional views	5	35	65	70	82	82	77
Line drawings							
Oldfield–Wingfield	22	45	57	68	—	74	52
Graded Naming Test	3	10	23	43	50	53	50
Model animals	15	20	35	65	65	60	45

a "DUSTER." Semantic errors included the "TAJ MAHAL" for a PAGODA and "PEGASUS" for the CENTAUR. Some errors could have been either visual or semantic, e.g., "DOOR HANDLE" for TAP and "FORCEPS" for TWEEZERS.

Jenny had always had particular problems with model animals. During the initial assessment, a set of 20 plastic model farm and zoo animals was used to assess recognition of animals. Jenny's ability to recognize them improved from 15% in April 1982 to 65% in 1985 and 1988. Her 1992 score was 60%. A list of animals and errors can be seen in Table 15.2.

Jenny's drawing from memory was reassessed on several occasions. She was always asked to draw a bicycle, an elephant, and a person. On some occasions she was also asked to draw a tree, a horse, a snail, a kangaroo, a bird, an airplane, a fish, and a camel. Her drawings of trees, horses, and people were always recognizable (see Figure 15.3).

Figures 15.1 and 15.2 show the changes in her drawings between March 1982 and May 1992. Although her elephant is much better drawn in December 1988 and May 1992, she gave it a mane and prick ears in 1988 and omitted the trunk in 1992. Her bicycle drawings improved until December 1988.

Jenny often provided a commentary when she was drawing. For example, when asked to draw an airplane in 1992 she first drew one with four legs and later drew another without wings, commenting at the same time, "Getting this to fly would be harder than getting a dodo to fly. Well here's the pilot . . . and the passengers . . . and the cargo. Would you like it jet propelled? Well, here's the propulsion." These two drawings of airplanes can be seen in Figure 15.4.

Table 15.2. Model Animals and Responses

ANIMAL	MAR./APR. 1982	NOV./DEC. 1982	FEB. 1984	JUL. 1985	APR. 1988	MAY 1992
Giraffe	Elephant or Kangaroo	Giraffe	Giraffe	Giraffe	Giraffe	Giraffe
Tiger	Bear	Tiger	Lion	Lion	Lion	Tiger
Rhinoceros	Lion	Cow	Bear	African pig	Rhinoceros	Bear
Kangaroo	Kangaroo	Ape	Kangaroo	Kangaroo	Kangaroo	Kangaroo
Polar Bear	Little dog	Lion	Polar bear	Polar bear	Polar bear	Polar bear
Ostrich	Kangaroo	Don't know	Ostrich	Stork	Ostrich	Gazelle
Camel	Camel	Indian elephant	African elephant	Camel	Camel	Camel
Horse	Horse	Horse	Horse	Horse	Horse	Horse
Elephant	Camel	Elephant	Cow	Elephant	Elephant	Elephant
Deer	Horse	Horse	Kangaroo	Deer	Kangaroo	Deer
Rabbit	Puppy	Puppy	Cat	Rabbit	Cat	Cat
Pig	Cow	Bull	Bull	Pig	Bull	Pig
Cow	Sheep	Bear	Cow	Cow	Cow	Pig
Bull	Dog	An herbaceous eater	Pig	Pig	Bull	Pig
Lion	Tiger	Wolf	Tiger	Lion	Lion	Lion
Penguin	Don't know	Seal	Sea bird	Road runner	Crane	Penguin
Goat	Don't know	Don't know	Deer	Deer	Don't know	Ram
Dog	Polar bear	Goat	Dog	Dog	Dog	Dog
Gorilla	Bear	Don't know	Gibbon	Rhino	Gibbon	Gorilla
Sheep	Lion	Cow	Cow	Sheep	Cow	Pig

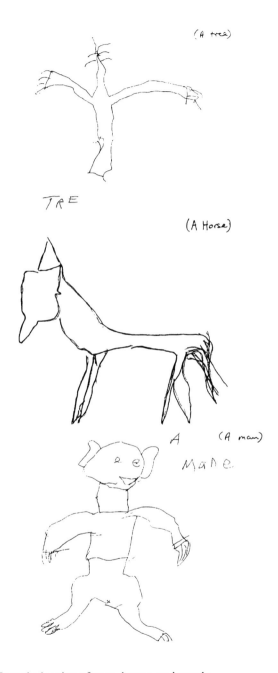

Figure 15.3. Jenny's drawing of trees, horses, and people.

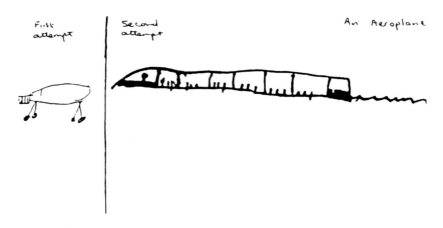

Figure 15.4. Jenny's 1992 airplane drawings.

DESCRIBING FROM MEMORY

Animals

In 1982, Jenny described a camel as having ". . . four humps and eight legs" although her initial reaction to the question, "What is a camel?" was to say it was, ". . . a ship of the desert." An eagle was defined as ". . . a carnivorous bird" but described as ". . . having lots of teeth, four legs, and a long tail." Although Jenny has improved in her ability to describe such animals as an eagle, a frog, and a snail, she still confuses different creatures. An elephant was described as ". . . having prick ears and a mane" (1992), a camel as "A little like a large cow, there are Indian and African ones. Both have long ears but the Indian has one hump and the African two. They are brown, I think. They have very long trunks and like shooting water at you" (1988).

One example from the 1992 assessment was a skunk. Jenny identified a model skunk as a "koala." When asked later to describe a skunk she said, "It's a small animal and when it's defending itself it turns its bottom to you, lifts up its tail and exudes a revolting smell." When asked to describe what a skunk looked like she replied, "I think they can be quite vicious." When asked its color she replied, "Dark brown, I think." These are examples of the difficulties, even resistance, demonstrated by Jenny when asked to describe physical characteristics of animals.

When she actually makes an attempt she frequently makes errors; this contrasts with her willingness to discuss other characteristics such as animal diets, their geographical location or the names of their offspring.

Non-living Things

The tendency to omit the description of physical characteristics was also apparent in Jenny's description of objects. She described the function of things rather than their appearance. Her description of a refrigerator for example, was "it uses a lot of CFCs, which are harmful to the atmosphere." However, she made no errors when asked if certain vehicles had wheels or not. It could be argued that wheels are physical characteristics as well as functional characteristics.

NAMING TO DESCRIPTION

Throughout the six assessments, Jenny's naming to description was good. On a set of 15 items (Coughlan and Warrington, 1978) she scored 100% on each occasion. In May 1992, however, she was given a set of 24 object descriptions loaned by Dr. John Hodges. Half of these were living creatures and half nonliving things. She made four errors, three of which were living creatures. These were: (1) "a small furry animal which lives in trees and has a long bushy tail" resulted in three answers: "a peacock," "a kookaburra," or "a fox"; (2) "a sea animal with a hard shell, large claws, and a tail" was called "a crab" (the correct answer is lobster); (3) "a fish-eating sea animal that has flippers and is hunted for its fur" was called "an otter" or "dolphin." (4) The only error for the nonliving things was "a musical instrument with a squeeze box and keys" that Jenny called "an organ."

   The results demonstrate that Jenny has shown considerable recovery over a period of 10 yr. Most of the recovery appeared to take place in the first 3 yr following her initial assessment. Her recognition of real objects is, with few exceptions, good. However, she still has some difficulty with photographs, line drawings, and model animals. The less the amount of information (such as in line drawings), or the more confusing the information (such as shadows in the photograph), the harder it is for her to recognize the objects. She continues to be a letter-by-letter reader, and her difficulty with famous faces remains. There is no evidence for any category specific impairment. Thus, even with the partial resolution of Jenny's agnosia over time, the impairments are still characteristic of associative agnosia.

IMPROVEMENT OF READING AND SPELLING

Jenny's reading continued to improve. Initially, she had been untestable on formal reading tests but by 1984 she was able to read 66 out of 100 words on one test and in the following year, on a different test, she was reading at the level of a $9^1/_2$- to 10 yr-old: very encouraging for someone who took 9 mo to learn 10 letters of the alphabet. In April 1988 Jenny was reading at the level of a 12 yr old—a performance that many adults in the general population do not achieve. Jenny was also able to read correctly all the numbers I presented to her but she still made errors in writing number from dictation, so that 103 was written as 1003 and 333 as 3033.

The errors Jenny made in reading were not absolutely typical of a person with surface dyslexia. She read, for example, APPLAUD as "APPLIED" and CALF as "CAVE." Other errors *were* more like those one might expect from someone with surface dyslexia, for example, DISEASED was read as "DECEASED," CONSCIENCE as "CONCISE," and CHOIR as "CHORE." She was also able to read some irregular words such as "SCINTILLATE," "MISCELLANEOUS," and "GUEST."

By 1983 Jenny had become a surface dyslexic and letter-by-letter reader. When reassessed in 1992, she was able to read 15 irregularly spelled words from the National Adult Reading Test (Nelson, 1982), and achieved a reading age of 11.5 to 12 yr on the British Ability Scales Word Reading List (Elliot et al., 1977). Her errors included "ORNT" for AUNT and "SAYED" for SAID. Her spelling remains very phonetic (e.g., "ORTOGRAF" for AUTOGRAPH and "CAUSHUS" for CAUTIOUS). She also makes homophone confusions (e.g., BREWS defined as if it were "BRUISE," and POUR defined as "PORE"). As expected of someone with surface dyslexia there is no "parts of speech" effect and she can read most nonwords, making only 2 errors from a list of 20 (GACE read as "GAKE," and BARCH read as "BORCH"). Because of the letter-by-letter reading, Jenny showed a "word length effect;" she read GAS and WAX within 1 sec but took 9 and 10 sec to read NEIGHBOR and ROUGHNESS.

CONCLUSION

Jenny currently earns a modest wage by giving talks to student nurses and other health service professionals about her experiences and personal views on the treatment of head injured people. Her ambition is to be an authoress and write books for adolescents. In many ways she has pulled through. She has never lost her strong personality, she can walk, talk, read, laugh, receive, and give pleasure to those who know her. Some physical and cognitive problems will always remain but Jenny has, as her parents always wanted, achieved a reasonable quality of life.

VI

PERCEPTUAL AND VISUOSPATIAL PROBLEMS

Four people are described in this section. All have severe problems with perceptual and/or visuospatial tasks. Perception is the process of integrating and organizing the information we receive from our senses. The process of perceiving includes the experience of sensations but also the cerebral interpretation of these sensations. Although adequate sensory functioning is a prerequisite of normal perception, impairment at the sensory level cannot be described as a perceptual impairment. Thus it would be incorrect to regard a blind person as someone with a visuoperceptual disorder or a deaf person as someone with a disorder of auditory perception (Wilson, 1987e). Although it is possible for both sensory and perceptual deficits to coexist, it is not possible to assess perceptual abilities when severe sensory impairment occurs in the same modality. These issues were addressed in the last chapter in the previous section on Jenny who showed a visual object agnosia in addition to her inability to read.

Paula, another person with poor object recognition is described in this section although Paula has a different kind of object recognition impairment than Jenny. Jenny had an associative agnosia whereby she could see adequately, match to sample and copy objects she could not recognize. Paula's deficit, however, was due to a simultanagnosia, i.e., an inability to see more than one part of a stimulus at a time. She showed characteristics of an apperceptive agnosia in that she could not match to sample, was considered to have poor vision, and (if she had not been quadriplegic) would probably have been unable to copy the objects she could not recognize.

Kirsty, the second person described in this section, also had object recognition difficulties more similar to those of Jenny (Chapter 15). Both Kirsty and Jenny appear to have a visual semantic memory disorder in that they can access semantics or meaning from words much easier than they can from pictures. Ratcliff and Newcombe (1982) suggest that if objects can be recognized by touch but not through vision, the underlying deficit is a disconnection syndrome whereas in people who cannot recognize objects by touch or by vision then the cause is a visual semantic memory disorder. Initially Kirsty was much better at tactile recognition than visual recognition although she now seems to have resolved into a person with a more clear-cut semantic memory disorder.

Richard, the third person in this section, sustained two hemorrhages in childhood and has enormous problems with face processing tasks. He recognizes very few famous faces, is severely impaired at unfamiliar faces, cannot tell if someone is looking directly at him or not, is poor at recognizing emotional facial expressions, and even has problems telling men from women by their faces. Despite this Richard is very socially skilled and popular with his peers. Ellis and Young (1997) say, "Other people's faces provide us with a wealth of social information," (p. 87). Obviously this information is unavailable to Richard so his social skills must all come from elsewhere. He is a good example of someone who uses his intact skills to compensate for his impairments.

The final person in this section, Dolly, showed a severe and classical unilateral neglect following a right hemisphere stroke. Neglect is now believed by most people to be an attentional disorder (see for example Halligan and Marshall, 1994) in which patients fail to attend to part of space. As Halligan and Marshall say, "There are very substantial numbers of neurological patients who after unilateral brain damage appear to live in a world that is spatially skewed," (p. 103). Robertson et al. (1998) remind us that unilateral neglect is notoriously difficult to rehabilitate although a few studies have found some therapeutic effects of intensive therapies such as scanning. This was the main treatment approach used for Dolly but as I say in the chapter about her, if I were treating her today, I would certainly have employed some of the newer treatment procedures such as limb activation (Robertson and North, 1993) and sustained attention training (Robertson et al., 1995). Rehabilitation of unilateral neglect is one of the major growth areas in neuropsychological rehabilitation.

16

PAULA: FEAR OF PHYSIOTHERAPY AND PROBLEMS RECOGNIZING OBJECTS AFTER A SEVERE HEAD INJURY

BACKGROUND

After leaving school at 18 yr old with good examination results, Paula obtained employment as a security officer in a factory. She was an energetic, happy young woman with a large circle of friends and a zest for life. With a busy social life Paula wanted her own transport and started to save for a motorcycle. Her only brother who was 2 yr older already had his own treasured Harley Davidson and Paula decided it would be less expensive to purchase a two-wheeled vehicle than a four-wheeled one. Tragically, when Paula was 19 yr old, her brother was killed in a road traffic accident. After the initial grief Paula's parents were extremely reluctant, quite understandably, for Paula to buy a motorcycle and offered to pay for car driving lessons. They also agreed to help purchase a car for Paula when she passed her test.

In due course, the test was passed and the car bought. Within 3 mo of the test in spring 1979 when she was 21 yr old, Paula, too, was involved in a very serious road traffic accident. No other car was involved and it appeared that Paula had lost control and crashed into a tree. She sustained very severe head injuries and, like Jenny in the previous chapter, was in a coma for 3 mo. Unlike Jenny, however, Paula survived with severe physical as well as cognitive difficulties. In addition to cortical damage, Paula had sustained brain stem damage, which resulted in a permanent spastic quadriplegia together with moderately severe dysarthria. These remained unchanged for the next 2 yr.

Following the accident Paula was admitted to a large hospital in a big city about 20 miles from her home. One of the staff at the hospital was a remedial gymnast. This profession no longer exists in the United Kingdom but until 1987, remedial gymnasts were found in many hospitals and, to some extent, were employed as partially trained physiotherapists. The senior remedial gymnast at Paula's hospital was interested in coma stimulation and frequently saw Paula to "stimulate" her with ice packs and steel wool. His approach was controversial and considered by some people to be ethically dubious. Eventually Paula emerged from the coma although there is no way of knowing, of course, whether or not the stimulation hastened the end of it. During the coma, Paula's family played tapes of her favorite music and tapes containing conversations and messages from people she knew. When she did come out of the coma, the local press reported on her "Miracle Recovery." Needless to say, there was no miracle recovery and Paula, like most people with a 3 mo coma (reflecting very severe brain damage) remained with significant problems despite showing some improvement over time.

The next stage in Paula's treatment was early rehabilitation and she was duly admitted to the rehabilitation department of the same hospital where she had received her acute care. The same remedial gymnast was involved in her rehabilitation and subjected Paula to some rather harsh treatment. Among other things he fitted her with hip-length calipers and "walked" her around the physiotherapy gymnasium. The physiotherapists who treated Paula later in her rehabilitation felt this was inappropriate. The aim of physiotherapy for brain injured patients is to encourage normal movement and posture and to let patients experience normal movement patterns. Hip-length calipers prevent normal movement such as bending at the knees. The reeducation of postural reactions such as balance should also be encouraged in physiotherapy. Once again hip-length calipers are inappropriate for achieving this. The calipers prevented Paula from tapping into movement patterns acquired prior to her brain injury. They certainly caused pain to Paula and this man's approach was almost certainly responsible for Paula's fear of physiotherapy, which had to be tackled when she was admitted to the postacute rehabilitation center almost a year after her accident. In fact, several other patients who had been "treated" by this particular remedial gymnast demonstrated behavior problems when admitted to the postacute center. Although it is true that behavior problems are relatively common after severe head injury and should be expected in a percentage of people referred for neuropsychological rehabilitation, we observed that almost *all* patients treated by this particular man and later sent to us, had disruptive or challenging behaviors.

Paula was admitted to our center in March 1980, 11 mo after her accident. She was now 22 yr old, alert, oriented, and sociable. Although dysarthric, her speech was always intelligible and none of the staff, other patients or visitors needed

Paula to resort to a spelling board or other supplementary forms of communication in order to understand her.

INITIAL ASSESSMENT

Soon after admission Paula was referred for a psychological assessment. Unable to do any tests involving motor control because of her quadriplegia, Paula's verbal IQ on the Wechsler Adult Intelligence Scale (WAIS) was in the low-normal range. Her verbal memory appeared to be adequate. She obtained an immediate score of 10 on the recall of the Anna Thompson story of the Wechsler Memory Scale (WMS) and a delayed recall score of 8. Her recognition memory for faces was also good and she obtained an age scaled score of 12 (i.e., above average) on the prepublication version of Warrington's Face Recognition Test. On tests of object recognition however, Paula showed noticeable impairment. Her performance varied according to the size, type, and category of the stimulus. She correctly identified 62% of real objects (excluding toys and models) on first presentation and her performance improved to 86% when these were rotated in front of her. With toy objects her performance dropped to below 40% correct and she identified correctly less than 25% of model animals. Her ability to recognize drawings and photographs ranged from 0% to 36%. Her poorest performance was on the Graded Naming Test (GNT) where she could not identify a single item. On Warrington and Taylor's (1978) unusual views she managed 15%. Even when photographs of the usual or prototypical views were presented, Paula could only identify 20%. When asked to match the unusual view with the usual view Paula made 7 (out of 20) errors. Her performance on line drawings was also poor. She identified 36% of the easy Oldfield-Wingfield (1965) drawings. These results can be seen in Table 16.1.

Paula's visual fields were assessed and found to be full. Her visual acuity was also adequate, so poor eyesight could be ruled out as an explanation for her object recognition deficit. In addition she had scored well on the Recognition Memory for Faces Test. Because of the quadriplegia we could assess neither drawing nor tactile object recognition. Paula could identify environmental sounds without error so there was no question of auditory agnosia.

When Paula was asked to describe the function of an object she had misidentified (her physical handicaps prevented miming) she invariably indicated the use of the object she had *named* rather than that of the object presented to her. For example when she was shown a picture of a BUOY she said it was a "TURNIP" and then described it as "a vegetable used in stews or given to cows to eat." Her errors were predominantly suggestive of visual rather than semantic confusions and on the Lexical Understanding with Visual and Semantic (LUVS) distractors test (Bishop and Byng, 1984) in which the subject has to point to a named object

Table 16.1. Paula's Neuropsychological Assessment Results

TEST/TASK	SCORES
Wechsler Adult Intelligence Scale	Age scaled scores
Verbal subtests	
Information	5
Comprehension	10
Arithmetic	4
Similarities	12
Digit span	4
Vocabulary	9
Verbal IQ	IQ = 85 (Low normal)
Performance IQ	Couldn't do
Unusual views	3/20
Usual views	4/20
Naming from description	13/15 (Plus 2 correctly recognized from a choice of 3)
Counting the number of dots on a card	0/10
Raven's colored matrices	Unable to do
Famous faces	5/10 Correct (Mild impairment)
National Adult Reading Test (words spelled to her)	Predicted premorbid IQ at least 94
Lexical decision (distinguishing words from nonwords)	78% Correct (Impaired)
Wechsler Memory Scale	
Personal and current information	100%
Orientation	100%
Mental control	Mildly impaired
Associate learning	Mildly impaired
Logical memory (prose recall)	Immediate recall = 10 (Average) Delayed recall = 8 (Average)
Warrington Recognition Memory Test (prepublication version)	
Words	Age scaled score = 13
Faces	Age scaled score = 12
Real objects	
Static	31/50 (62%)
Rotated	43/50 (86%)
Toys/miniature objects	6/16 (37.5%)
Model animals	6/26 (23%)
Photographs	
Unusual views	3/20 (15%)
Usual views	4/20 (20%)
Line drawings	
Wingfield-Oldfield	11/30 (36.6%)
Graded Naming Test	0/30 (0%)

in an array that includes either semantically or visually confusable distractors, her errors were invariably from the visually confusable items. The errors themselves were sometimes intriguing. For example, the line drawing of a KANGAROO from the GNT elicited the response "TOILET." Paula could neither point to nor trace an outline of the object to support her interpretation but she was asked to try to explain her responses. This occurred with the kangaroo. I said to her, "Are you sure it's a toilet?" she replied, "Yes, there's the toilet bowl," and she nodded her head towards the back of the kangaroo. With a little imagination one could just about "see" a toilet bowl. Another bizarre error occurred with a photograph of a hand-held drill. Paula looked at it carefully and said, "It's a beefeater." A beefeater is a soldier in a distinctive costume at the Tower of London. Beefeaters wear black hats and I assume Paula saw the black handle of the drill as the beefeater's hat. Sometimes she verbally described a picture in an attempt to cue herself. This did not always work. In the GNT there is a drawing of a thimble above a finger. Paula focused on the thimble, she said, "It's white and bumpy, it must be a cauliflower."

From these and other errors, it is clear that Paula, despite full visual fields, was not attending to the whole stimulus. If pushed she could describe a number of the individual features of the objects presented. For example, with the kangaroo, once she had offered the name "toilet bowl" I asked her to describe what she could see. She said, "There are two long things at the bottom—it might be a handle." (These were the kangaroo's feet.) "What else can you see?" I asked once again. "There's another long thing. Is it another handle?" (This was the kangaroo's tail.) So Paula could see all (or most) of the picture yet could not integrate her impressions into a whole. She had simultanagnosia, i.e., an inability to see two stimuli or more than one part of one stimulus at a time. The term itself was first coined by Wolpert (1924) to describe a condition whereby patients could identify individual details or elements of pictures and objects yet could not appreciate the overall meaning.

Farah (1990) in her interesting book on visual agnosia says there are two distinct forms of simultanagnosia namely dorsal simultanagnosia and ventral simultanagnosia. People with the former condition are typically unable to identify objects and their perception has a "piecemeal" quality to it, i.e., "they may recognize some part or aspect of an object and guess the object's identity of the perceived feature" (p. 16). People with ventral simultanagnosia however, can usually recognize a single object but do poorly with more than one object or with complex pictures. Paula fits the typical picture of someone with the former type, i.e., dorsal simultanagnosia. She had full visual fields yet could only appear to see part of a picture at a time. There are similarities between simultanagnosia and Balint's syndrome (see Sarah: Chapter 22) in which patients demonstrate an inability to direct their eye movements voluntarily, are unable to reach for or point to visual targets, and can only perceive one stimulus at a time, i.e., they have a ventral simultanagnosia. It was not possible to assess Paula's reaching because of her severe physical limitations. However, she was unlike other people with Balint's syndrome (Wilson et al., 1997) in that she had a dorsal simultanagnosia and was not able to identify single objects.

Perhaps not surprisingly, Paula's simultanagnosia extended to reading. She was able to read a few words if I pointed to one letter at a time but she frequently omitted a letter, for example she read METAL as "M–E–A–L, MEAL." She also made mistakes with individual letters reading X as "Z" and G as "C." When shown cards containing a number of large black dots—and asked how many dots there were—she failed completely even when there were only two dots present. She failed every item, even the practice ones, on the Ravens Coloured Matrices being unable to attend to the central stimulus and to the six choices available. It will be remembered that Ron (Chapter 12) with his severe tunnel vision, could do this task reasonably well.

Paula's performance on a variety of simultaneous and delayed visual matching tasks was very poor. She was given one task using Attneave shapes (Ratcliff, 1970). These are silhouettes of nonsense shapes. One item was shown to her and then removed. Immediately afterwards a set of four shapes were presented with Paula being required to select the first stimulus shown from the array. She scored 7 out of 20. Even when the first stimulus was left in front of her Paula could only achieve 10 out of 20. This is a poorer score than that of any of the men with right hemisphere missile wounds studied by Ratcliff (1970).

There was no evidence of dysphasia (apart from her inability to identify visually presented objects). On a naming to description task Paula correctly identified 13 out of 15 objects described and correctly identified the remaining two items when given three choices. The nature of her errors and the decline in her scores when presented with less realistic material strongly suggested a perceptual rather than a naming disorder. Following discussion with her therapists and with Graham Ratcliff, an attempt was made to improve Paula's object recognition. At the same time Paula's physiotherapist was expressing concern over Paula's behavior in her physiotherapy sessions. The treatment programs for these two problems will be described separately in the order they were treated in the clinical psychology department.

Fear of Physiotherapy

I was approached by Paula's physiotherapist within 2 wk of Paula's arrival and asked if I could do anything for Paula's extreme fear of her physiotherapy sessions. I knew our physiotherapists were kind and sensitive and also experienced in working with brain injured people. For them to ask for help meant the problem was an unexpected one. When clinical psychologists are referred patients exhibiting extreme fear, they are usually faced with patients exhibiting an emotional disorder. Desensitization programs, for example, can be very effective for those with phobias such as an extreme fear of spiders or fear of the hydrotherapy pool (Wilson, 1991b). Sometimes the fear is secondary to a cognitive difficulty such as fear of walking because of loss of depth and distance perception (ibid.). In Paula's case, however, the fear seemed to have resulted from pain and inappropriate earlier treatment. She appeared to have learned to be afraid of her physiotherapy exercises and consequently her fear manifested itself as a behavior problem. When asked to engage in a difficult exercise she screamed, cried, shouted, and trembled. Without her physiotherapy, her contractures would get worse and her quality of life severely restricted. She needed to be flexible enough for her parents to be able to take her to the toilet, get her dressed, and get her in and out of the car or else she would probably have to remain in institutional care for the rest of her life.

Following some preliminary observations and discussions with Paula's physiotherapist, it emerged that three exercises caused particular problems in physiotherapy, namely trunk rotation, long sitting (sitting with one's legs straight out), and bridging (lifting one's bottom from the floor with bent knees). We decided to take baselines on how much time Paula spent on each exercise before making a fuss. This turned out to be a few seconds in each case. We also noticed during the baseline recording that there was one exercise Paula actually enjoyed. This was head balancing. We felt she enjoyed this because it was easy for her and caused no pain.

The treatment plan we devised was to use a multiple baseline across behaviors design (Wilson, 1987e) and tackle one problem exercise at a time. We would record the time taken on all exercises but during the first week only ask Paula to increase the time spent on the trunk rotation exercises. The procedure would be to (1) tell Paula how long she had spent on this exercise the previous session, (2) ask her to try to beat her previous record, (3) if she succeeded in beating her previous record she could spend a few minutes on head balancing exercises (we were using the Premack Principle here, i.e., using a desired activity to reinforce an undesired activity), and (4) give visual feedback in the form of a graph (although we realized Paula probably would not be able to interpret the graph because of her simultanagnosia, we felt that the attention she received in making and explaining the graph would be positively reinforcing).

The time Paula spent on trunk rotation increased steadily during the week. At the start of the 2nd wk, we applied steps 1–4 (above) to long sitting (in addition to trunk rotation) and once again, Paula's time gradually increased. Bridging was tackled in week 3 and, again, Paula spent longer and longer at this exercise. This shaping approach together with the staggering of the treatment for each exercise resulted in Paula's spending an appropriate amount of time on her physiotherapy exercises. Furthermore, she quickly came to enjoy her physiotherapy session, her contractures decreased, and she was easier for her family to transfer from one place to another and easier to dress.

Object Recognition

Once Paula was engaging in her physiotherapy sessions, treatment for her object recognition problems began. Dr. Graham Ratcliff designed this program with me. Initially, a simple pilot study was carried out to compare five different treatment conditions. Twenty line drawings that Paula had named incorrectly were selected and randomly assigned to one of five conditions.

PILOT STUDY

Condition 1:   The original stimuli which Paula had failed to recognize were laid aside and several alternative examples (between 20 and 30) of each stimulus were collected. These were held up in front of Paula about 12 inches from her face and she was told "this is a (kangaroo)" giving the name of the stimulus. The original stimuli were not exposed during this treatment stage.

Condition 2:   This was similar to Condition 1 except that only one alternative picture of the stimulus object was used.

Condition 3:   Several different examples of the incorrect responses to drawings were collected, shown and labeled as in Condition 1. For example, she had erroneously called a pair of tweezers an airplane so she was shown 30 different pictures of airplanes and these were verbally identified for her. The original stimuli were not exposed.

Condition 4:   The original stimuli were exposed *once* only and labeled as in Condition 1.

Condition 5:   No form of training was given on one subset of stimuli to check for spontaneous improvement.

Treatment began 2 mo after the first assessment. Paula was seen at this stage for 1 h per day, 5 days a wk, for 2 wk. The pictures from Conditions 1 and 3 were shown in every session. Pictures from Conditions 2 and 4 were shown on the 1st day only.

RESULTS

The results are shown in Figure 16.1. There was little or no improvement on the control stimuli (Condition 5) or in Conditions 2 and 3. Condition 1 led to a 50%

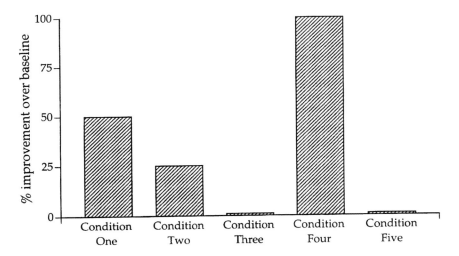

Figure 16.1. Paula's improvement over baseline in a pilot study comparing four different treatment methods and a no-treatment control condition.

improvement but was very time consuming. Condition 4, in which she was simply told the name of the original stimulus on a single trial, led to correct identification of all the stimuli.

Because the preliminary experiment suggested that simple labeling of the stimulus was a quick and effective way of teaching Paula to recognize objects, this method was selected as the main treatment. We now wanted to determine how many such labels she could learn and how long she could retain them.

LABELING METHOD OF TEACHING OBJECT RECOGNITION

During the next 6 mo, over 10 sessions, Paula was shown 93 drawings that she had previously failed to name and these were named once only in the same manner as Condition 4 in the pilot study. Three pictures were exposed on the first occasion, a further three on the second, four on the third, seven on the fourth and fifth, twelve each on the sixth and seventh, and fifteen each on the eighth, ninth, and tenth sessions. From session 3 onwards she was tested, at each session, for recognition of all the pictures that had been presented up to that time. Thus, at session 10 she was tested on all 93 pictures.

A further series of 52 control drawings which she had also failed to name were presented (between 3 to 7 each session) but were not labeled. At the end of the training period she was presented with alternative examples of 20 of the objects for which she had learned names in order to determine whether or not she could generalize the names she had learned.

RESULTS

The results are shown in Figure 16.2. At the end of the training period Paula was able to name 89 of the 93 objects on which she had been trained, but only 6 of the 52 control stimuli. She was able to learn at least 15 labels during any one session (this being the maximum number attempted) and retain them for 10 wk between initial presentation and first recall for a total period of 6 mo. Unfortunately, however, she correctly named only 6 of the 20 alternative pictures indicating that her learning was specific to the training stimuli and did not generalize to other examples of the objects in question. Nevertheless, as I have discussed elsewhere, generalization can be taught or built into rehabilitation programs.

The results of the labeling method suggest that Paula was learning names for specific visual patterns as specific new paired associates rather than being cued by provision of the correct object name or learning to recognize objects as examples of their class. If this were so, one would expect that Paula would show equal facility in learning the incorrect name for any object that she did not recognize and be able to learn names for nonsense shapes.

Accordingly, towards the end of the 6 mo treatment period, Paula was shown 10 line drawings of objects which she had previously failed to name and these were labeled with *incorrect* object names. The names used were also the names of objects that Paula had failed to recognize in the past. She was able to remember six of these names and associate them with the "correct" stimulus both on immediate recall and when retested 2 days later.

At the same time she was given three consecutive learning trials in which she was required to learn 10 labels (object names) for 10 meaningless shapes using a procedure similar to that of the Associate Learning Subtest (ALS) of the WMS. She remembered 4 out of 10 on trials 1 and 2, and 7 out of 10 on trial 3. If we regard this task as analogous to learning the difficult pairs on the WMS-ALS, then Paula would achieve the very respectable score of 15 in Wechsler's terms.

While the results of these two tasks confirm that Paula was good at learning unrelated visual–verbal paired associates, her scores of 60% correct on the object task and 70% correct after three training trials on the nonsense figure task are clearly inferior to her performance on the task in which she was required to learn the *correct* name for an object that she did not recognize when she performed at a level of approximately 95% correct. There were at least three possible reasons for this dissociation. First, it is very likely that the nonsense figures are less discriminable than the line drawings we used in other tasks. Second, although she was unable to name all the line drawings we used in our attempts to teach her incor-

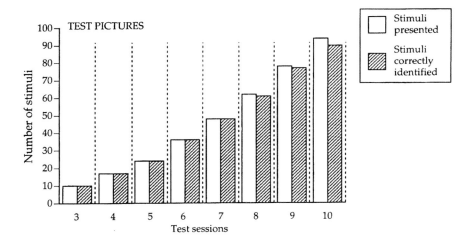

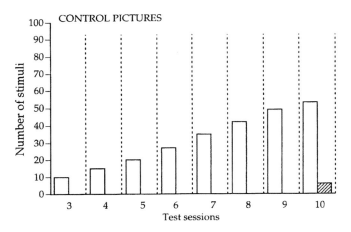

Figure 16.2. Number of stimuli presented and correctly identified after Experiment 2.

rect object names, she was satisfied in several instances that the name we gave her was indeed incorrect. Thus she may have rejected some labels as being inappropriate names for the objects to which they were attached that, in turn, may have interfered with her learning of the labels. Third, it may be the case that her excellent performance in learning the correct name for objects was not entirely the result of learning a new, arbitrary label for the stimulus but, on some occasions, the result of being cued in by the provision of the correct name.

Paula's ability to associate names with line drawings suggests that an ability to recognize visual patterns could not have been the sole cause of her impaired object recognition—had she been unable to discriminate the drawings she would presumably have been unable to learn names for them. This is of interest in view of her very poor performance on some visual matching tasks mentioned earlier. These tests typically used stimuli (in our case random shapes), which are more difficult to discriminate than line drawings of object. It follows, therefore, that poor performance on such tasks, while it may indeed indicate that presence of a perceptual deficit, does not constitute a sufficient explanation for failure to recognize objects. In view of this and her poor performance on Warrington and Taylor's (1978) Unusual Views Test it is tentatively suggested that the main cause of Paula's failure to recognize objects is an impairment at a later stage of perceptual processing—perhaps at the level of "perceptual classification" (Warrington and Taylor, 1978) or the information of a "3D model representation" (Marr, 1982; Ratcliff and Newcombe, 1982).

From the point of view of rehabilitation, our results might be considered disappointing. Although Paula learned a very high proportion of the object names we attempted to teach her, the learning was largely specific to the particular representation on which she was trained and thus unlikely to be of practical use to her outside the laboratory. Nevertheless, it was possible to teach her the names of some objects present in her everyday life, and we planned to tackle the generalization problem by (1) presenting Paula with the same object (or picture) in many orientations and (2) gradually moving from the original stimulus to others very similar and then less similar. Given that (1) this kind of generalization works well with learning disabled people (Yule and Carr, 1987) and (2) Paula learned very rapidly in the labeling procedure, we would have expected to be able to "teach" generalization. Before we could implement this program, however, Paula's father discharged her from the rehabilitation center against the advice of all the staff. Although able to accept Paula's physical handicaps, her father had never come to terms with her cognitive problems and had refused to accept the findings from our cognitive assessment. Like Jenny's father in Chapter 15, he lost a son prior to his daughter's accident and was, not surprisingly, quite possessive of his only surviving child.

FOLLOW-UP

Despite many attempts over the next 14 yr, Paula's father refused to let us see her again or provide information about her current situation. We believe she is still alive but have no information at all on whether or not she continued to improve, remained the same, or deteriorated.

17

KIRSTY: A CASE OF OPTIC APHASIA, ASSOCIATIVE AGNOSIA, OR SEMANTIC MEMORY IMPAIRMENT?

BACKGROUND

Kirsty was almost 17 yr old in September 1982. She was school captain, she had 7 "O" levels, and was planning to go to University. Described as "happy, sociable, strong-willed and rebellious," her life was to change drastically following a car crash in which her father was killed. Her parents had separated 2 yr earlier, Kirsty lived with her younger sister, younger brother, mother, and her mother's partner. Early in September Kirsty spent the weekend with her father who was driving her home when the accident occurred.

Kirsty sustained a very severe head injury and was unconscious for several weeks. A CT scan carried out during this period showed no focal changes, enlarged ventricles, contusion, and areas of infarction in the left temporal lobe. There was also some suggestion of optic nerve atrophy. She remained in the hospital for over 4 mo before spending 2 wk at home and then a further 4 mo at a rehabilitation center.

On admission to the rehabilitation center Kirsty was described as having a hemiplegic right arm and weakness of the right leg although she was able to walk with a stick. She had reduced visual acuity in her right eye and suffered from petit mal seizures that were controlled with anticonvulsants. Emotionally Kirsty was described as passive and labile and still grieving over her father's death.

Soon after admission Kirsty was referred to clinical psychology for an intellec-

tual assessment. Having already been assessed by the speech therapist and occupational therapist, the severity of Kirsty's cognitive problems was obvious. The
speech therapy report said Kirsty had a mixed dysphasia with both comprehension and expressive difficulties. She also had specific word finding problems and
frequently made syntactic errors. All these areas were thought to be improving.
In addition, Kirsty had severe reading, writing, and calculation impairments. The
occupational therapist said Kirsty had significant memory and calculation difficulties and was unable to read numbers.

INITIAL ASSESSMENT

Because of Kirsty's severe cognitive problems the WAIS was not considered to
be appropriate. The British Ability Scales (BAS) and the Raven's Standard Progressive Matrices (RSPM) were used to assess her general intellectual functioning. Mental age scores on these tests ranged from 5.5 yr for digit recall to 8 yr for
the BAS matrices. On the RSPM Kirsty performed at the 7.5-yr-old level. Her
basic perceptual skills appeared to be reasonably intact as she could count the
number of items on a page, match (but not name) colors, copy and match shapes,
and even copy the Rey-Osterreith Complex Figure. On higher level visuoperceptual tasks however, she was impaired. She scored in the abnormal range on both
Unusual and Usual Views (Warrington and Taylor, 1978) and on a face perception task (Benton et al., 1975). On an unpublished test designed to elicit visual
and semantic errors (similar to Bishop and Byng's 1984 Lexical Understanding
with Visual and Semantic distractors [LUVS] test), Kirsty made both visual and
semantic errors although far more of the latter. Scores on both immediate and delayed memory tasks were poor although Kirsty appeared to recall incidental
events and episodes relatively well. Her naming of pictures and objects was very
impaired. She named only four pictures from the Oldfield-Wingfield test (an easy
naming test) and only one of seven real objects. She was unable to name any
shapes or colors and she could not name from description. She was, however,
able to mime the use of some of the objects and could name a few real objects
when asked to identify them by touch.

Kirsty's reading was virtually nonexistent. She could not read aloud any words
from the Schonell Graded Word Reading Test nor could she read any individual
letters in upper or lower case. She could, however, recite the alphabet and could
also copy letters and words without error. On a lexical decision task, i.e., deciding whether a printed word was a real word or a nonsense word, her performance
was at chance. We felt the mild visual sensory deficit (reduced acuity in her right
eye) could not explain the reading and naming difficulties given her adequate
performance on the basic perceptual tests. Kirsty's results from this and later assessments can be seen in Table 17.1. The main conclusions from this initial assessment were as follows:

Table 17.1. Results from Kirsty's Assessments in 1983, 1984, and 1993

TEST	Results (Age level or number correct)		
	1983	1984	1993
British Ability Scales			
Speed of information Processing	7 yr 3 mo	6 yr (possibly due to anxiety)	—
Matrices	8 yr	10 yr 6 mo	— (Improved)
Similarities	6 yr 9 mo	7 yr	—
Recall of digits	5 yr 6 mo	5 yr 6 mo	—
Digits from Wechsler Adult Intelligence Scale	Aged scaled score 3 (Impaired)	Age scaled score 4 (Well below average)	Age scaled score 8 (Marked improvement)
Raven's Standard Progressive Matrices	7 yr 6 mo	11 yr 6 mo	—
Visual tasks			
Counting dots on a page	All correct	All correct (Seemed to be much faster)	—
Counting lines on a page	All correct	—	—
Color matching—10 color squares and 10 colored circles	All correct	—	—
Perceptual			
Copying and matching shapes	All correct	—	—
Rey-Osterreith Copy	30/36 (Unimpaired)	—	—
Recall	0/36 (Impaired)		
Benton four choice matching task	6/10 (Impaired)	7/10 (Still impaired)	—
Same/different faces	13/20 (Impaired)	9/20 (Some decline)	—
Unusual views	7/20 (Impaired)	7/20 (Unchanged)	5/20 (Little change /slightly worse?)
Usual views	10/20 (Impaired)	14/20 (Slight improvement)	14/20 (No change)
Benton Face Recognition	8/13 (Impaired)	—	—
Drawing from memory (tree, man, bicycle)	All recognizable	—	—
Learning on Seguin form board	Trial 1 = 56 sec Trial 4 = 44 sec (Evidence of learning)	—	—
Reading			
Schonell Graded Word Reading Test	Unable to read any words	Reading age 6 yr 3mo (Poor but improved)	—

(continued)

Table 17.1. Results from Kirsty's Assessments in 1983, 1984, and 1993 (*continued*)

| TEST | Results (Age level or number correct) | | |
	1983	1984	1993
Reading single letters			
Upper case (visual condition)	0/26	All except B,E,V,J,Q	—
Lower case (visual condition)	0/26	—	—
Reading tactile letters	4/26	All except X,Q	—
Reciting alphabet	No errors	—	—
Easy lexical decision	10/24 (Chance)	—	—
Copy letters and words	100% correct	—	—
Numbers			
Identifying and copying digits	100%	—	—
Naming digits	50% Correct	100% Correct	—
Naming and Language			
Oldfield-Wingfield	4/18 (Impaired)	11/18 (Improved)	17/36 (Improved)
Naming from description	0/15 (Impaired)		—
Naming objects	1/7 (Impaired)	4/7 (Improved a little)	—
Tactile naming	5/7 (Probably OK)	6/7 (Improved a little)	—
Naming colors	0/20 (Impaired)	11/20 (Improved)	
Fluency			
"S"	0	—	—
"Animals"	3 (Plus 4 perseverative errors)	—	—
Visual Agnosia Test	31/60 (Impaired)	50/60	47/60 (Little change)
(unpublished but similar to LUVS, see Bishop & Byng, 1984)	Errors: Visual = 9 Semantic = 18 Random = 2	Errors: Visual = 9 Semantic = 18 Random = 0	Errors: Visual = 9 Semantic = 4 Random = 0
Apraxia (Left hand only)			
Gesture with limbs	3/6 (Impaired)	—	
Manipulation with limbs	2/6 (Impaired)	—	
Bucco facial	100% Correct	—	

1. Presumably Kirsty was probably of above average ability given her educational achievements.
2. Her current general intellectual functioning would appear to be at the level of a 7–8-yr-old.
3. The slight visual sensory loss with somewhat reduced visual acuity in her right eye does not seem to be sufficient to explain her problems with object recognition, naming, and reading—given that she can match colors and shapes and can count the number of items on a page.
4. Kirsty has difficulty in the recognition of objects and complex patterns such as faces. Her tactile recognition of objects would appear to be better than her visual recognition.
5. She has some language difficulties in that she is unable to name objects although on occasion she is able to mime their use.
6. The problems outlined in 4 and 5 suggest Kirsty might have optic aphasia. This is a modality specific condition whereby people are unable to name visually presented objects but (a) are able to show recognition by indicating or miming use of the object and (b) show preserved auditory and tactile naming. Kirsty, of course, has diffuse cognitive difficulties so it is not possible to be sure about the optic aphasia. However, we plan to investigate this in greater detail.
7. Staff may wish to capitalize on Kirsty's superior tactile recognition in certain circumstances. Meanwhile, the clinical psychology department will see her on a regular basis to (a) investigate the optic aphasia in more detail, and (b) try to improve her reading skills.

INVESTIGATION OF OPTIC APHASIA

Optic aphasia is a term introduced by Freund (1889) to describe one of his patients with a right homonymous hemianopia and dysphasia following a left parietal tumor (see Rubens, 1979). The term is used currently to describe patients who manifest an inability to name visually presented objects although they are able to name the same objects when these are presented through another modality or who can demonstrate recognition by pointing or through pantomime. Lhermitte and Beauvois (1973) described a patient with optic aphasia who could point to objects on command and indicate the use of objects. He could also *write* the name of the object despite being unable to *say* the name. Rubens (1979) notes two of his patients whose pattern of deficits resolved from associative visual agnosia in the first few months to optic aphasia in the chronic period.

Farah (1990) discusses the similarities and differences between associative visual agnosia and optic aphasia. She points out that some researchers believe the two conditions differ in degree rather than in kind. She said (p. 85),

The distinction . . . has not always been made clearly in the literature, and there is disagreement over the relation between the two syndromes. Some authors have theorized that associative agnosia is nothing but optic aphasia (Geschwind, 1965). Others have assumed a less extreme, but also less clear position, stating that optic aphasia is equivalent to a *mild* associative agnosia (e.g., Bauer and Rubens, 1985; Kertesz, 1979). Still others have suggested that optic aphasia is a *type* of associative agnosia, in which perception is truly normal (Humphreys and Riddoch, 1987).

Based on Farah's (1990) discussion of the similarities and differences between the two conditions I have drawn up a table comparing and contrasting optic aphasia and associative visual agnosia (see Table 17.2).

Table 17.2. A Comparison of Similarities and Differences Between Optic Aphasia and Associative Visual Agnosia

	OPTIC APHASIA	ASSOCIATIVE VISUAL AGNOSIA
Naming of visually presented objects	×	×
Copying of objects	√	√
Indication of visually presented objects through pointing or miming	√	×
Naming of objects when presented in another modality	√	√
Naming to description	√	√
Semantic errors made in naming	√	√ (but not as frequent as visual errors)
Visual errors made in naming	Rare	√
Location of lesion	Left posterior possibly occipital	Bilateral occipito–temporal lesions
Handicapped in everyday life	Tend not to be	Often are
Sensitivity to visual quality of stimulus	×	√

×, cannot do well.
√, can do well.

Farah concludes that optic aphasia and visual associative agnosia are distinct syndromes, although, as she notes, it is quite possible for patients to have a combination of the two conditions.

In order to help determine whether or not Kirsty had an optic aphasia, we investigated her ability to recognize objects and letters through the visual and tactile modalities. The procedure was as follows:

1. Visual modality. (a) Objects: Ten real objects were selected and presented one at a time. First Kirsty was asked to name the object. The object was then rotated and again she was asked to provide the name. Third, Kirsty was asked to demonstrate use of the object. (b) Letters: All 26 upper case plastic letters about 1″ high and ¼″ thick were presented in random order, one at a time. First Kirsty was asked to name the letter or to say the sound the letter made. Second, the letter was rotated and she was asked to provide the name or the sound.

2. Tactile modality. (a) Objects: The same 10 objects were presented one at a time behind a screen. Kirsty was asked to place her hands in the slot at the front of the screen and manipulate the object with her left hand only, as she could not use her right hand, and then to say the name. If she failed to provide a response or made the incorrect response, she was asked to show how the object would be used. (b) Letters: All 26 plastic upper case letters were presented one at a time behind a screen and Kirsty asked to name the letter or provide the letter's sound.

On the object recognition task Kirsty scored 1/10 correct in the visual condition, 8/10 correct in the tactile condition, and at least 7/10 when asked to demonstrate the use. It is possible she actually scored even higher but two responses (to onion and comb) were ambiguous. Rotating the object did not help. With regard to letters, she was unable to identify any in the visual condition and four in the tactile condition. These results can be seen in Table 17.3. Thus, although not perfect, she was certainly better in the tactile condition. Of course, some people with associative visual agnosia can identify by touch. Ratcliff and Newcombe (1982), suggest that agnosic people who can identify by touch have a disconnection syndrome and those who cannot (like Jenny in Chapter 15) have a visual semantic memory disorder. What people with associative agnosia cannot do however, is indicate use of the objects they are unable to name visually.

Another characteristic of optic aphasia according to Farah, is that visual errors made in naming are rare while semantic errors are common. On a test involving pointing to target pictures with visual, semantic, and random distractors (described above), Kirsty was correct on 31/60 items, she made 9 visual errors, 18 semantic errors, and 2 random errors. In this area therefore, she made rather a high number of visual errors and thus did not quite fit the picture described by

Table 17.3. Kirsty's Results on Visual and Tactile Recognition of Objects and Letters

OBJECTS	VISUAL–STATIONARY NAMING REQUIRED	VISUAL–ROTATED NAMING REQUIRED	MIMING USE MIMING REQUIRED	TACTILE NAMING REQUIRED
Onion	Carrots	Beans	? Peeling	For dinner
Coin	For buyings thing	No response	Paying money √	Money √
Comb	Brush hair	Brush?	? Brush or comb	√
Toy horse	Horse √	Horse √	Riding √	√
Candle	No response	No response	Lighting it √	√
Tin opener	No response	No response	Opening tins √	Can opener √
Pen	Use it	(Pointed to psychologist's pen)	Writing √	√
Matchbox	For lighting	You light it	Striking a match √	√
Plate	Saucer	For cup of tea	Putting cup on saucer	Saucer
Spoon	Fork	For cup of tea	Stirring tea √	√
Total	1	1	7	8
Letters	Visual			Tactile
26 Upper case letters presented	Failed all letters			Identified A K M T

√, correct response.

Farah. Nevertheless, she made more than twice as many semantic as visual errors. In retrospect, I wish we had asked Kirsty to draw from memory the objects she could not name. As it was, we asked her to draw only three objects from memory (a man, a tree, and a bicycle). All these were easily recognizable.

The location of the lesion as identified by the CT scan did not confirm the typical areas involved in optic aphasia or in associative visual agnosia. Kirsty's primary lesion was in the left temporal lobe although the length of her coma suggested a diffuse head injury in addition to the left temporal damage.

Our conclusions in light of (1) superior tactile over visual naming, and (2) her ability to mime or demonstrate the use of some visually presented objects she was unable to name, suggested she showed at least some of the characteristics of optic aphasia. We recognized, however, that this was not a pure or clear-cut syndrome.

REMEDIATION OF LETTER RECOGNITION

Given that it is sometimes easier for brain injured people to read through the tactile route than the visual route (see Derek, Chapter 14), we decided to capitalize on Kirsty's slightly superior tactile ability and use this to teach her to recognize letters. We hoped this would then provide a means for her to read again.

A pilot study was carried out in one session to see if it were possible for Kirsty to learn new letters through the tactile route. Three 1" high and $^1/_4$" thick plastic letters (B, H, O) were placed in Kirsty's left hand, one at a time. She was (1) asked not to look at the letter, (2) encouraged to note the distinctive features of the letter (e.g., O is perfectly round with no corners or breaks), and (3) asked to try the name of the letter several times. During one session lasting $1^1/_4$ hr all three letters were presented nine times and then tested after a 10-min delay. In the testing condition, the three practiced letters were interspersed with three untrained letters (N, C, X). Kirsty named all three of the trained letters but none of the untrained ones. These same six letters were then presented visually. Kirsty failed to name any of them.

These results suggested that Kirsty could indeed learn in the tactile condition. Following the pilot study she was seen for a further eight sessions over a 4 wk period. The distractor letters from the pilot study were selected for treatment together with seven other randomly selected letters making 10 in all. The letters taught were C, D, G, L, N, R, S, U, W, and X. Three letters were taught in the first session, then another added in the second, and so on. The procedure adopted was identical to that used in the pilot study. Following training Kirsty was tested on all the letters she already knew at the start of the study (i.e., A, K, M, T) plus the three learned in the pilot stage. She appeared to find this reinforcing and we wanted to increase her self-esteem by ensuring success. Following this, Kirsty was tested with the letters taught so far. Each taught letter was presented three times in random order. In order to be recorded as "successfully learned," the letter had to be named correctly on three consecutive presentations. She never saw the letters during training, all training was achieved through touch.

Following the eight training sessions, Kirsty was assessed 2 days later on all 26 letters of the alphabet, i.e., both trained and untrained letters and in both visual and tactile conditions. In the tactile condition she had learned 8 of the 10 trained letters, and remembered the original 4 letters and the 3 taught in the pilot study. With the remaining two letters (introduced in sessions 7 and 8) she was correct on one of the three occasions for both L and U. In the visual condition she was only correct with two letters, O and X. These results can be seen in Figure 17.1.

Kirsty was obviously able to learn fairly quickly with this method. We wanted to extend the training program to teach her the remaining letters of the alphabet through the tactile method and also to see if we could teach her to recognize let-

Letters		Initial assessment	Treatment Sessions								Final assessment
			1	2	3	4	5	6	7	8	
Letters recognised	A	✓	✓	✓	✓	✓	✓	✓	✓	✓	✓
initially and	K	✓	✓	✓	✓	✓	✓	✓	✓	✓	✓
rehearsed each	M	✓	✓	✓	✓	✓	✓	✓	✓	✓	✓
session	T	✓	✓	✓	✓	✓	✓	✓	✓	✓	✓
Letters taught in	O	✓	✓	✓	✓	✓	✓	✓	✓	✓	✓
pilot and rehearsed	H	✓	✓	✓	✓	✓	✓	✓	✓	✓	✓
each session	B	✓	✓	✓	✓	✓	✓	✓	✓	✓	✓
Letters trained	W	✗	✗(2)	✗(2)	✗(1)	✗(2)	✗(1)	✗(2)	✗(2)	✗(2)	✓
during eight sessions	S	✗	✓	✗(1)	✗(2)	✗(1)	✓	✓	✗(2)	✓	✓
	D	✗	✗(1)	✗	✓	✓	✓	✓	✓	✓	✓
	C	✗	—	✗(1)	✗(2)	✗(0)	✗(0)	✗(0)	✗(0)	✓	✓
	R	✗	—	—	✓	✓	✓	✓	✓	✓	✓
	X	✗	—	—	—	✓	✓	✓	✓	✓	✓
	G	✗	—	—	—	—	✓	✓	✓	✓	✓
	N	✗	✗	—	—	✗	—	✓	✓	✓	✓
	L	✗	✗	—	—	✗	—	—	✗(1)	✗(2)	✗(1)
	U	✗	✗	—	—	✗			✗(1)	✗(1)	✗(1)
Untrained letters	E	✗	—	—	✗	—	—	—	✗	—	✗
	F	✗	—	—	✗	✗	—	—	—	—	✗
	I	✗	—	—	✗	—	—	—	—	—	✗
	J	✗	—	—	—	✗	—	—	✗	—	✗
	P	✗	—	—	—	✗	—	—	—	—	✗
	Q	✗	—	—	—	✗	—	—	✗	—	✗
	V	✗	—	—	—	—	✗	—	—	—	✗
	Y	✗	—	—	—	—	—	✗	—	✗	✗
	Z	✗	—	—	—	—	✗	—	—	✗	✗

Key: ✓ = 3 correct responses
✗ = 0/2 correct responses
— = not tested
⌐ = Training started

Figure 17.1. Results of the tactile reading program for Kirsty.

ters through the visual route. Unfortunately, Kirsty was very reluctant to stay at the rehabilitation center which was a $3^1/_2$ h drive from her home. She had been in the hospital or rehabilitation for most of the 9 mo since her accident and wanted very much to return home. The staff agreed this might be the best thing for her and suggested she return again for a follow-up period in about 6 mo time.

REASSESSMENT

In fact it was 9 mo before Kirsty returned for an assessment. Her mother had now remarried and agreed with Kirsty that this time she would only spend a week at the center. Kirsty enjoyed being at home and wanted to be away from her family as little as possible. We were able to readminister many of the tests given the year before and noticed considerable improvement on some tests as can be seen in Table 17.1.

Kirsty was cheerful and relaxed during the assessment and seemed to be feeling more positive about herself than she had the previous year. She was careful about her appearance and appeared to be proud of how much she had achieved since returning home 9 mo earlier. Her speech was more fluent, her word-finding difficulties were less obvious, she completed tasks faster, and concentrated for longer periods of time before needing a break.

Although Kirsty's short-term memory as assessed by forward digit span had not changed a great deal, her mother reported that at home Kirsty appeared less forgetful. Her perceptual difficulties were perhaps a little better than before but were nevertheless still significantly impaired. The main area of improvement was in the area of language. Kirsty could read a few words, and could identify most letters of the alphabet and more of the real objects. There was little evidence to suggest optic aphasia although she was still marginally better at identifying letters of the alphabet by touch than through vision.

Kirsty's mother was, on the whole, pleased with the progress Kirsty had made. She had arranged private physiotherapy for Kirsty and private tuition from a remedial teacher supervised by a speech therapist. She felt Kirsty not only enjoyed these sessions but also had gained in confidence as a result.

We recommended a further assessment in a year's time but in fact it was to be nearly 9 yr before I saw Kirsty again.

FOLLOW-UP IN 1993

In January 1993, I visited Kirsty at her home for one of my follow-up studies. I was interested to see how she was getting on and wanted to readminister some of the earlier tests and perhaps give her other tests which had not been appropriate or available for her in 1983 and 1984.

As with all the follow-up subjects, I began by asking Kirsty what she now saw as her main problems. She replied, "I don't think I have many. I don't have much use of my right hand so I can't do certain things. If I have to do something with two hands I ask other people." Her mother said Kirsty was rather like a tape, bits of which have been erased. "I wouldn't leave her alone," she continued, "because she doesn't have any fears." "Are there any other problems?" I asked. Kirsty's mother said, "If I ask her to get the shampoo she'll spend ages and then get the wrong thing. She can't go out alone, she wouldn't know what bus to get or where to go. If we're on holiday she gets confused." Kirsty chipped in here saying, "I can remember everything from before the accident but I get lost easily now." Her mother added "She's good at ironing and make-up but she can't be self-sufficient."

I went on to ask what Kirsty had been doing since I last saw her in 1984. I learned that she had attended a community center for a while. The Department of Health and Social Security (as it was then) paid for Kirsty's taxis to and from the center. "It didn't work out," said her mother who added, "there's very little help for people of Kirsty's age. We saw centers for people with Down's syndrome, for blind people, and for physically handicapped people but I wouldn't allow her to go there. I paid for private physiotherapy twice a week and arranged for her to help out with children at a local kindergarten. That was more a social thing really. We didn't join Headway (the National Head Injuries Association) as I didn't think they would offer much. She's at home now and doing voluntary work 2 mornings a week in the kindergarten. There are 30 children there between 3 and 5 yr old. Kirsty helps with painting, writing, and naming and she keeps an eye on them, she does picture puzzles and can walk there. I would have liked her to get more education but now I think we don't want to push her anymore. She's comfortable here."

"Is Kirsty in touch with any friends she had before her accident?" was my next question. I learned that Kirsty writes regularly to one friend and another friend comes to visit once a year. When I asked if she had made new friends, I was told by Kirsty that she had three friends of her own age and had gone on holiday with one of them. Her mother added, "She doesn't have a good social life though."

Kirsty was able to get out of the house every day and she belonged to a swimming club where she was the youngest member. Her mother thought Kirsty got on better with older people. Her greatest pleasure was to listen to music and do the ironing at the same time. She ironed impeccably with her left hand, having been right-handed before her accident. She also enjoyed going out if she could find a companion. She was envious of her sister who was always going out and who was usually reluctant for Kirsty to go with her. Kirsty found it difficult to meet people of the opposite sex and did not have a boyfriend.

I wanted to know whether Kirsty had epilepsy. Apparently in the hospital immediately after the accident, she had a seizure every few minutes. The frequency decreased and stopped altogether before she left the hospital to go to the rehabilitation center. She was still on a small dose of anticonvulsants.

Before readministering any tests, I asked both Kirsty and her mother about specific cognitive difficulties. They showed little agreement on this as can be seen in Table 17.4 They were, however, in complete agreement on the noncognitive items.

I administered only one test on this occasion (the unpublished visual and semantic errors test given in 1983) as we had spent most of the afternoon talking and completing the questionnaires. I was able to return a few weeks later though to readminister a few other tests and these results can be seen in Table 17.1. In addition, I administered the Corsi Blocks on which Kirsty's forward span was 5, i.e., in the normal range. I also asked her to write "The quick brown fox jumps over the lazy dog," which she did in a beautiful neat hand and with no errors. In addition, after administering the Oldfield-Wingfield test of picture naming, I asked her to define the names of the pictures she had been unable to name, e.g., she thought the picture of a horseshoe was a hair clip although when asked later, "What is a horseshoe?" she said, "It's on the bottom of a horse's foot so he can walk properly—it's

Table 17.4. Responses from Kirsty and Her Mother about Current Cognitive and Other Problems

PROBLEM AREA	KIRSTY'S RESPONSE	MOTHER'S RESPONSE
Attention or concentration	No	Yes
Memory	No	Yes—short-term memory
Thinking things through or working things out	No	Minor problems
Finding the right word	No	Yes
Reading	No	Yes
Writing	No	Yes—it's very basic and very phonetic
Understanding what you see	Yes	Yes
Sleeping	No	No
Bladder or bowels	No	No
Finances	No	No
Anything else	No	No

like half a circle." In fact she unambiguously identified 10 of the 14 verbal names with one more probably correct. Thus for "tuning fork," she said, "Is it a long thin thing for pianos? He takes the top off and tunes it high or low."

Again, although Kirsty had shown very little improvement on the perceptual tasks, she had improved in her recall of digits and her naming of the Oldfield-Wingfield pictures.

Because Kirsty appeared to have some semantic memory problems and I was now working in Cambridge, I arranged for her to be admitted to a Cambridge hospital for a few days to be assessed by Dr. John Hodges, one of the world's leading experts in semantic memory. He arranged for Kirsty to have an MRI scan during her admission. In the summer of 1993 Kirsty's stepfather brought her to Cambridge where she was to spend 3 days.

FURTHER ASSESSMENT AND INVESTIGATION OF SEMANTIC MEMORY: SUMMER 1993

The relative rarity of semantic memory disorders following traumatic head injury is, perhaps, partly due to a lack of awareness of the characteristics of semantic memory impairments by neuropsychologists who routinely assess head injured patients. Although a typical neuropsychological assessment includes tests of language, memory, and perception, i.e., skills through which semantic knowledge is established, such knowledge is not always considered in its own right. Yet in a follow-up study of 50 severely head injured people originally seen several years earlier (Wilson, 1995b), at least three could be described as having disorders of semantic memory using the criteria of Patterson and Hodges (1995). These criteria are:

1. Selective impairment of semantic memory causing anomia, impaired single-word comprehension (both spoken and written), reduced generation of exemplars on category fluency tests, and an impoverished fund of general knowledge,
2. Relative sparing of other components of speech production, notably syntax and phonology,
3. Unimpaired perceptual skills and nonverbal problem solving abilities, and
4. Relatively well-preserved episodic memory.

Wilson (1997) describes four patients with semantic memory disorders, two of whom had herpes simplex encephalitis and two a severe traumatic head injury, one of these was Kirsty.

Kirsty was assessed on a number of tests in an attempt to confirm or disconfirm semantic memory impairment. She also had an MRI scan.

The MRI scan showed severe yet selective damage to the anterolateral portion of the left temporal lobe and, to a lesser extent, the inferior parietal region. The hippocampal formation was relatively well preserved and the right side looked normal. The primary lesion location is consistent with the claim made by Patterson and Hodges (1995) that the temporal neocortex appears to be the crucial region for semantic memory impairment.

What about Kirsty's performance on other tests? Did this confirm semantic memory impairment? She was given the semantic memory battery described by Hodges et al. (1992b) and Hodges et al. (1992a). (This battery is described in more detail in Jason's chapter [Chapter 9]). As can be seen in Table 17.5, Kirsty's performance was, on the whole, worse than that obtained from people with moderate Alzheimer's disease and far worse than young controls or elderly controls.

Like a number of patients reported including Jason (Chapter 9), Kirsty had more difficulty with living than with man-made items. These results can be seen in Table 17.6.

As in the assessment a few months earlier, Kirsty continued to find the definition of words easier than the recognition of pictures. In the 1993 assessment she recognized 17/36 pictures on the Oldfield-Wingfield test but could give a good definition of 30/36 words. On the more difficult Graded Naming Test (McKenna and Warrington, 1983), she recognized only 3 pictures yet could define 16 words. This ability to access information more easily via one route (verbal) than another (visual) suggests the semantic memory difficulty is because access to the system is damaged rather than damage to the system itself (Hodges et al., 1992a; Wilson, 1997d). In contrast, Jason in Chapter 9 had problems both in defining words and in naming pictures suggesting that in his case, the system itself was damaged.

To what extent did Kirsty fulfill the criteria for semantic memory impairment outlined earlier? The first characteristics included anomia, impaired single-word comprehension, reduced fluency, and an impoverished fund of general knowledge. Kirsty's naming, fluency, and comprehension were all poor as can be seen from the results in Tables 17.5 and 17.6. In addition she achieved an age scaled score of 4 on the WAIS-R information subtest (a test of general knowledge) which, once again, is in the impaired range.

Relative sparing of other components of speech production, notably syntax and phonology was the second characteristic. Kirsty spoke clearly, pronouncing words very well with no evidence of poor phonology. Her syntax, too, was apparently normal. For example, when asked to define "syringe," she said "It's something doctors have when they want to draw some blood."

The third characteristic described unimpaired perceptual skills and nonverbal problem solving abilities. As we saw earlier, Kirsty's basic perceptual skills were intact. In 1993, the Visual Object and Space Perception Test (Warrington and James, 1991) was administered to provide further evidence about her perceptual functioning. She scored at ceiling on the basic screening test and on all the space

Table 17.5. Kirsty's Responses on Subtests from the Semantic Memory Battery (Hodges et al., 1992 a + b)

SUBTEST	KIRSTY	MEAN FOR DAT SUBJECTS (n = 22)	MEAN FOR HODGES ET AL. CONTROLS (n = 25)	MEAN FOR YOUNGER CONTROLS (n = 8)
Fluency				
Animals	10	9.9	19.7	21.6
Birds	0	5.4	14.1	16.5
Water creatures	3	4.4	13.0	14.5
Dogs	5	3.2	10.2	12.7
Household items	10	9.1	19.8	21.5
Vehicles	9	6.9	13.9	14.2
Musical instruments	4	6.5	14.0	15.8
Boats	4	4.4	11.6	11.6
Naming				
Total correct (Max = 48)	17	35	46.5	46.6
(A) Living items (24)	7	17.1	23.3	23.0
Land animals (12)	4	8.3	11.6	11.8
Water creatures (6)	1	4.1	5.9	5.8
Birds (6)	2	4.7	5.8	5.4
(B) Man made items (24)	10	18.3	23.2	24.0
Household items (12)	7	9.7	11.9	12.0
Vehicles (6)	7	4.9	6.0	6.0
Musical instruments (6)	1	3.7	5.1	6.0
Picture–Word Matching				
Total correct (48)	41	43.1	47.9	48.0
Living items (24)	17	21.8	23.9	24.0
Man made items (24)	24	22.2	24.0	24.0
Naming to Description				
Total Correct (24)	11	7.9	22.5	22.3

perception items. She could not identify the objects of course because of her semantic memory disorder. Furthermore she achieved an age scaled score of 9 (average range) on the Block Design subtest of the WAIS-R, i.e., her nonverbal problem solving skills do not appear to be affected.

The fourth characteristic was relatively well-preserved episodic memory and here Kirsty with poor memory differed from the semantic memory patients with progressive conditions described by Hodges et al., (1992ab); and Patterson and

Table 17.6. Differences between Living and Man Made Items on Four Tasks: Number Correct

TASK	LIVING	MAN MADE
Fluency	18	30
Naming	7	10
Word–picture matching	17	24
Naming to description	6	5
Totals	48	69

Hodges (1995). Nevertheless, she did not perform like severely amnesic patients such as Jay (Chapter 4), Clive (Chapter 6), and Jason (Chapter 9). Kirsty was by now able to recall 13 of the 36 items of the Rey-Osterreith Figure after a 40-min delay. This is still poor but amnesic patients typically remember nothing. She scored 4 out of 12 items from the Rivermead Behavioural Memory Test, i.e., in the moderately impaired rather than the severely impaired range. On the recall of the stories from the WMS-R Kirsty recalled a total of 11 items on immediate recall and 5 items after a 20-min delay. While not good, these results suggest her episodic memory is not as severely impaired as someone with an amnesic syndrome and the poor scores are, at least in part, secondary to her semantic memory disorder. She certainly has reasonable recall of day-to-day events.

Patterson and Hodges' semantic memory patients also have a surface dyslexia (so too does Jason in Chapter 9). What about Kirsty's reading? It will be remembered that initially she was completely alexic. Dr. Hodges' team administered the reading tests during Kirsty's admission to Cambridge. He wrote, "her surface dyslexia is only apparent on the low-frequency-exception words but like many of our patients she is much worse on writing than reading, again showing an effect of regularity."

In conclusion, Kirsty appears to have changed over the course of time into someone with fairly clear-cut semantic memory problems. After her return home I wrote to her trying to explain in fairly simple language her main areas of difficulty. This is an excerpt from the letter.

> Dear Kirsty,
>
> I hope you were not too tired after your trip to Cambridge. We certainly enjoyed having you with us, and were very impressed with your persistence and cooperation with the testing.
>
> I have scored all the tests you did with me. You should be hearing from Dr Hodges about the MRI scan and the other tests in 2 or 3 weeks time.
>
> As I expected you have a particular problem with recognising objects. This cannot be explained by poor vision as you were able to do other tests requiring vision with absolutely no trouble. It is because the "object processing centres" in your brain were affected in the accident. The difficulty with colours is part of this picture. So

too, are the reading problems. You have learned to read again but have particular difficulty with irregularly spelled words (or non-phonetic words). The same is true of your spelling, you spell words as they sound. This works fine for some words but not for those which are spelled in an irregular way.

The difficulty with reading is called "surface dyslexia" and the difficulty with spelling is called "surface dysgraphia." The object recognition problem is called "visual object agnosia." You also have a tendency to recognise man-made things better than living things such as animals. One of my tests, for example, where you had to name model plastic animals was particularly hard for you.

Another reason for believing your problem is not due to poor eyesight is that you have difficulty describing what things look like—particularly animals. This is done by getting a mental picture inside your head so you do not need vision for this.

However, you still have a great deal of information available about animals and objects. You can tell me if they can be eaten or not, if they are normally found in Britain or not, if certain substances smell and so on. It is just the physical appearance of certain things (not all things) which cause you problems.

Despite all these difficulties, Kirsty, you have lots of strengths. In addition to your strength of character which is impressive, you were very good on a number of my tests. On spatial tests (e.g., judging which number in one square corresponded to a dot in another square), you scored as well as anybody else your age would. On a spatial reasoning task where you had to work out how many blocks would be needed to complete a pattern, you scored 100%. You learned a new short route in one go and remembered it after a 20 minute delay. You were able to copy a complex spatial figure. On a short attention test you obtained maximum points. You also scored perfectly on a test of planning a route to search a field where you, supposedly, had lost your keys. Finally you showed good insight and awareness of your problems and behaviour on a questionnaire I asked you to complete.

So, all-in-all, Kirsty, you have considerable ability and, given the severity of your accident, have done remarkably well.

If you want to discuss any of these results with me then please telephone.

With very best wishes to you and your mother.

Yours sincerely,

(Dr) Barbara A Wilson

A BRIEF EXPERIMENT ON ERRORLESS LEARNING

During one of the sessions Kirsty spent with me during her stay in Cambridge I decided to see if she could relearn some animal names and carried out a brief experiment using the errorless learning procedure described in Chapters 6 and 9.

Kirsty had been asked to name 32 model plastic animals. She was correct on 7 (dog, cow, kangaroo, skunk, lion, antelope, and sheep). Of the remainder I selected 15 animals and allocated these to 3 groups: 1 group of 5 animals was to be taught in an errorless way, 1 group in an errorful way, and 1 group would be untaught. The procedure for the errorful and errorless learning was virtually identical to that used to teach Jason (Chapter 9) the names of pictures. So in the errorless condition Kirsty was shown the animal, told the correct animal name, and

Table 17.7. Results from a Brief Experiment Comparing Errorless and Errorful Learning to Reteach Animal Names

	INITIAL RESPONSE	RESPONSE FOLLOWING TRAINING	SCORE
Errorless Stimuli			
Carthorse	Fox	Carthorse	1
Otter	King Kong	Otter	1
Brown Bear	In America	Bear	1
Goat	Fox	Goat	1
Deer	See them at Christmas	Deer	1
Total			5
Errorful stimuli			
Palomino	Antelope	Horse	$1/2$
Ostrich	On farms—a duck	Duck	0
Polar Bear	Squirrel—have them in our garden	Bear	$1/2$
Pig	Antelope	Sheep	0
Lamb	Fox	Wolf	0
Total			1
Untaught stimuli			
Rhinoceros	Bull	Elephant	0
Tiger	Lion	Lion	0
Gorilla	Half man and half human—a monkey	Monkey	0
Foal	Wolf	Fox	0
Kid	Fox	Deer	0
Total			0

asked to write it down. We went through all five animals in random order for five trials. Then Kirsty had a 10-min break. After the break I showed her the animals one at a time and asked her to tell me what the animal was. For the errorful procedure I showed an animal and asked Kirsty to have three guesses at what the animal was. After three guesses I told her the correct name which she wrote down. Again we followed this procedure for five trials, changing the order of presentation each time. Once again we had a short break before the test during which each animal was presented once and Kirsty asked to identify it. Finally, after another short break in which we chatted for about 10 min, the untaught animals were presented one at a time for Kirsty to identify. The results can be seen in Table 17.7.

Thus, at least in the short term, Kirsty would appear to be able to relearn new animal names using errorless learning. If she lived nearer, I would certainly have tried to employ this method to extend new learning and to ensure generalization

by testing her at gradually increasing intervals, i.e., adopting an expanding rehearsal approach similar to that used with Laurence (Chapter 11).

KIRSTY TODAY

Kirsty was very reluctant to come back to the hospital again and her mother and
stepfather felt she had been through enough and should be left to get on with her
life as best she could. Consequently I have not seen her since 1993. She still lives
at home, still helps out at the kindergarten, and continues to have private physiotherapy. She showed considerable recovery after a lengthy period of coma. When
I first knew her she showed some signs of optic aphasia although it was not possible to be absolutely certain of this condition. Nine yr later though, when she
had recovered sufficiently to be examined with additional tests, her condition appears to have resolved into a more clear-cut semantic memory disorder.

18

RICHARD: A SOCIALLY SKILLED YOUNG MAN DESPITE SEVERE MEMORY AND PERCEPTUAL DIFFICULTIES

BACKGROUND

Richard was born in August 1973, the youngest of three children. Following a normal pregnancy and delivery his first few weeks passed uneventfully. When he was 10 wk old, however, he woke his parents in the early hours of the morning and was obviously unwell. For the following 4 days he was crying and irritable and vomited frequently. He was admitted to a nearby children's hospital, a lumbar puncture was performed, and the results suggested a recent intracranial hemorrhage. Richard remained unwell, vomiting after feeds, and at 13 wk was referred to a neurological center. On admission, there was evidence of rising intracranial pressure with a tense bulging fontanelle and prominent lamdoid sutures. Richard continued to be irritable, he was also anemic but there were no other abnormalities noted. Over the next few days he became less irritable but his head circumference was increasing rapidly. He began vomiting again and a ventriculogram showed a communicating hydrocephalus with no obvious cause. A shunt was inserted on November 11, 1973. Following this operation Richard progressed well. He began feeding normally and his head circumference reduced.

No underlying etiology was determined during this admission although it was suggested that an angiography be performed in the future to see whether Richard

279

had a surgically remedial lesion. Apparently this procedure was not carried out until several years later.

Over the next few months Richard was seen regularly in the neurosurgery outpatients department. In July 1974, at 11 mo old, he was readmitted to the neurological unit because of vomiting and listlessness. There seemed to be problems with the valve of his shunt although this sorted itself out after a few hours. Richard was kept in the hospital for 5 days of observation during which time the valve appeared to be functioning quite normally. The neurosurgeon in charge of Richard's care felt that although the valve was probably "sticking" at times, he should leave matters alone for the present because Richard remained reasonably well and he did not want to stir things up. Richard's mother was concerned about the possibility of the shunt sticking or blocking but the neurosurgeon told her that even if it did "stick," nothing catastrophic would happen immediately and there would be plenty of time to get Richard to the specialist unit.

Richard remained well and continued to be seen regularly in neurosurgery. The consultant did not wish to interfere with the shunt as Richard was doing so well. In fact all did go well for several years until the 30th of September 1983 when Richard was 10 yr old. At this time he developed a severe occipital headache and neck stiffness. Vomiting followed and Richard was admitted to the children's ward of the local hospital. At first it was not clear whether he had another hemorrhage or was suffering from a viral or meningitic illness. A CT scan showed an intraventricular bleed and an angiography a few days later showed an arteriovenous malformation in the parietal region of the right hemisphere. At midnight on October 6th Richard had a sudden onset of rigidity and arching of his back. A respiratory and cardiac arrest followed and he had to be resuscitated. A further CT scan revealed he was suffering from another bout of hydrocephalus. Bilateral parietal burr holes were performed and a right ventriculo-peritoneal shunt inserted. Richard was transferred to the intensive care unit where he slowly improved and several weeks later was well enough to be sent back to the children's ward.

Richard remained in the hospital for over 3 mo. His neurosurgeon felt it was too dangerous to excise the angioma. So negotiations began between Richard's local health authority and a hospital in Sweden. The plan was to send Richard to Stockholm for stereotactic radiotherapy treatment to seal his blood vessels and prevent further bleeds. Although now available in the United Kingdom, this treatment was then available only in Stockholm.

FIRST PSYCHOLOGICAL ASSESSMENT

In December 1983, some $2^1/_2$ mo after his second hemorrhage, 10-yr-old Richard was referred to the pediatric psychology department for an assessment of his cognitive functioning. Some subtests from the British Ability Scales were administered. Richard was below average on matrices (a nonverbal reasoning test) and immediate and delayed visual recall. He was within the average range for similarities (a verbal reasoning test) and digit recall. His visual recognition was estimated to be at a $3^1/_2$-yr-old level and his naming ability at a $7^1/_2$-yr-old level.

The psychologist who assessed Richard wrote in the report that physical and articulatory problems made the assessment difficult. Although friendly and cooperative, Richard became frustrated when he could not make himself understood. He was also distressed over his physical difficulties.

The psychologist went on to say that Richard was fully oriented in time and situation. He described his family and his school, knew his age, and the ages of his siblings. The test results showed very wide discrepancies between his auditory and visuomotor abilities with his verbal memory and verbal reasoning remaining relatively intact and his spatial reasoning, visual perception, and visual memory all severely impaired.

In January 1984, the neurosurgeon noted, "there has been very great improvement. Richard is now fully continent, his walking has improved, his speech has improved, he is a happy child who speaks with a slight dysarthria. His vocabulary is extensive." Richard's vision at this time was described as follows: "To confrontation there is a marked constriction of both visual fields. Acuity is normal."

An educational psychologist also saw Richard in January 1984 to assess him prior to advising on school placement. She administered the Wechsler Intelligence Test for Children-Revised. These results can be seen in Table 18.1.

Richard's verbal IQ was estimated to be 85 (low average) and his performance IQ less than 45 (severely impaired).

The educational psychologist recommended Richard attend a special school and start as soon as possible. She felt he had "massive educational and psychological needs" that should be addressed without delay.

Meanwhile negotiations were completed with Stockholm and Richard went with his parents in February 1984 for just over 2 wk. All expenses were paid by the National Health Service. He was readmitted to neurosurgery in May 1984 for an overnight stay to have an angiography. This showed "no evidence whatsoever of any residual vascular malformation." The treatment then was successful and Richard has had no further hemorrhages.

Following his return from Sweden Richard went first to a day school and then to a boarding school—both schools were for children with special needs.

The neurosurgeon continued to see Richard every year. In 1987, when Richard was 13, with concerns about his transition from school to adult life beginning to emerge, Richard was referred to the rehabilitation consultant. In 1988, he was also referred to me for assessment of his memory and perceptual functioning and advice on rehabilitation. I first saw him in August 1988 just before his 15th birthday.

Table 18.1. Richard's Results on the Wechsler Intelligence Scale for Children-Revised January 1984 (Aged 10 yr)

	RAW SCORE	SCALED SCORE
Verbal Tests		
Information	12	8
Similarities	10	7
Arithmetic	8	5
Vocabulary	32	11
Comprehension	13	7
Verbal IQ = 85		
Performance Tests		
Picture completion	3	1
Picture arrangement	2	1
Block design	0	1
Object assembly	4	1
Coding	0	1
Performance IQ = less than 45		

FIRST NEUROPSYCHOLOGICAL ASSESSMENT

Richard came to see me twice during the summer holiday and I arranged to see him again during the Christmas holidays when he was home from boarding school. The results of the August assessment can be seen in Table 18.2.

I noted that Richard was very cooperative, he appeared to enjoy doing the tests, and as far as I could tell carried them out to the best of his ability.

Neuropsychologically Richard was a very interesting young man showing a pattern of deficits consistent with a right hemisphere cerebral vascular accident, which indeed he had sustained twice, at the age of 10 wk, and 10 yr.

I felt his visuoperceptual and visuospatial problems were not due to poor eyesight or to visual sensory loss as he could identify some complex material. He attempted perceptual or spatial tasks by trying to verbalize the task. His ability to recognize famous faces was extremely poor. When shown a photograph of Billie Jean King, the tennis player (whom I thought Richard might be too young to identify), he said to me, "Is it you?" I did not reply so he looked again and said, "It *is* you, isn't it?" I still did not reply so he looked a third time and said to me, "Do you wear glasses?" I told him I did not wear glasses whereupon he said, "Oh well it can't be you then can it?" Nobody else has ever thought I resembled Billie Jean King. He also scored poorly on tests of unfamiliar faces. On the Behavioural Inattention Test (Wilson et al., 1988) Richard had particular problems on those subtests where detailed scanning was expected and where the density of the stimuli was high.

I did not assess Richard's memory in as much detail as I would have wished because we were restricted to two sessions owing to his return to school. Although I thought it possible that some of his memory problems might result from faulty perception, I had little doubt that he had severe memory problems over and above this. It is possible that some of the memory deficits were due to anoxic brain damage sustained at the time of his respiratory and cardiac arrest. My conclusions to this report were as follows:

1. Had he not had the hemorrhages, Richard would probably have been of at least average ability—judging by the evidence of the Graded Naming Test and his overall vocabulary.
2. Currently, he has considerable visuospatial and visuoperceptual deficits which cannot be explained by poor eyesight or visual field loss.
3. Some of these perceptual problems are:
    a. Poor and erratic scanning—he may jump a line, start scanning from the right or in the middle of a page, and omit sections of a page. This makes reading, writing, and copying slow, difficult, and full of errors.
    b. He finds face perception tasks difficult. This is true for both famous faces and for unfamiliar faces. It is not clear how far this is a problem in real life but he thought two photographs of famous people (Margaret Thatcher and Billie Jean King) were photographs of me.
    c. He was unable to identify photographs of common objects when these were taken from an unusual view. He had no difficulty with the same objects taken from a conventional or usual view. This demonstrated Richard could *see* adequately and he was not hampered by *naming* problems. (Indeed his naming to verbal description was good.)
    d. He is sometimes unable to reach objects accurately or judge accurately where someone is pointing—for example he went to the wrong door when I pointed out the toilet to him.
4. These deficits are all associated with right hemisphere (and in particular right temporo-parietal) damage.
5. Richard's immediate verbal memory span is normal. He has difficulty retaining information after a delay or distraction. It is possible that some of these memory problems are secondary to perceptual deficits.

Before I saw Richard again during the Christmas holidays, I saw a copy of a letter from the school psychiatrist asking the rehabilitation consultant if there could be "a neurological reason" for Richard's memory problems, his inability to read a timetable, and his problems finding his way around the school. The psychiatrist had assumed Richard's problems were emotional in origin but wanted to be sure. It is hard to believe how Richard's early neurosurgical history could have escaped notice!

Table 18.2. Richard's Neuropsychological Assessment Results

TEST	SCORE (1988)	COMMENT	SCORE (1994)
British Ability Scales Word Reading List	Reading age = 8 yr	Although well below average for his age, some of the errors were due to scanning problems and to omitting letters within a word	Reading age = 10.5 yr
Graded Naming Test	Raw score = 13	Probably within average range for his age	Raw score = 17 (Improved—average range)
Rivermead Behavioural Memory Test	Screening score = 0/12 Standardized profile score = 2/24	Severely impaired range	
Immediate Memory Span	Digits forwards = 7 Digits backwards = 3 Corsi blocks = 3	Average Below average Below average	5 (Low average) Backward = 3 Corsi = 5 (Average)
Naming to Description	14/15	Within normal limits	
Unusual views	2/28	Severely impaired	7/28 (Still impaired)
Usual views	27/28	Normal	27/28 (Normal)
Same/different Faces	9/20	Chance. Impaired	13/20 (Still impaired)

Famous Faces		
Without context	2/29	Ronald Reagan and Princess Diana
With context	5/29	Elvis Presley, Margaret Thatcher, Daley Thompson, Princess Diana, and the Queen
Identifying person from name	13/29	Probably within normal limits for his age
Behavioural Inattention Test		
Conventional tests	Total score = 132/146	Evidence of neglect on star cancellation and figure/shape copying
Behavioral tests	Total score = 62/81	Evidence of neglect on picture scanning, article reading, telling and setting time, coin sorting, and card sorting
Rey-Osterreith Complex Figure	Copy = 12/36 Recall = 0/36	Severely impaired
Grooved Peg Board	Right hand 5 min 43 sec Left hand—unable to do	Extremely slow Could only lift peg with left hand and then transfer to right hand
		Still evidence of neglect on star concellation

His end-of-term school report provided further information on Richard's progress and difficulties. His class teacher reported examples of his memory lapses and confusion between the period September–December 1988. She said he frequently turned up in class at the wrong time especially in the afternoons. He had great difficulty in locating his pen, pencil, ruler, and other belongings even when his pencil case containing these items was in front of him. He had problems copying from a work card or text book to a piece of paper or transferring numbers into a calculator. On one occasion when returning to school from a visit to town, Richard failed to recognize the building where he lived thinking it was a newly built house.

Richard's physiotherapist also noted that despite working hard, Richard's memory often let him down and he needed frequent reminders about the task in which he was currently engaged. He also forgot instructions in the swimming pool, which could be dangerous if he were not properly supervised. The care staff said he could not follow lists of any kind and appeared to be increasingly frustrated at his inability to remember things. He was extremely slow getting dressed, he often called out to the staff but when someone came Richard would forget why he had called. He was unable to cross the road safely, seemed unaware of the passing cars, and was often lost.

These examples graphically illustrate how Richard's memory, perceptual, and visuospatial impairments caused problems in his everyday life. He was always a popular boy and well liked by just about everyone who knew him. His school report said, "[he] has a charming, easygoing personality." Nevertheless there appeared to be a serious misunderstanding of his perceptual and spatial problems. The fact that he was easily lost, could not follow lists, find his belongings, or transfer work from one place to another, was unaware of cars and had problems getting dressed, are all readily explained by his spatial disorientation, inattention, scanning problems, and so forth. The memory problems were easier to understand but even these were thought to be due to emotional causes especially as Richard's parents had recently divorced and his mother was about to remarry. I am sure this did not help Richard but his significant cognitive problems were without a doubt due to the intracranial hemorrhages sustained several years earlier.

The one person who did have some understanding of the nature of Richard's difficulties was his speech therapist. She wrote that his language skills continued to be affected by his visuoperceptual difficulties and memory problems. Although he had a good understanding of concepts and vocabulary, his comprehension for both visual and verbal material was compromised by his poor memory. His ability to use visual aids as a memory prompt was affected by his perceptual problems which prevented him from locating a detail in a chart, text, or illustration. Despite a laborious reading rate Richard's reading age had progressed by a full 12 mo during the past term but his reading was frequently hampered by his tendency to lose his place and question the accuracy of words he read correctly in the first place. The speech therapist concluded her report by saying that Richard's expressive skills were basically sound in relation to vocabulary and syntax although he sometimes had difficulty organizing what he wanted to say largely due to recall problems, which affect his memory for names, events, and information. To me this seemed a sensible and accurate summary of Richard's functioning.

I saw Richard once again just before Christmas while he was on holiday from school. I wanted to look at his visual short-term memory in more detail. Did he have a straightforward deficit in his visuospatial span or did he also have problems with visual imagery, i.e., "seeing with the mind's eye?" I knew from the previous assessment that his Corsi span was poor. He could manage only a sequence of 3 blocks whereas most people, even those with brain damage, can manage 5 blocks (Wilson, 1996). On a visual short-term memory (VSTM) recognition test based on one by Phillips (1983) and described in Chapter 11 on Laurence, Richard made failures on the 3×2 matrix, i.e., he was very impaired in comparison with amnesic patients. He also had problems with certain tasks dependent on visual imagery. He was poor at describing the kind of tails certain animals had, saying a greyhound had a bushy tail and a monkey had no tail. He was able to indicate the color of most things presented to him, and which of two objects was the larger. Richard was given the Manikin Test (Ratcliff, 1979), a test of right–left discrimination dependent on mental rotation. In this task, several drawings of a manikin are presented. In each drawing the manikin is holding a black circle in either the right or left hand. The manikin is presented sometimes facing the subject and sometimes with its back to the subject. In addition the manikin may be upright or inverted (see Figure 18.1).

The task is to say whether the manikin is holding the circle in the right or the left hand. Richard was at chance on this task whether the response was oral or whether Richard lifted his own right or left hand to indicate the answer. Another task dependent on visual mental rotation, the Flags Test (Thurstone and Jeffrey, 1956) caused Richard such difficulty that it had to be abandoned. It would appear then that Richard had a visuospatial sketchpad deficit in addition to his other difficulties.

ADVICE ON MANAGEMENT

During the December 1988 visit, Richard's mother expressed her concern at the school reports. She had recently remarried and knew Richard might have been upset by the divorce and the new arrangements but nevertheless felt the school was being too critical of Richard and mistaken in the belief that he had deteriorated. I felt it was more likely that his problems had become more apparent as demands on his cognitive skills increased. Although I could not offer direct rehabilitation to Richard I agreed to write to the school to see if I could arrange a visit

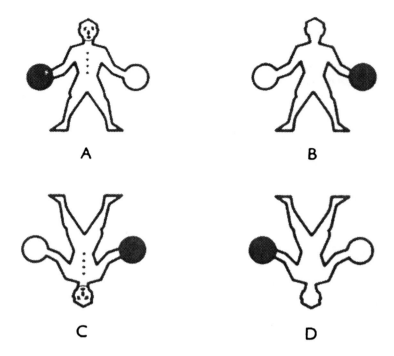

Figure 18.1. An example from the Manikin test (Ratcliff, 1979).

to try to explain Richard's cognitive difficulties and how these might affect his day-to-day functioning. I wrote in January 1989 explaining that in addition to his memory difficulties he had severe visuospatial and visuoperceptual problems that prevented him from making efficient use of lists and instructions and would cause him problems in finding his way around. I said that people with right hemisphere damage often respond poorly to rehabilitation and this might be the reason Richard appeared to "stand still." I offered to visit to try to discuss any problems with the staff.

While awaiting a reply, Richard's neurosurgeon wrote to ask if I thought he would ever be able to obtain paid employment. I replied that I thought his chances of employment on the open market were slim and that he would probably always need sheltered employment.

I eventually visited the school in May 1989. I talked to a group of staff involved in Richard's care and found it informative to see how the neuropsychological deficits manifested themselves in his everyday life. Richard recognized me straight away but whether from my voice or my face it was hard to say. He had been told I was coming and told I was there when he was brought to see me, so his recognition could have been due to a number of factors. He had problems showing me around, he could not find his mug in the kitchen (among an array of 8 mugs), his work books were untidy, and he was very slow at most tasks. The main reason for my being there was to try to convey to the staff that Richard's problems were not due to laziness, emotional distress, or to his being difficult, but were the result of cognitive impairments caused by his strokes in early childhood. It is often hard for people to understand perceptual and spatial difficulties. Typically they interpret these as meaning poor eyesight but it was not Richard's eyes or visual acuity at fault. He simply had difficulty interpreting or making sense of certain things, he was unaware of certain parts of the spatial scene, could not attend to all aspects of an array, and had problems understanding the spatial relationships of components of a figure or array. I did my best to convey the nature of Richard's problems and make some suggestions about compensating for his difficulties, e.g., make his mug a very distinctive color and shape from the other mugs so it would be easier to identify; try to encourage him to use the same route from one part of the building to another as he did not have an overall spatial map and use verbal cues, e.g., "go in the door by the window box" rather than "turn right at the end of the building." As Richard was nearing the end of his stay at this school and due to move to a college for youngsters with physical handicaps in September, I felt I was unlikely to change the behavior or attitudes of the staff to any great extent.

I saw Richard for a few more tests and a further discussion before he moved on to the college. He was impaired on the Benton et al. Face Recognition Test (score 36/54), on the Rey-Osterreith copy and recall (16 and 0 respectively), on cube counting (9/16), position discrimination (9/16), and the Hooper Visual Organisation Test (8/30). These results simply confirmed what we already knew, that Richard had very severe problems with these kinds of tasks.

Richard's mother was concerned about the move to the college. I knew the college well and thought it would suit Richard. The staff I had met were familiar with brain injured youngsters and the atmosphere was good. I sent my report from August 1988 and a letter explaining Richard's everyday problems.

I visited Richard at the college a few weeks after he started. His housemother talked to me and showed me Richard's bedroom and the living area. I was impressed with the way she had tried to circumvent Richard's visuospatial difficulties. The problem with his mug had surfaced as soon as Richard started at the college. He was unable to find his own mug along the shelf. This problem was solved very easily. The hook for Richard's mug was placed on a higher, separate shelf just above the other student's mugs. Now that Richard's was the only mug on the shelf, he found it easily. Another problem was finding his clothes. If he wanted clean pajamas, he could not retrieve these from the drawer. There was no shortage of storage space in Richard's room so his housemother placed pajamas in one drawer, socks in another, and so forth. She labeled the drawers and Richard found it much easier to find the clothes he needed. He was still slow and still got lost easily on the college grounds but I felt the staff saw Richard's problems as a challenge to be solved and not something he should be blamed or criticized for. I felt much happier about Richard's situation and knew the college had a tradition of trying to ensure a smooth transition from education to work or alternatives to work. For the next few years I lost touch with this young man who had always been a pleasure to work with. He was cheerful, good tempered, witty, entertaining, and socially skilled despite his massive memory, perceptual, and visuospatial problems. He had learned to read despite his scanning and attention difficulties, and his general knowledge was good despite his memory problems. He was the kind of person who brought out the best in others. His poor performance on formal tests belied his sophisticated social behavior and basically good performance in everyday life.

FOLLOW-UP

In October 1994 I had a telephone call from an occupational psychologist asking if I would reassess Richard who was undergoing an assessment for employment at a center in the south of England. I had often wondered how he was getting on so I arranged to visit with Andy Young, a colleague from Cambridge who had a great interest in face processing problems. I told Andy of Richard's earlier performance on face perception tests so we went to the Employment Rehabilitation Center to see him together.

We repeated several of the tests from 1988 and, as can be seen in Table 18.2, Richard had improved on several. He was also given some new tests including a test of motor neglect (Richard showed no evidence of motor neglect) and a new test of Famous Faces. Richard recognized and named only 5/30 (Noel Edmonds, John Major, Margaret Thatcher, Terry Wogan, and Prince Charles). On a Names test in which Richard had to say whether or not names were familiar he correctly chose 30/30 famous names as familiar and 10/10 nonfamous names as unfamiliar. He was able to provide sufficient identifying information for 26 of the 30 names and failed on four. Andy Young felt this was consistent with a memory problem but was not sufficient to explain his face recognition deficit.

Another task Andy Young gave was to show Richard pairs of photographs with the eyes of each face in each pair either looking straight at the subject or slightly averted. Richard had to identify the face looking directly at him. The eye-gaze of one of the pair of photographs deviated by 5°, 10° or 20°. Richard found this task difficult particularly with the smaller angles. His overall score was 13/18 correct (2/6 correct at 5°, 5/6 correct at 10°, and 6/6 correct at 20°).

On a test of facial expression (selecting which of six emotions was being expressed: happiness, sadness, fear, anger, surprise, and disgust), Richard made 4/6 errors in the practice items so the test was abandoned for the time being.

We both found it hard to believe this young man was so socially skilled and well adjusted given his very significant handicaps in just about all aspects of face perception and processing. I felt unable to advise the occupational psychologist about work but I wished Richard was living locally so I could try out some strategies with him. I felt he seemed less happy than when I had last seen him. He did not like being at this occupational rehabilitation center although he tried to put on a brave face. He took us to his room (after a few false starts) and made us a cup of tea despite finding this task an obvious struggle.

Andy Young went to see Richard in his own home on three further occasions in February, April, and June 1995. Richard was now living at home and attending special classes in a college near his home for 2 days a week. His mother was trying to find something more permanent for him. The results from Andy's assessments can be seen in Table 18.3.

Richard is unusual in having such a severe face processing problem. Of more than 30 gunshot wound cases reported by Newcombe (1996), none were so impaired as Richard. He is also unusual in having the onset of such problems in childhood. It seems likely that these problems dated from the hemorrhage sustained when he was 10 yr old, given that he seemed to make a fuller recovery from the hemorrhage at 10 wk.

At the time of Andy's last visit in June 1995, Richard's mother asked him about further rehabilitation. Andy checked with me and I was able to put Richard's mother in touch with Dot Henry, an occupational therapist who worked a few miles away from Richard's home. Dot agreed to see Richard and decided to tackle some of the practical problems reported by his mother. His mother said that Richard often needed to be reminded to wash, clean his teeth, and shave. His memory for facts was very selective, he was often outspoken and sometimes stood too close to people in social situations. When asked what she saw as the main problem, she thought it was to do with his grooming and self-care skills. Richard was now almost 22 yr old.

Dot asked Richard's mother to keep a chart and write down the things to do with his self-care that he forgot over a 2 wk period. Certain problems were highlighted, namely leaving clothes on the bathroom floor, forgetting to wash his face, comb his hair, gel his hair, and clean his teeth. Dot then worked out a checklist to be placed over the hand basin in his bedroom to check when he had completed these activities. She also put a notice on the bathroom door telling Richard to take his clothes out when he left. I asked Dot how Richard had managed with the checklist when this had caused such difficulty at one of his schools. She said, "The checklist was on a whiteboard in huge writing with boxes for the checks. Richard needed frequent prompting at first to check each activity but soon became familiar with it." I suspect the checklists failed at school because they were too small and Richard was not helped to establish a routine through prompting. Memory impaired people need time and teaching to fill in questionnaires or

Table 18.3. Performance of Richard and Means and Standard Deviations (SD) for 20 Control Subjects of Comparable Age

	Richard		Controls	
	10.17.94	2.8.95	MEAN	SD
Object recognition				
Living		18/20	19.35	0.88
Nonliving		16/20***	19.50	0.95
Handled		20/20		
Not picked up		19/20		
Identification of Buildings				
Famous buildings				
Recognized as familiar	17/20		17.10	2.88
Correctly identified	7/20*		13.95	4.06
Unfamiliar buildings				
Correct rejections	7/10***		9.50	0.61
Identification of Familiar Faces				
New (1991) Faces Line-up				
High familiarity faces				
Recognized as familiar	12/30***	13/30***	29.45	1.28
Occupation	6/30***	8/30***	27.65	2.39
Name	5/30***	8/30***	27.65	2.39
Unfamiliar faces				
Correct rejections	8/10**	10/10	9.45	0.60
New (1991) Names Line-up				
High familiarity faces				
Recognized as familiar	30/30	30/30	30.00	0.00
Occupation	26/30***	26/30***	29.95	0.22
Unfamiliar names				
Correct rejections	10/10	10/10	9.95	0.22
Unfamiliar Face Matching				
Benton test	Unable to complete		49/15	3.69
Gaze Direction				
Forced-choice				
5 degrees	2/6***	3/6**	4.95	0.83
10 degrees	5/6***	4/6***	6.00	0.00
20 degrees	6/6	6/6	6.00	6.00
Overall	13/18***	13/18***	16.95	0.83
Facial Expressions				
Matching		8/18***	16.95	0.83
Recognition	Unable to complete		22.00	1.97

RT aged 21 yr; control mean = 29.50 yr, SD = 5.82; mean NART-R predicted IQ = 111.55, SD = 8.72 (Asterisked scores are significantly impaired in comparison to the performance of controls: *z > 1.65, $P < 0.05$; **z > 2.33, $P < 0.01$; ***z > 3.10, $P < 0.001$).

checklists as doing so involves memory. Thus they should not be expected to re-member straight away. This, together with his perceptual difficulties meant an even greater need for prompting and practice.

Another problem Richard's mother reported to Dot was her worry about letting Richard go out to the local shops alone. Mostly he was fine but sometimes he be-came disoriented and lost. Dot constructed an official looking identification card with Richard's photograph on it and an explanation concerning his memory prob-lems. His home address and telephone number were printed on the card and Richard kept the card in his wallet. He never actually used it but both Richard and his mother felt better knowing he *could* use it in an emergency.

RICHARD TODAY

In January 1996, Richard went to a privately run training center for young dis-abled people. It promotes and facilitates independence in self-care and life skills to the maximum ability of the person concerned. It provides a safe and consistent environment for Richard to socialize and develop freely. Richard has lived there for almost 2 yr with funding to remain until at least March 1998. Both he and his mother seem happy with the arrangements. Richard sometimes confabulates (no doubt unintentionally), he might forget to eat a meal or have a wash but says and thinks he has done these things. He sometimes loses his wallet, forgetting where he has put it, and could be vulnerable in a less protected situation. He responds better in a structured environment and needs time to learn new routines. He uses an electronic organizer to store important dates and telephone numbers but needs assistance to program some of the functions. He still uses the checklist Dot Henry prepared for him.

His favorite activity at the center is gardening. This has been a consistent plea-sure for many years even though it has not been easy for Richard to cope with the visuospatial requirements of gardening and horticulture. He works better in a small group and can get upset or lose concentration if there is a change in his rou-tine or there is too much noise or too many people around.

In February 1997, Richard's mother got in touch again as she had heard about our NeuroPage project (Wilson et al., 1997) described in Chapter 5 about Alex. Initially I thought the pager would not be suitable for Richard because of his scanning difficulties and slow reading, but his mother was keen for him to try. I suggested she ask the staff at the center to refer Richard and a few weeks later Richard came to the Oliver Zangwill Center for Neuropsychological Rehabilita-tion in Ely, Cambridgeshire, where the NeuroPage project is now sited. His mother and his key worker also came and Richard was duly entered as a subject on our NeuroPage project. He responded well showing an improvement in remembering to carry out tasks when he had the pager in comparison with a baseline period before the pager was provided.

I last saw Richard and his mother in October 1997 to talk to them about this chapter. We talked first about Richard's early years, Richard's mother thought the neurosurgeon considered her to be fussy as she took Richard into neurosurgery whenever he had a headache or vomited. This seems unsurprising behavior given Richard's early history. I asked Richard what he could remember about the time before his second hemorrhage when he was 10 yr old. He remembered his primary school days and told me about an occasion when he climbed a tree and hid there until it was dark so his parents could not find him.

"What about the time you were in hospital, when you were so unwell," I said, "can you remember anything about that?" Richard said, "I can remember when I was poorly Russ Abbott (a television comedian) came to the hospital and said, 'don't worry Richard you'll get better soon.' That will stay in my heart for the rest of my life. He's a kind and caring man."

I talked to Richard's mother about the time when Richard left school. When he first left school he attended a special unit at a college as a day student for 3 yr. He did all sorts of things like Health and Hygiene, English, and even attended some lessons in Japanese for which he was awarded a certificate.

From this college, Richard went to a Garden Training Center for a year. Most of the people there were developmentally learning disabled rather than brain injured so it was not ideal for Richard although he liked the gardening and continues to enjoy gardening and horticulture. He then returned to the previous college for 2 days a week where he stayed until going to his present residential center in March 1996. At present he is funded by social services until March 1998 and they are trying to secure further funding to keep him on for longer. He is very happy at the center that was set up in the late 1980s as a center for people with learning difficulties to learn about horticulture. It is set in the most beautiful countryside with about 17 learning disabled people staying for periods of time ranging from 6 mo to 5 yr. Richard appears to be a popular member of the group with lots of people his own age and a good social life. Richard, like the other residents, has to share in the housekeeping tasks. He also spends time each day in the gardens. He does some shopping, cooking, and banking. He spends time on the computer which he particularly enjoys. He goes on trips and has recently been sailing. He took part in the Special Olympics where he competed in the shot put and the 100 meters. He has his own music center which he listens to in the evening. Sometimes he goes bowling or to the cinema, or to the pub.

Richard's mother thought that sometimes he feels at loose ends and finds it difficult to amuse himself although, for the most part, she thinks the center an excellent place for Richard to be.

I spoke to a member of staff about Richard. He said, "Richard is not the only one here with brain damage. Every one of them has a problem, we try to help them cope with their problems. Richard is very even tempered, he's witty. He's never moaned about his problem, never once said, "I wish this hadn't happened."

"Do you ever think about what happened in the past?" I asked Richard's mother. "Yes," she said, "it's very sad what happened, but it's happened and you've got to carry on, you've got to look to the future. He's very loving and easy to get on with. There's nothing you can do about what's happened—you've got to go on. Because of his personality Richard's done very well. He has his good days and his bad days but the bad aren't really bad."

Richard's final comment when asked if there was anything he wanted me to say to the readers of this book was, "You shouldn't make fun of people with disability. They've got to live their lives—like anyone else."

19

DOLLY: LEARNING TO ATTEND TO
THE LEFT SIDE OF SPACE

BACKGROUND

In June 1983, at the age of 62 yr, Dolly was a busy, active woman who worked part time in her husband's business. She was a church warden, helped with the women's voluntary service, and had a wide circle of friends. One morning Dolly woke up and heard the alarm clock ringing. She tried to reach the clock to turn the alarm off but could not reach it. Her right arm flailed around but, try as she might, Dolly could not locate the clock. She tried to get out of bed and found herself on the floor. Her left arm and leg would not work. She could, by now, see the clock but found she could not tell the time, the numbers and hands no longer made any sense to her. Fully conscious but almost helpless, she called out and her husband who was downstairs came upstairs. It appears that he did not hear her fall because he had been in the garden at the time. He called an ambulance and Dolly was taken to her local hospital. She had obviously had a stroke. A CT scan carried out the following day showed a right parietooccipital infarct. She also had a left homonymous hemianopia and poor motor power in her left arm and leg. Her leg improved a little over the next few days. She remained in the hospital for 3 wk where she received daily physiotherapy and twice-weekly occupational therapy. After discharge from the hospital Dolly went to a private nursing home where she remained for 4 mo. At this time, Dolly's husband retired and felt he might be able to look after his wife at home. Consequently in October 1983, Dolly was admitted for rehabilitation to see if we could sufficiently improve her self-care and cognitive abilities to enable her to return home.

INITIAL ASSESSMENT

On admission Dolly was assessed by the rehabilitation team. The main findings were left hemiplegia with spasticity (the arm was more densely affected than the leg and she could walk with a leg brace), left homonymous hemianopia, unilateral neglect of the left side, diminished perception of touch, and loss of proprioception in both her left arm and left leg, i.e., she was unaware of the position of these limbs in space when her eyes were closed. She was reported to have poor insight into the nature of her difficulties and appeared to have little concern about her problems. She was referred for a psychological assessment to determine the nature and extent of her cognitive difficulties.

Dolly was given a fairly extensive assessment following which I decided to offer rehabilitation for her unilateral neglect. She had a normal verbal IQ, an impaired performance IQ, and a huge verbal–performance discrepancy. Her verbal recall was above average and her verbal recognition in the low-average range. Her visual recall and recognition were both very impaired. On the Rivermead Behavioural Memory Test she scored in the moderately impaired range. She had problems with the Wisconsin Card Sorting Test and particularly severe problems with all tests of visuoperceptual and visuospatial functioning. Her results can be seen in Table 19.1

In my report I noted that Dolly, like many right hemisphere stroke patients, was rather expressionless but, nevertheless, cooperated well. Her left inattention was very marked: She tended to sit at the extreme right of the table. Whenever she stood up she turned to the right to leave the room although the door to exit was on the left. For most tests the material was placed towards Dolly's right (her "good" side) unless the instructions precluded this, in which case the material was taped in the center and Dolly's chair placed centrally. The results were considered to be reliable estimates of her current levels of functioning. My conclusions were:

1. Premorbidly Dolly was probably functioning in the average to bright-average range of ability.
2. Her verbal IQ is currently in the average range. Any slight decline is probably due to problems with mental arithmetic and backward digit span both of which involve spatial as well as verbal skills.
3. Her performance IQ is in the retarded range of ability. This would appear to be partly due to her unilateral neglect and partly due to more widespread visuoperceptual difficulties.

Table 19.1. Dolly's Psychological Test Result

TEST	OCT. 1983	DEC. 1983

Wechsler Adult Intelligence Scale

Verbal IQ 99 (Average)	Age Scaled Scores	
Information	10	
Comprehension	11	
Arithmetic	6	
Similarities	10	
Digit span	10	
Vocabulary	12	
Performance IQ 62 (Retarded)		79 (Borderline)
	Age Scaled Scores	Age Scaled Scores
Digit symbol	3	7
Picture completion	6	8
Block design	3	8
Picture arrangement	6	3
Object assembly	1	6

National Adult Reading Test

Errors	14	
Raw Score	36	
Predicted premorbid IQ 116 ±7 (Bright average)		

Raven's Standard Progressive Matrices

Raw score	14	
Below 1st percentile		

Naming Objects | 15/15 (Normal) |

Wechsler Memory Scale

Logical Memory (Prose recall)		
Immediate recall	13.5 (Average)	
Delayed recall	10 (Within normal range)	

Recognition Memory Test | Age Scaled Scores |

Words	6 (Low average)	
Faces	3 (impaired)	

Rey-Osterreith Figure

Copy	10/36 (Severely impaired) (see Figure 19.1)	16/36 (Severely impaired but some improvement)

(continued)

298

Table 19.1. Dolly's Psychological Test Result (*continued*)

TEST	OCT. 1983	DEC. 1983
Recall	6/36 (Normal as percentage of copy) (i.e., perceptual difficulties rather than severe memory impairment)	6/36 (No improvement)
Rivermead Behavioural Memory Test	Screening score 8/12 (Moderately impaired) (Failed immediate route, delayed route, delivering a message, and orientation)	
Benton Visual Retention Test	Number correct 2 Number of errors 16 (Severely impaired)	
Unusual and Usual Views		
Unusual	7/20 (Severely impaired)	
Usual	19/20 (Normal)	
Same/Different Faces	10/20 (Chance)	
Benton and Van Allen Face Recognition	Converted score 34 (Severely impaired)	
Hooper Visual Organisation Test	2/30 (Severely impaired)	
Visual Object and Space Perception Battery (prepublication version)		
Dot counting	2/20 (Severely impaired)	
Position discrimination	13/20 (Severely impaired)	
Cube counting	3/10 (Severely impaired)	
Benton Multiple Choice Form Matching Test	22/32 (Impaired)	
Cancellation		
"H"	63 Errors (at 12th percentile for right CVA patients)	6 Errors (at 60th percentile for right CVA patients)
"C and E"	80 Errors (at 9th percentile for right CVA patients)	13 Errors (at 63rd percentile for right CVA patients)
Line Bisection	Mean deviation from centre 6.5 mm (at 30th percentile for right CVA patients)	Mean deviation from centre 3 cm (at 75th percentile for right CVA patients)

(*continued*)

Table 19.1. Dolly's Psychological Test Result (*continued*)

TEST	OCT. 1983	DEC. 1983
Drawing from Memory	Severe left inattention (see Fig. 19.2)	Improved
Reading		
Wide range achievement test	34 Omissions (Severe neglect)	4 Omissions
Reading a prose passage	23 Omissions (Severe neglect)	0 Omissions

4. The huge verbal–performance discrepancy is almost certainly due to the stroke she sustained 4 mo ago.
5. On almost all tests of visuoperceptual and visuospatial functioning Dolly's scores fall within the impaired–severely impaired range. She presents with a classic picture of unilateral neglect although this is severe even in comparison with other right CVA patients. (Some examples of Dolly's attempts at visuoconstruction tasks can be seen in Figure 19.1.)
6. Her memory does not seem to be particularly impaired, the poor scores on Recognition Memory for Faces, the Rey-Osterreith Figure recall and the Benton Visual Retention Test are compromised by her visuoperceptual and visuospatial difficulties.
7. Problems with the Wisconsin Card Sorting Test suggest difficulty with tasks involving the frontal lobes although there is little doubt that the greatest area of damage is the right parietal lobe.
8. Some improvement may be expected over the coming weeks and Dolly will be seen by the clinical psychology department in an attempt to reduce the problems caused by her unilateral visual neglect.

Unilateral visual neglect refers to a heterogeneous and often transitory phenomenon commonly associated with right hemisphere strokes (Heilman and Valenstein, 1985). People with this condition fail to report, respond, or orient to objects or situations in the space contralateral to a cerebral lesion. Patients with this disorder may behave as though one side of space has lost its meaning. They may collide with objects, ignore food on one side of the plate, and attend to only one side of their bodies. Typically they have problems with reading, writing, and drawing (Wilson et al., 1987). About 40% of right hemisphere stroke patients show evidence of visual neglect (Diller and Gordon, 1981). People with left hemisphere strokes may also exhibit unilateral visual neglect but less frequently and less severely. Cerebral tumor and head injury can also give rise to neglect.

The condition has serious effects on both recovery and the rehabilitation

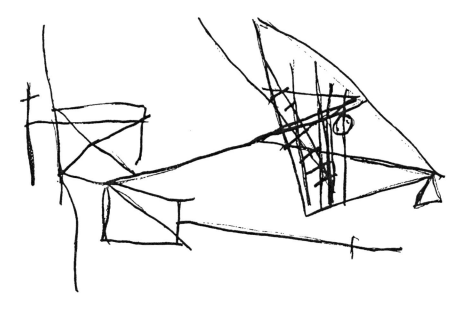

a

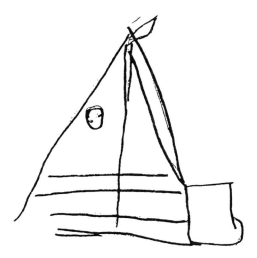

b

Figure 19.1. Dolly's Rey Osterreith complex figure: Copy and recall in October 1983 (**a** and **b**), copy and recall in December 1983 (**c** and **d**), and drawing of clock in October and December 1983 (**e** and **f**). (*continued*)

301

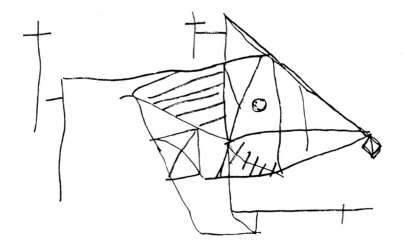

c

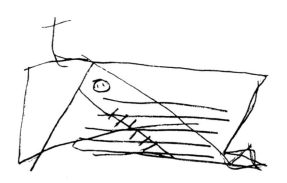

d

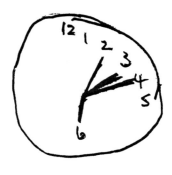 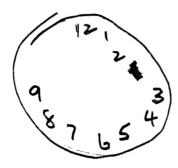

e   f

Figure 19.1. (*continued*)

prospects of patients. It is one of the major disruptive factors impeding functional recovery and rehabilitation success (Denes et al., 1982; Kinsella and Ford, 1980).

One of the first people to offer systematic rehabilitation to patients with neglect was Leonard Diller in New York. Diller and his colleagues (Weinberg et al., 1979) were a major influence in the rehabilitation of neglect patients in the 1980s. Consequently Dolly's program was, to a large extent, modeled on some of the strategies described by the New York team.

REHABILITATION

Dolly's unilateral neglect was tackled in two ways. First, we decided to try to reduce the neglect through exercises designed to improve her visual scanning. For this we were very much influenced by the work of Diller and his colleagues (Diller and Gordon, 1981; Weinberg et al., 1979). They argued that the basic underlying problem in unilateral neglect is poor scanning. It is certainly true that patients with severe neglect have scanning difficulties—they "jump" around the page missing lines and sections of lines and do not show systematic left-to-right scanning. We adopted some of the Diller group exercises for improving scanning to see if Dolly's visuospatial performance would improve. The second approach was to tackle some of her specific everyday problems such as transfers, route finding, and reading and try to find solutions for these specific difficulties.

General Training for Improving Neglect

We used two exercises to try to improve Dolly's scanning:

1. Practice in scanning using a scanning board, and
2. Practice in cancellation tasks.

1. Scanning board

We used a piece of apparatus modeled on one described by Diller and his colleagues and built for us by a group of engineers and rehabilitation workers. The wooden board was rectangular and measured about 2 meters by 1 meter. At evenly spaced intervals around the board were 32 lights each clearly numbered 1–32. A cross (the fixation point) was painted in the center of the board. Subjects are seated about 3 feet away facing the board and in front of the cross (see Figure 19.2). They are told that a tone will sound and immediately following the tone, one of the lights will be switched on. The subject is requested to indicate the number of the light as soon as possible by calling out the number and pressing a hand-held button. The tone and lights are controlled by the experimenter who also records the response latency.

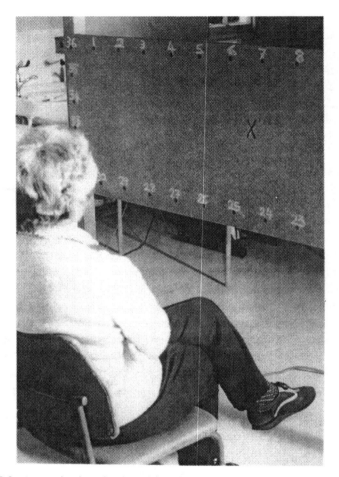

Figure 19.2. A scanning board (adapted from Weinberg et al., 1979).

Following a baseline of 20 trials, treatment consists of first teaching the patient to find an anchor point and second, giving practice in finding the anchor point and systematically scanning the board to find which light is switched on. Feedback is also given on time taken to detect each light. In Dolly's case the anchor point was a red strip at the edge of the board. In the baseline period Dolly's mean time for the detection of lights on the left side of the board was 15.36 sec, on the right side the mean time was 8.62 sec, and for lights in the central part of the board it was 9.21 sec. This information was fed back to Dolly, and the "anchor" point explained to her. She was told that part of her problem was her failure to scan systematically and the board would probably help to improve her scanning. She must find the anchor point first, i.e., the red strip at the extreme edge of the board, and then check from one light to the next to see which was switched on. It was stressed that she must go from left to right and not the other way round. She would be told how quickly she identified each light and also how fast the sum total was for lights on the left and lights on the right. Dolly was seen three times a week for 3 wk for the scanning training. She spent about 15 min each session on the scanning training and the remainder of the session (45 min) on other tasks. Dolly became progressively faster at identifying lights on the left side. The mean times for baseline and weeks 1, 2, and 3 can be seen in Figure 19.3.

Thus it can be seen that Dolly sped up her scanning over the 3 wk. What we could not establish, however, was whether this improvement generalized to other activities. Had we not been training her on cancellation tasks at the same time, we could perhaps have used performance on this as a measure of generalization, although any improvement could simply have been spontaneous recovery. We knew Dolly's everyday problems with route finding, activities of daily living, and reading persisted so we were fairly certain that the scanning board improvement had not generalized to these everyday tasks.

2. Practice in cancellation tasks

In the initial assessment Dolly had made 63 out of a possible 104 errors (60.6%) when asked to cancel one letter (H) and 80 of a possible 105 errors (76%) when asked to cancel two letters (C and E). For the training sessions we borrowed some cancellation sheets from occupational therapy with different letters, digits, or symbols to be cancelled. We excluded the original tasks from the assessment. Three baselines were taken of Dolly's omissions on a variety of cancellation tasks. The percentage of omissions in each baseline were 45%, 68%, and 66% respectively. Variability is common among patients with unilateral neglect, depending on such factors as fatigue, position of tester, and whether there are any strong stimuli (such as a red curtain) to draw attention to one side or another.

Once again, the training consisted of an "anchor" point along the lines suggested by Diller and his colleagues, practice, and feedback. A thick red line was drawn on the left side of the stimuli to be cancelled. Dolly was told once again

	Baseline	Week one	Week two	Week three
Left-hand lights	15.36	11.9	9.64	8.86
Central lights	9.21	10.6	6.4	6.25
Right-hand lights	8.63	6.1	6.4	5.5

Figure 19.3. Results on mean response times (sec) to lights appearing on scanning board.

that we wanted to help improve her scanning, and that practice at this task along with the scanning board should improve matters. She was to find the thick red line before attempting to cancel any stimuli and work along each line using a ruler and her finger to help her. At the end of each line she was to return to the left side, find the red line, move the ruler down one line, and proceed as before. Once again she had 3 wk of training and spent about 15 min three times a week on the cancellation tasks. In week 2, however, she was required to manage without the ruler and in week 3, the line was reduced in thickness and the color was changed, so a narrow black line was used as the anchor point instead of a thick red line, in other words the prompts were gradually faded out. The percentage of errors in weeks 1, 2, and 3 were 5.7%, 4.3%, and 4.3% respectively. Dolly was then reassessed on the original cancellation tests and made 6 errors (5.7%) when cancelling 1 letter (H) and 13 errors (12.3%) when cancelling 2 letters (C and E). This put her at the 60th and 63rd percentile for right CVA patients, i.e., a considerable improvement on her earlier scores. Again this could have been due to natural recovery although she had had severe neglect for 4 mo before our training. Many patients with neglect recover in the first few weeks. Those who do not may remain with neglect for years (Denes et al., 1982). Dolly was receiving considerable stimulation from her full rehabilitation program in physiotherapy and occupational therapy, so the improvement could have been due to nonspecific factors.

For the remaining $^1/_2$ h in her thrice-weekly sessions in Clinical Psychology, Dolly worked on other tasks recommended by Diller and his colleagues. These included estimating the length of plastic rods by placing pegs the same distance apart as she estimated the rod to be. Having made her guess, the rod was placed on top of the pegs so that Dolly could see instantly whether she had under- or overestimated. She had also practice and feedback in line bisection. All of this extra activity could have helped with her improvement on the visual scanning board and the cancellation tasks.

Dolly had now been at the rehabilitation center for 6 wk and it became clear that some of the everyday problems were not improving in her other therapy sessions so we felt it was time to deal with these head-on. Following a case conference with Dolly and her physiotherapist, occupational therapist, nurse, social workers, physician, husband, and myself, we decided to target three problems, namely route finding, reading, and walking through doorways.

Route Finding

One of the problems that the rehabilitation staff found irritating was Dolly's difficulty in getting from one department to another. Although independently mobile, she seemed unable to find her way around, was late for her sessions, and always seemed to be lost within the rehabilitation center. As this problem seemed to cause most trouble at lunch time when Dolly left physiotherapy to go to the ward for her midday meal, we decided to tackle this first. The neuropsychological assessment suggested that Dolly's problem resulted from her unilateral neglect and visuospatial difficulties. We knew her verbal memory was relatively intact so decided to try to help her use her verbal strengths to try to teach her the way to the ward. Following a baseline in which we observed what happened when Dolly left physiotherapy to go to the ward on six occasions, we implemented the teaching procedure. During the baseline Dolly had to be "rescued" by one of the nursing staff on two occasions and she asked one of the other patients on four occasions. The treatment was as follows: I met Dolly at the end of her physiotherapy session and gave her an audio tape recorder. As I led the way to the ward I asked Dolly to describe what was happening. I suggested that she try to avoid giving spatial descriptions, such as, "left and right," and, instead, use verbal ones such as, "I am going along the brick wall by physiotherapy," and "look for the yellow hollyhocks." Dolly recorded the landmarks as we proceeded to the ward. The following day, I met Dolly again at the same time, gave her the tape recorder and said she should switch it on when she was ready, listen to the directions, and find the ward. She was successful and reached the ward without taking any wrong turns or getting lost. After 3 days of finding the ward by listening to the taped instructions, Dolly thought she could manage without the tape recorder. She was right. From then on she never got lost going from physiotherapy to the ward.

The next stage was to teach her the route from the ward to occupational therapy, using the same procedure. Once again she learned very rapidly. Finally we taught her the way from occupational therapy to physiotherapy. By now Dolly was more oriented around the center and rarely got lost. The program almost certainly succeeded because we were capitalizing on Dolly's verbal strengths to overcome her visuospatial weaknesses.

Reading

Although Dolly could read individual words and had no problems with comprehension, she nevertheless, did not read for pleasure because her neglect caused her to omit so many words that the text did not make sense. As usual she was unperturbed by this. As noted in the original assessment she omitted 34 out of a possible 75 words on the Wide Range Achievement Test (WRAT) (Jastak and Jastak, 1965) and 23 of a possible 53 words on a simple prose passage. On the prose passage the text was meaningless when so many words were omitted, but instead of expressing surprise or commenting that the text did not make sense, Dolly said nothing. When asked how she thought she had done on reading the passage, Dolly said that she thought she needed new glasses.

Once again we decided to adopt Diller et al.'s scanning procedure to try to improve Dolly's reading given that Weinberg et al. (1979) had used this successfully with their right hemisphere patients with neglect dyslexia. For the baseline the original prose passage and the WRAT were each administered to Dolly on three more occasions. Errors ranged from 17 to 23 on the passage and from 32 to 41 on the WRAT. Several short passages of similar length to the original were prepared for the training sessions. In stage 1, a thick red line was drawn vertically down the left side of the passages. This was to be the "anchor point" as described in the scanning board training above. In addition, each line in the passage was numbered with the number drawn to the left of the red line and at the end of each line (see Figure 19.4).

Dolly was prompted to find number 1, then the red line, then read the first line until she came to the number 1 at the end of this line. Next she was to return to the left, find the number 2, and repeat the procedure until she had completed the passage.

Following 3 days practice stage 2 was introduced. This involved omitting the numbers at the end of each line. Dolly followed this procedure for a further three training sessions. Stage 3 involved omitting the numbers at the beginning of each

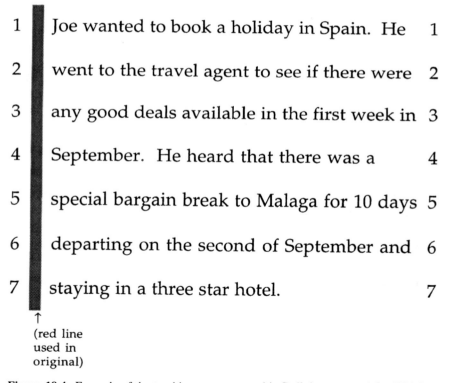

Figure 19.4. Example of the teaching passages used in Dolly's program (after Weinberg et al., 1979).

line, stage 4, reducing the thickness of the red line, and stage 5, reading without the line.

Then came the posttreatment assessment whereby Dolly was given the original prose passage and the WRAT which she had not seen for over 3 wk. She made 3 errors on the prose passage and 12 on the WRAT, i.e., a considerable improvement on her pretreatment performance. Furthermore, her husband reported that for the first time since her stroke, Dolly was reading the newspaper at home even though the layout of the newspaper was very different from the layout of the prose passage.

Walking Through Doorways

Dolly frequently misjudged distances particularly when leaving or entering a room. She often bumped into the left side of a doorway, apparently unaware of where the doorpost was. Because of the success of the scanning procedure, a red strip of ribbon was pinned vertically on the left side of two of the doorways used regularly by Dolly. She was observed going through these doorways and through two other doorways with no red ribbon. She bumped into far fewer of the doors with the ribbons.

Other Problem Areas

Because of the success with the anchor point procedure, we extended the strategy to cover (1) the telephone (a red strip was placed to the left side of the dial), (2) using the stove in occupational therapy (once again a red strip was placed to the left side of the top of the stove), and (3) writing (a thick red felt tip margin was drawn on Dolly's writing paper). Although no detailed records were kept, the staff generally felt that Dolly's neglect was less of a problem once these measures were introduced.

Had Dolly been referred in the 1990s rather than the 1980s, there is little doubt we would have employed other strategies. Robertson and North (1993) used limb activation as a way of reducing neglect. They found that encouraging movement in the left arm of patients with neglect reduced neglect. Many neglect patients, of course, are hemiplegic but even so might have some residual movement in a shoulder or finger. Even slight movement like this can reduce neglect (ibid.). If all else fails, moving the hemiplegic arm with the good arm can do the trick provided the left arm is moved on the left and not the right side of space.

Another strategy used by Robertson and his colleagues to improve the functioning of neglect patients is sustained attention training (Robertson et al., 1995). Neglect, they say, is a deficit of sustained attention so treatment should be aimed at improving this deficit. They employed a procedure partly based on the self-instruction procedures of Meichenbaum (1977). Initially as the neglect patient is working at a task, the experimenter (or therapist) knocks loudly on the desk every 20–40 sec and calls out, "attend" in a loud voice. Not surprisingly this alerts the subject. In a later stage the subjects takes over the alerting procedure himself or herself. Then the "attend" is said subvocally, next the "knocking" is carried out in the imagination. Robertson et al. have produced good results in neglect patients. We would almost certainly have tried both limb activation and sustained attention training with Dolly had we known about the procedures at the time.

POSTTREATMENT NEUROPSYCHOLOGICAL ASSESSMENT

Two months after her admission Dolly was reassessed on several of the original measures to see if she had improved. These results can be seen in Table 19.1.

There is little doubt that Dolly had improved. I noted in my report, "Dolly was cooperative and appeared to do the tests to the best of her ability. The most marked change since her last assessment was the way she tackled the tests. Her scanning was normal, she showed only a little evidence of missing the left-hand side of the page and appeared to be compensating well." In my conclusions I wrote:

1. There has been considerable improvement in the unilateral neglect since the last assessment. However, this is not entirely resolved and is particularly likely to reappear if in a complex or demanding situation.
2. There is still evidence of visuospatial problems. For example on the copy of the Rey-Osterreith Complex Figure (Mrs. _) continues to have great difficulty.
3. I should like to reassess (Mrs. _) in 6 mo time.

Dolly was discharged just before Christmas and went home to live with her husband. The plan was for her to attend the day center attached to the rehabilitation hospital for 2 days each week.

Sadly however Dolly had another stroke early in the new year and was admitted to a nursing home where she died a few months later.

VII

BEHAVIOR AND
SELF-CARE SKILLS

The final three people described in this book have a mixture of problems. Jim exhibited concentration and behavior problems following a severe head injury. Angela, a young mother, became virtually unable to do anything for herself after encephalitis damaged her brain stem, and Sarah sustained massive brain damage as a result of an anesthetic accident that left her able to walk and talk but able to do little else.

Behavior problems or conduct disorders are one of the common sequelae after traumatic brain injury. Among the most common behavior problems are yelling, shouting, and swearing, but it is physical violence and sexually offensive behavior that are likely to cause most distress and anxiety for relatives and staff. These problems are often the major reason for admission to long-term psychiatric care where, unfortunately, a sizeable proportion of head injured people are eventually placed. Fortunately, Jim's behavior problems were not so severe as to exclude him from the rehabilitation center and he responded well to a behavior management program.

Psychologists employing principles from behavioral medicine have an important role to play in the management of behavior problems. Growing awareness of the importance of behavior programs and the subsequent growth of these over the past 30 yr are reflected in increasingly sophisticated publications. Ince (1969) employed the Premack principle (whereby a desired activity is used to reinforce an undesired activity) to teach two stroke patients to attend speech and occupational therapy sessions. Both patients enjoyed physiotherapy so these sessions were used as reinforcers for attendance at other sessions. This principle was used with Paula (Chapter 16) in the previous section. She liked head balancing exercises but not other physiotherapy exercises. Consequently the head balancing exercises were used as a reward for engaging in exercises such as trunk rotation and bridging.

Since Ince, many others have reported the use of behavioral principles in neuropsychological rehabilitation, e.g., Taylor and Parsons (1970), Booraem and Seacat (1972), Lincoln (1978), Wilson (1981), Wood (1984), and Alderman and Ward (1991).

The number of strategies available in behavior therapy provide a rich source of ideas for treatment of neurologically impaired people even though the strategies may have to be adapted or modified for brain injured clients as opposed to the psychiatric or learning disabled clients for whom they were originally designed (Wilson, 1989d). Positive reinforcement, shaping, modeling, systematic desensitization, prompting, and fading have all been used successfully with neurologically impaired people.

Another behavioral technique adapted for use in brain injury rehabilitation is *Portage,* a home-based teaching technique originally designed for preschool children with learning disabilities (Cameron and White, 1987). A home advisor works with the parents of the children and visits weekly. Following an initial assessment on five developmental scales (motor, language, self help, socialization, and cognition) developmental gaps are pinpointed and treatment centered around these gaps. The home advisor and the parents select one or two tasks each week. These should be small enough to ensure that the child is almost certain to achieve the goal within the week, following which further tasks are set.

I have been using a modified version of Portage with brain injured adults since the early 1980s (Wilson, 1985) and also used this approach with Paula in the previous section. Therapists have stood in for parents although relatives could also be engaged in the programs in certain circumstances. In this section an adapted Portage approach was the method of choice for Angela to improve her self-care skills and, indirectly, her motivation and engagement in rehabilitation.

Sarah, the final person to be described in this book, had extremely severe self-care deficits probably due to a combination of apraxia and Balint's syndrome. She responded well to another behavioral strategy based on chaining whereby tasks are broken into small steps and the steps taught separately. We adjusted this method with Sarah, teaching all the steps in a sequence. She is a good example of how behavioral assessment and behavioral treatment are often hard to disentangle. Our fine-grained assessment of Sarah's problems, in drinking from a cup or putting on her coat, was also the method of treatment. Thus we could not say where assessment stopped and treatment began.

Behavioral psychology has contributed a great deal to neuropsychological rehabilitation. It has provided clinical psychologists and other therapists with a technology of learning based on careful observation and a concern for gradual increments in behavior. The combination of measurements and treatment, and the development of single case experimental designs typically found in the behavioral approach has provided us with some powerful strategies. Provided we recognize that emotional and social issues also need to be addressed in rehabilitation, we are unlikely to abuse these powerful tools.

20

JIM: IMPROVING CONCENTRATION AND REDUCING BEHAVIOR PROBLEMS

BACKGROUND

On the referral form sent out by the rehabilitation center, Jim's social worker described him as "a bit of a drifter and a loner." He had left school at 16—apparently of average ability—and for the next 10 yr held a succession of short-term jobs on building sites, at supermarkets, and in garages. He lived with his elderly widowed mother and had never married. In 1979, when he was 26 yr old, Jim was involved in a motorcycle accident, sustained a very severe head injury, and was in a coma for 3 wk. Soon after the accident Jim developed epilepsy.

Four months later, in 1980, Jim was admitted to the rehabilitation center. He had numerous problems, including ataxia, dysarthria, acquired dyslexia, and perceptual and reasoning difficulties. Each day, for the first month, Jim spent two sessions in physiotherapy, two in occupational therapy (OT), and one in speech therapy. He seemed to cope well with speech and physiotherapy, but was very disruptive in OT. His conduct caused such problems to staff and patients that he was referred to clinical psychology for help with his disruptive behavior. His occupational therapist also asked for help in improving Jim's concentration.

The notes from the referring hospital did not mention any behavioral problems, and Jim's physiotherapist, at the rehabilitation center, said he was unsteady on his feet, because of his ataxia, but that he cooperated well with his physiotherapy sessions. His speech therapist said Jim had severe reading difficulties and some dysarthria, but that his other language skills were unimpaired.

Thus, Jim was only causing concern in OT. His therapist there said, "he is unable to concentrate and he's very disruptive. He keeps getting out of his seat, wanders around, swears, shouts, and throws things on the floor." Prior to starting treatment I arranged to see Jim:

1. For a neuropsychological assessment; and
2. To observe him in several therapy sessions.

INITIAL ASSESSMENT

The neuropsychological assessment took $4^1/_2$ h, over three sessions. Although, he needed short breaks, every 20 min or so, Jim cooperated fairly well. On the Wechsler Adult Intelligence Scale (WAIS) Jim's verbal IQ was estimated to be 79 (borderline range), his performance IQ was 48 (impaired range), and his full scale IQ was 64 (mildly retarded range). The huge discrepancy of 31 points suggested greater damage to the right hemisphere than the left. On the verbal subtests his best age scaled score was vocabulary (9) indicating that he was probably functioning in the average range premorbidly.

The indication of greater right hemisphere damage was supported by Jim's performance on other visuoperceptual and visuospatial tasks. For example, on a test in which he was asked to identify objects photographed from an unusual view (Warrington and Taylor, 1978), he scored only 6 out of 20, even though he identified 80% of the objects when they had been photographed from a conventional angle. This suggested Jim's poor performance on the unusual views could not simply be explained by poor eyesight or a naming disorder. Furthermore, he was unable to copy or draw from memory any visual designs, although he could accurately describe the designs verbally, both when the designs were present and from memory. He was unable to write and could read only a few simple words. He could identify letters of the alphabet, both upper and lower case, provided these were presented one at a time. A normal reader before the accident, Jim now appeared to have what Shallice and Warrington (1977) described as *attentional dyslexia*. People with this condition can name individual letters, but typically make errors when strings of letters are presented.

Jim was oriented in time and place. His forward digit span was five, i.e., just within normal range. His backward span of three was poor for his age. His immediate and delayed recall of a prose passage were both within the normal range, and he was 100% correct on the easy pairs of the paired-associate learning task from the Wechsler Memory Scale (although he only managed to learn one hard pair). These results can be seen in Table 20.1.

Table 20.1. Jim's Psychological Test Results

TEST	JAN. 1980	FEB. 1981
Wechsler Adult Intelligence Scale		
Verbal IQ	79	84
Performance IQ	48	60
Full scale IQ	64	72
Subtests	**Scaled scores**	**Scaled scores**
Information	6	6
Comprehension	8	13
Arithmetic	3	2
Similarities	8	
Digit span	6	4
Vocabulary	9	10
	—	—
Digit symbol	0	0
Picture completion	4	5
Block design	0	7
Picture arrangement	5	4
Object assembly	1	3
Wechsler Memory Scale		
Personal and current information	1 (Severely impaired)	
Orientation	3 (Low average)	
Mental control	0 (Severely impaired)	
Logical memory mean for 2 passages immediate	10.5 (Within normal range)	
Logical memory delayed	8.0 (Within normal range)	
Associate learning	10 (Impaired but could learn easy pairs)	
Memory Quotient (M.Q.)	59 (Impaired)	
Unusual views	6/20 (Severely impaired)	
Usual views	16/20 (Below 5% cut off)	
National Adult Reading Test	0 (Severely impaired)	
Famous Faces	3/10 (Severely impaired)	
Recognition Memory		
Words (Words were read to Jim)	Raw score 45/20 Scaled score 6 (Below average)	

(continued)

Table 20.1. Jim's Psychological Test Results (*continued*)

TEST	JAN. 1980	FEB. 1981
Faces	Raw score 30/50 Scaled score < 3 (Severely impaired)	
Fragmented Pictures and Words (Perceptual priming/implicit memory task)	Failed to score (Severely impaired)	
Wisconsin Card Sorting Test **(Nelson's modified version)**	Perseverative errors 7 (Impaired)	

Cognitive Estimates	Error score 13 (Indicative
	  of frontal lobe damage)
		Error score 17
		(Indicative of frontal
		  lobe damage)

Naming from Description	14/15 (Within normal range)	
Dot Counting (From 5–9 dots on 10 cards)	Unable to do (Severely impaired)	
Fragmented Letters	Unable to do (Severely impaired)	
Graded Naming Test	9/30 (Predicted vocabulary scaled score = 8)	
Raven's Standard Progressive **Matrices**	Unable to do (Severely impaired)	

BEHAVIOR DURING ASSESSMENT

In my report of Jim's assessment I said,

> Jim was cooperative on the whole, although he appeared anxious on the first occasion. At times he seemed to be physically uncomfortable shifting around in the chair and breathing rapidly. This seemed to coincide with tasks he found particularly difficult. Another noticeable piece of behavior was his tendency to grimace on the left side of his face whilst holding his hand over his face and going red. At first it looked as if he was stifling a laugh, but said he had those 'turns' and could do nothing about them. They may have been minor motor seizures and occurred approximately three times every half an hour. He also became tired easily, apparently finding the assessment exhausting. However, as he is unable to concentrate for more than a few minutes at a time in OT, his behavior was better than might have been expected.

CONCLUSIONS ABOUT THE ASSESSMENT

Jim is obviously a very severely handicapped young man. He is functioning in the mentally retarded range as far as his overall general intellectual level is concerned and in the severely retarded range with visuospatial tasks. His verbal skills are somewhat less impaired, but still nowhere near the average level of the general population. As he was once a grammar school boy, there has, no doubt, been marked cognitive deterioration over the past year.

Because Jim has poor eyesight it was necessary to exclude this as a reason for his poor performance on some of the visuospatial tests. It was possible to demonstrate that the difficulties were not solely due to impaired vision as:

1. In the unusual and usual views tests, photographs of familiar objects are shown from an unusual and a usual angle. The photographs are the same size, so ability to recognize the usual view but not the unusual shows a cognitive or perceptual difficulty rather than poor vision. Although Jim's performance was below normal with both usual and unusual views, he was much more severely impaired on the unusual views, which strongly indicates deficits of parietal lobe functions. Some examples of Jim's responses on the unusual views include:

    (a) He called a SAUCEPAN "a CUP OF COFFEE";

    (b) an IRON "a SHOE"; and

    (c) a GUITAR "a PEN."

    With all these examples, he correctly named the usual view, so the difficulty was not a linguistic one either.

2. When asked to reproduce the Wechsler designs from memory, he was unable to do so. He was then asked to *copy* the design that was placed in front of him but was unable to do so. This could have been the result of his poor sight again; however, when the card was removed and Jim was asked to *describe* what he'd seen, rather than draw it, he did so adequately. Thus, he had "seen" the card although he was unable to draw it.

3. He did much better on the Picture Arrangement subtest of the WAIS than on Block Design although the materials in the former are more difficult to see than the latter. Again, his difficulties are not the result of bad eyesight, nor are they due to language problems. Apart from his ability to name correctly more of the usual than unusual views (which he would not have been able to do if he had severe word-finding problems) he was able to name objects from description normally.

His memory is impaired although his auditory memory for some verbal material is normal (he had normal scores on both immediate and delayed logical memory passages). He has some problems with other verbal material though, e.g., his Associate Learning and Recognition Memory scores were below average. The real difficulty is with nonverbal memory, e.g., memory for faces and memory for designs and this may not be a true memory problem at all. The scores may simply reflect his inability to correctly perceive or interpret what his eyes see.

In short, this young man is severely impaired intellectually and particularly with visuospatial tasks. He is not able to interpret what he sees correctly and this cannot be explained by poor eyesight. His language functions are intact although his speech is hurried at times and difficult to understand. His auditory perception and memory are much less impaired than his visual perceptual abilities. His ability to learn new material is reasonable, given his overall level of functioning, provided this is presented in an auditory rather than a visual mode.

PLANNING TREATMENT

How did these results help us to understand Jim's problems as witnessed in OT and how did we use the information to plan his future treatment? Jim's general intellectual functioning was impaired and he had particular problems with visuospatial and visuoconstructional tasks. His reading and writing skills were severely compromised, yet his verbal memory skills were relatively unimpaired. One hypothesis was that the tasks set in occupational therapy had been too difficult for him and that this caused or exacerbated his behavior problems. I thought maybe Jim had poor attentional skills, but his relatively normal digit span and recall of prose passages suggested adequate attention at least for verbal material.

When planning Jim's treatment program, we needed to bear in mind his limited intellect, his poor perceptual visuospatial and visuoconstructional skills, and his almost complete inability to read. Further analysis of his reading was planned as this problem was thought to be due to his visuospatial difficulties. Considering Jim's cognitive strengths, it was noted that he could learn new material if this was presented verbally and he could remember new verbal information.

OBSERVATIONS OF THERAPY SESSIONS

Jim arrived on time for his physiotherapy sessions and appeared to understand what was required. He was guided through his exercises and was able to work alone for up to 15 min. For his session in OT, Jim arrived 10 min late and was then asked to do some typing. The therapist realized Jim could not write but assumed he could identify individual letters and tap the keyboard. She was thus trying to give him tasks within his capabilities. Jim complained that OT was stupid, he sat down, shouted, picked up some paper, screwed it up, threw it on the floor, stood up, walked round the room muttering to himself, before leaving to go to the toilet. He returned 10 min later. The therapist sat with him at the typewriter and talked to him about his school, jobs, and his mother. (His mother found it difficult to get to the rehabilitation center, although she was in regular contact with the social worker. There were no other relatives in contact with Jim.) Jim remained seated and talked appropriately to the therapist for 15 min until she left to see another patient. Jim then wandered off to the canteen to wait for 15 min for his midmorning tea break.

After further discussions with the occupational therapist, it was decided to operationally define "poor concentration" as "the inability to work for more than 5 min at any one task set in OT." Behavior problems were defined as:

1. Swearing;
2. Leaving his seat before finishing a task; and
3. Throwing material on the floor.

A chart was drawn up to record the date, time of day, task set, and length of time spent on a task before a behavior problem occurred. There was also space for comments and space to write how many people were present in the room at the time. Another chart was used to record the frequency of Jim's behavior problems.

A clinical psychology student acted as an independent observer and recorder. She observed Jim during his two occupational therapy sessions each day for 5 days. On two of those occasions I also observed Jim independently as a reliability check. Although I recognized that independent observers may change the behavior they are interested in, I thought this unlikely in Jim's case, as:

1. He was not aware he was the focus of attention in OT; and
2. Visitors to the center were numerous, so the student was probably taken to be just another visitor familiarizing herself with the work of the center.

THE TREATMENT PROGRAM

The five-day baseline was completed just as the neuropsychological assessment came to an end. The information obtained from the two different assessments was integrated and used to plan the program. The behavioral-observational assessment showed that on tasks where Jim was expected to work alone, he typically spent no longer than 3 min working and often refused to start the task at all. He swore between 0 and 6 times per session and left his seat between 3 and 7 times per session, but only threw things on the floor twice during the whole week. Interrater reliability ranged between 88% and 99% for behavior problems; ratings for time spent on tasks differed by only a few seconds. These baselines can be seen in Figure 20.1.

Jim and I met with his occupational therapist, physiotherapist, speech therapist, social worker, nurse, and one of the medical doctors to draw up the treatment program. Although the occupational therapist had recognized the fact that Jim was intellectually handicapped as a result of his head injury, she had not realized the full extent of his problems. Many of the tasks required of Jim in OT were beyond his abilities. His reading was almost nonexistent; he could not write, draw, or copy; he could not fit paper into the typewriter, or easily find the right key.

Further assessment was required before deciding on a plan to help with Jim's reading deficits. Meanwhile, we were able to agree on goals for improving his concentration (as operationally defined above) in OT. Our long-term goal was for Jim to work for 15 min before leaving his seat. Our short-term goal was for him to work a little longer in each session than he had the previous session. Our objectives for his disruptive behavior were to eliminate all swearing, throwing of material, and leaving his seat during a task.

Jim agreed with these objectives and a program was typed up and given to each department. The plan was as follows:

1. The occupational therapist was to identify tasks that Jim could manage on his own (e.g., looking at motorcycle magazines to identify particular models, sorting colors, listening to audio tapes, and sequencing cards;
2. The occupational therapist would also identify tasks Jim had difficulty with, such as loading the typewriter with paper and completing a simple jigsaw puzzle or block design tasks (these tasks were to be divided into small steps that could be used at a later stage in the program);
3. Jim was to be given a task he could manage on his own and asked to work at this for 30 sec. A timer was set to sound so that Jim would know when he had succeeded;
4. The interval for this task was to be increased by 5 sec every time Jim succeeded in reaching his goal;
5. Each time Jim succeeded in reaching his target, he was to be praised, given feedback, allowed to get up and walk around for 3 min, and encouraged to appraise his progress by means of a visual record kept on a wall chart. (We expected that even though Jim might not understand the chart, he would be reinforced by the attention surrounding the filling in of the chart and by its very presence.)
6. When Jim was able to work on tasks that he could manage alone for 15 min, those tasks were to be alternated with more difficult tasks, which Jim would be asked to work on for 2–3 min. Jim was to be taught the more dif-

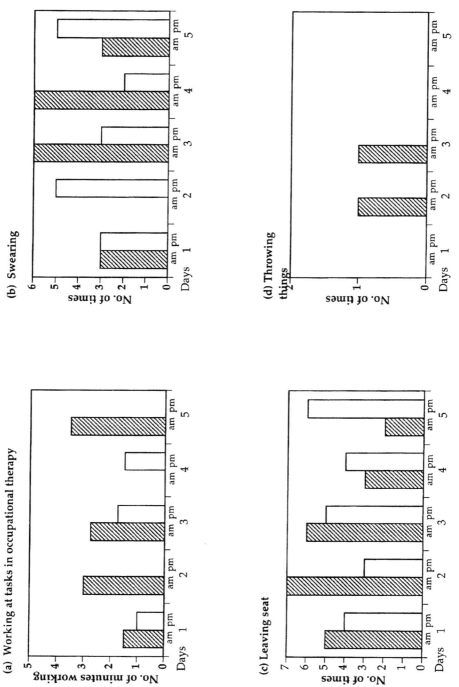

Figure 20.1. Baselines for Jim's disruptive behavior.

ficult tasks one step at a time in the presence of a helper who would supply prompts, demonstrations, and reinforcement when necessary;

7. Treatment for the behavior problems would be postponed in order to see whether our hypothesis (i.e., that the behavior problems resulted from the fact that Jim was given tasks beyond his abilities) was correct;

8. Records were to be kept as follows: the occupational therapist, or her colleagues, were to record (a) the duration of the interval set for each session; (b) whether or not Jim succeeded; (c) transfer information to the wall chart; and (d) any episodes of swearing, throwing, or leaving his seat prior to the timer sounding;

9. We agreed to review the program weekly. Although we were aware of Jim's epilepsy and he was taking anticonvulsants, his seizures were not particularly disruptive to his rehabilitation sessions.

The program was immediately successful. Jim's behavior problems ceased once he was given tasks within his capabilities. The program had been tailored to Jim's individual problems as they occurred in his environment. Complementary information was obtained from both neuropsychological and behavioral assessments. The neuropsychological investigations highlighted the severity of his cognitive deficits as well as his relative cognitive strengths. His occupational therapist had been expecting too much from him, had not been capitalizing on his strengths, and had not taken into account the nature of his limitations. The behavioral assessment allowed us to identify Jim's problems in his therapeutic environment and to tackle them directly. We needed to address the issue of generalization. If generalization occurs spontaneously in rehabilitation then this is a bonus. We are safer in assuming it will not occur and that we should build it in to our rehabilitation programs. Research in cognitive psychology has demonstrated the principle of *encoding specificity* (Tulving, 1983) which means retrieval is enhanced when the original encoding situation is reinstated at the time of recall. Similarly, *context specificity* principles (Godden and Baddeley, 1975) suggest that material learned in one context is recalled best in that context. To overcome *context specificity*, patients should be taught in a variety of contexts, with different cues, different environments, different people present, and so forth. In Jim's case, certain aspects of the environment were regularly adjusted or else were changing naturally, so different tasks were tackled; patients were changing from day to day and week to week and staff changed according to different schedules, patients programs, annual leave, and so on. Because Jim worked in the same room for the first few weeks, it was decided to set some of his tasks in different rooms for the remainder of his program. Thus, he spent some sessions in the work assessment area and some in the woodwork department. Jim saw this as "promotion" and an indication that he was improving, so it helped his morale.

READING ASSESSMENT

A month or so later, I saw Jim again to carry out a more detailed reading assessment. He appeared to have improved a little, although still had significant problems. He was able to read both upper and lower case single letters without error. On a single-letter-pair cross-case matching task (e.g., Aa, Gh) where Jim had to say whether the two letters were the same or not, he was 100% correct. Thus, he could certainly cope with two letters at a time without making mistakes.

On a simple lexical decision task, where he was shown 25 real words and 25 nonsense words, one at a time in random order, and asked to say "yes" to the real words and "no" to the nonsense words, he was correct with 82% of the stimuli. He made seven false positive responses and two false negatives.

Furthermore, Jim was able to read all 25 real words from the lexical decision task without error. These were all regularly spelled words. When asked to read aloud nonsense words however, he made a significant number of errors and showed many regularizations (e.g., MUN read as "MUM" and EKT as "EAT"). People with phonological dyslexia and with deep dyslexia show these kinds of errors. When asked to read aloud irregularly spelled real words, Jim again had problems although many of his errors were strange and not like those one might see in someone with surface dyslexia. Thus, Jim read AUNT as "GAWK" and SUBTLE as "STREET." Once again, it appeared as if he had attentional dyslexia or approximate visual access. Like Jenny, in Chapter 15, Jim's reading errors were of several different types.

I had hoped to implement a reading program with Jim along similar lines to the program designed for Derek and for Jenny. As Jim was already able to read individual letters correctly he would have had a head start on Derek and Jenny. This was not to be however, as the medical director decided it was time for Jim's discharge and he returned home to attend a day center twice a week.

FOLLOW-UP

One yr later Jim came back for a 1 day assessment. He was seen in physiotherapy, OT, speech, and clinical psychology. This meant I had only $1^1/_2$ h with Jim. I decided to readminister the WAIS. I also had time to give him the Cognitive Estimates Test (Shallice and Evans, 1978) as a quick frontal lobe measure. Jim's WAIS scores had improved as can be seen in Table 20.1 with a verbal IQ of 84, a performance IQ of 60, and a full scale IQ of 72. He still appeared to have considerable frontal lobe and reasoning problems as assessed by the Cognitive Estimates Test, where his error score was 17 (mean for normal control subjects = 3). He thought, for example, that race horses galloped at $^1/_2$ mile per hour and the length of an average man's spine was 12 feet.

During this 1 day assessment he cooperated well in occupational therapy and there was no evidence of the disruption seen the previous year.

Jim had responded well to the treatment program designed for him. Driven by patient and staff need, it might be easy to miss the theoretical influence behind the rehabilitation plans. Indirectly, however, strong theoretical influences were behind the program. As far as the assessment went, neuropsychological localization models enabled us to identify right hemisphere deficits as possible explanations of Jim's unsocial behavior. Models of attention, reading, and memory influenced our selection of assessment procedures, and of the way we conceptualized, understood, and explained his disorder.

Perhaps the most influential model in Jim's case, and in other cases in which behavioral assessment is carried out to plan and monitor treatment, is Kanfer and Saslow's (1969) SORKC model. This stands for stimulus, organism, response, contingency, and consequence. According to Ciminero et al. (1977), *stimulus* refers to the antecedent events or discriminative stimuli that trigger problem behaviors; these events, or stimuli, can be physical, social, or internal. *Organism* refers to a person's biological condition and to individual differences resulting from previous experiences. *Response* refers to the behaviors of concern; these can be motor, cognitive, or physiological behaviors. *Contingency* refers to schedules of reinforcement in operation. *Consequence* refers to events that follow behavior and these can be physical, social, or self-generated.

This behavioral analysis prescribed treatment by taking into account the effects of Jim's head injury, the resulting cognitive weaknesses, and residual strengths. The analysis alerted us to the fact that Jim's behavior was being maintained through continuous or partial reinforcement (the latter being more resistant to extinction than the former). Thus, in order to reduce or eliminate the problem behavior, we needed to set tasks within Jim's capabilities, avoid reinforcement of inappropriate behavior and strengthen appropriate behavior. Knowledge of behavioral treatment strategies such as shaping, and chaining together, with an appreciation of the importance of feedback, rest, and praise as powerful reinforcers in rehabilitation (Ince, 1976; Lincoln, 1978; Wilson, 1989d) enabled us to implement the program effectively.

SINCE 1981

For 12 yr I lost touch with Jim, and then in 1993, I tried to contact him for a long-term follow-up study. For a while I could not find out anything about him, but finally, I had a letter from a medical doctor involved in his care. She told me that Jim had died in 1991. His mother came downstairs one day to find Jim dead in the sitting room. Apparently, he had died of a seizure.

21

ANGELA: IMPROVING THE SELF-CARE SKILLS OF A WOMAN WITH QUADRIPLEGIA AND DYSARTHRIA

BACKGROUND

Angela was 30 yr old, married to a farmer, and the mother of two boys—one 6 yr old and the other 3 yr old, when she succumbed to encephalitis. She felt unwell one morning, became worse during the day, went to bed early in the evening, and could not be roused the following morning. Her husband called for an ambulance and Angela was admitted to her local hospital. The following day she was sent to a hospital specializing in neurological diseases where she was diagnosed with brain-stem encephalitis. The virus was not identified but it did not appear to be herpes simplex encephalitis which Clive and Jason (Chapters 6 and 9) had. Angela was in a deep coma for 10 days and initially was not expected to live. She gradually emerged from the coma, but had quadriplegia and severe dysarthria. Thus, she had very little movement in any of her four limbs and her speech was unintelligible. The speech problem was caused by loss of muscular control and not by damage to the language areas in the cortex.

Some slight improvement occurred over the next few weeks, but Angela was dependent on others for all her physical needs and her only means of communication was to try to point to letters on a board to spell out a few words. Because of her restricted mobility, this was extremely slow. Angela was tearful for much of the time.

Two mo after her illness, Angela left the hospital for a rehabilitation center about a 2 h drive away from her home. She was to spend several months at the rehabilitation center, although she did go home for most weekends.

I was not involved in Angela's care until 2 mo later, i.e., 4 mo since her illness. Meanwhile, Angela spent two sessions a day in physiotherapy, two in occupational therapy, and one in speech therapy. The speech therapist provided her with a Canon® communicator—a small calculator sized communication aid on which words could be typed one letter at a time. The words then emerged from the machine on a piece of ticker tape. Still with little control over her movements, Angela found this method of communication slow and tiring, although it had the advantage of providing a permanent record, unlike the letter board.

Angela's therapists asked me to assess her cognitive functioning. Although it was generally believed that no cognitive deficits had occurred owing to the fact that the brain damage was confined to the brain stem, the therapists were not entirely convinced of this. Angela's poor motor and communication skills together with her low mood, meant it was difficult to ascertain her level of cognitive functioning. Consequently, I arranged to see Angela for a neuropsychological assessment.

INITIAL ASSESSMENT

By the time I began seeing Angela, she had gained a little more control over her limbs although she was ataxic and her movements were jerky and unsteady. I was unable to understand much of her dysarthric speech, so Angela frequently resorted to the Canon® communicator. She told me, "[she was] frightened of her illness." She had also expressed suicidal thoughts, so was being seen by a psychiatrist. Many verbal tests were impossible because of the dysarthria and excessively slow response times. Motor tests were very difficult because of the ataxia. I was able to administer three tests that required a pointing response (the Ravens Standard Progressive Matrices, the Leiter International Performance Scale, and the Recognition Memory Test) together with a test of orientation, and a perceptual test (unusual and usual views) which Angela named using the Canon®. I saw her four times altogether for a total of 6 h. The results of these tests can be seen in Table 21.1.

All results were in the normal range. In the conclusions to my report, I said that the findings should be taken as the minimum level of Angela's current intellectual functioning, given the difficulties encountered in assessing her. Present results suggested that intellectually there were no serious problems: her reasoning was at least in the low-average range, her perception apparently normal and her recognition memory above average. I felt there could have been some decline in Angela's cognitive abilities, but it was impossible to be precise given her current speech, motor, and emotional problems. The findings were fed back to Angela and her therapists shortly before Christmas 1981. The center closed for the Christmas holiday and I did not see Angela again until January 1982.

Table 21.1. Angela's Test Results in 1982 and 1994

TEST		Results 1982	Results 1994
Ravens Standard	Raw score	34	31
Progressive Matrices	Predicted IQ	89	91
Leiter International Performance Scale	Passed	All tests up to 9-yr-old level 3/4 tests at 9 yr 2/4 tests at 10 yr old level 3/4 tests at 12 yr (Older tests not available)	
Orientation and personal information		100%	100%
Unusual and usual views	Raw score	Unusual 17/20 Usual 20/20	18/20 20/20
Recognition Memory Test	Words raw score	49/50	48/50
	Words Age scaled score	14	13
	Faces raw score	46	48
	Faces Age scaled score	12	15
Rivermead Behavioral Memory Test		NA	Standard profile Score 20/24 Screening score 10/12

NA, not administered.

Soon after the new year Angela's physiotherapist and occupational therapist asked me if I would see Angela to "improve her motivation." I felt reluctant to do this because the request was somewhat nebulous and the motivation hard to define. Nevertheless, because of my training and its emphasis that (1) the role of clinical psychologists is to use psychological knowledge to solve health related problems; and (2) no patient is untreatable, I agreed to get involved in Angela's rehabilitation.

ADAPTING PORTAGE TO IMPROVE SELF-CARE SKILLS

In an interview with Angela and her therapists in January 1982, I deduced that the "poor motivation" described by the therapists was another way of saying that Angela was despondent because she felt she was not improving. Initially, she had expected to recover from the illness, but now that almost 6 mo had passed and she was still severely disabled, she felt hopeless. How would she be able to return home, look after the house, and care for her two young sons, when she could do so little? I decided that one approach might be to demonstrate to Angela that she *was* improving, albeit slowly, and that if this change was documented and made obvious to Angela, then she would feel less hopeless about her condition, increase her involvement in the rehabilitation process, and perhaps change her belief that she was not getting any better.

I decided to modify the *Portage* approach to select goals, plan treatment, and monitor effectiveness. The rationale for this was previous success with an even more disabled patient a few months earlier (Wilson, 1984).

The Portage method is named after the town Portage in Wisconsin, USA, where it was developed as a home-based teaching technique for the parents of children with developmental learning disabilities. Bluma et al., (1976) the originators of Portage, began with some basic operational premises, e.g., that parents care about their children and want them to reach their maximum potential— whatever that might be; that parents can learn to be effective teachers of their own children; and that precision teaching is the preferred model as feedback is provided daily to parents to reinforce their efforts. It was also postulated that home-based learning avoided problems of generalization, tackled more functional problems, was more likely to involve the whole family, and would better equip parents for dealing with problems that might arise in the future.

A home advisor makes contact with the parent(s) to explain the Portage approach. An assessment is then carried out, using developmental checklists of behavior occurring from birth to 6 yr of age. The checklists cover five areas:

1. Self help,
2. Motor,
3. Socialization,
4. Language, and
5. Cognitive skills

The parent(s) and home advisor can then identify any delays or deficits in the child's development and attempt to remediate these.

In the next stage the home advisor and parent(s) decide on certain skills to be taught. Each skill may need to be broken down into a series of smaller steps or tasks, and one or two of these are selected for treatment each week. The guiding principle here is to try to guarantee success. The tasks should be small enough so that there is a high likelihood of their being reached within a week, thus providing reinforcement for the parent(s) and possibly the child. The teacher models the teaching procedure, written instructions and recording charts are provided and baselines taken. Monitoring and evaluation of the process are essential aspects of Portage. In fact the whole procedure closely resembles many behavioral approaches to treatment.

Both the assessment and treatment stages can be incorporated into neurological and neuropsychological treatment programmes. The five developmental checklists can provide an assessment of even very severely intellectually disabled adults and were the impetus for the development of somewhat similar assessment scales for severely head injured patients (Wilson et al., 1994). Portage checklists can give an objective measure of the developmental stage reached in each of the five areas. This kind of assessment may also prove useful in monitoring improvement over time. Some people (e.g., Eson et al., 1978) recommend using developmental scales to assess progress following very severe head injury, and Portage provides more detailed check-lists than many others available, as well as separating the items into different subscales.

Physiotherapists, occupational and speech therapists, nurses, and others can administer the checklists with minimal training. Shortly before seeing Angela, I was asked to assess a woman who had sustained hypoxic damage during an anesthetic accident, which left her blind, dysphasic, hemiplegic, and apraxic. I was asked to inform the rehabilitation team of the woman's level of intellectual functioning. Given that she could not see, could not speak, and had problems with voluntary motor control, all the tests I would normally administer were inappropriate. Although there are tests that can be administered to people without sight, speech, or motor control, there are no tests as far as I am aware that can be administered to people with *all* of these deficits. For such people checklists seem to be the only answer and I used both Portage and the Vineland Social Maturity Scale (Doll, 1953) to assess the woman with hypoxic brain damage. We used the failures on the Portage checklists to identify our goals for treatment and managed to teach her some basic self-care activities. Inevitably some Portage checklist items are inappropriate for neurologically impaired adults: for example, they include behaviors that are too childish, e.g., "waves good-bye in imitation of an adult," others involve vision so could not be included in the assessment of the blind, hypoxic patient.

Further modification of the Portage procedure is required for the treatment stage. First, parents are not always available or, indeed, appropriate as teachers. In a residential, or day rehabilitation program, therapists, nurses, or others may be more suitable. Second, the tasks selected for treatment may not come from developmental delays on the checklists, but from failures in other more adult oriented activities. Third, patients can be more involved in the selection of target skills than learning disabled children.

Certain essential features of Portage may remain, however. These include:

1. The selection of specific tasks;
2. The establishment of pre- and postbaselines;

3. The specification of how, where, and when to teach the task;
4. The provision of information about procedures to follow, if the trainee succeeds or fails; and
5. The monitoring and evaluation of progress.

It is the structure that seems to be important, rather than the particular teaching method selected.

The structure and rationale were explained to Angela and her therapists. We agreed to meet each Monday morning to select a goal for the coming week, take baselines, and prepare the record chart. The physiotherapist and occupational therapist were the teachers. The overall aim was to increase Angela's independence by teaching her to carry out a number of tasks by herself. We were, of course, constrained by her physical limitations, so our desire to extend her capabilities had to be realistic and possible for Angela to achieve.

The first goal selected was for Angela to drink half a cup of tea alone. She could lift half a cup, but not a full cup. The plan was for Angela to practice the task twice a day (at morning and afternoon tea breaks) in the canteen. The procedure was as follows:

1. Angela was to sit at a bench in the canteen;
2. She was to wear a protective bib;
3. Half a cup of tea was to be placed in front of her;
4. Angela was to reach for the tea and drink alone;
5. She could stop and start whenever she wanted, but had to be finished within 15 min.

Completion of the task was thought to be sufficiently reinforcing. If Angela appeared to be failing, we decided to first try encouragement, second, use a weighted cuff to steady her hand, and, third, if both of these failed, we would guide her hand as necessary. Thus, Angela would not be allowed to fail. The recording procedure was to give two check marks if she completed the task alone, give one check mark if she needed help, and add 1, 2, or 3 if necessary, i.e.,

1 = Encouragement provided;
2 = Weighted cuff; and
3 = Guidance of hand provided.

The record sheet can be seen in Figure 21.1.

At the end of the 1st wk Angela was drinking half a cup of tea alone, with verbal encouragement. We felt we needed to continue the task for another week by

	Week beginning	25.1.83		Success	✔
	Name	Angela		Abandoned	
	Therapist	Carrie O.T.		Change	
				Continue	

		Base-line	M	T	W	T	F	Post base-line
Task	To drink half a cup of tea without help	am						
Number of times	Twice a day - 10.30 am and 3.15 pm	3✔	3 ✔	3 ✔	3 ✔	1 ✔	1 ✔	1 ✔
Directions	1. Angela to sit at bench in canteen					✔	✔	✔
	2. Half a cup of tea to be placed in front of her (Put bib on)	pm						
	3. Angela to reach for tea and drink it alone. She is allowed to stop and start	3✔	3 ✔	3 ✔	3 ✔	1 ✔	1 ✔	1 ✔
	4. To be finished by end of teabreak					✔	✔	✔
Reinforcement	Success at task. Feedback charts							

Correction procedure

1) Try encouragement first

2) If this fails use weighted cuff to steady hand

3) If this fails guide hand through procedure

Recording procedure

✔✔ = success alone

1✔✔ = success with encouragement

2✔ = success with weighted cuff

3✔ = success with hand guided

Figure 21.1. Record sheet for first task selected for treatment for Angela.

which time she was managing without encouragement. Meanwhile, another task was selected by Angela and her therapists. This second task was to remove her shoes. The laces were to be undone and Angela was required to remove her shoes by any means possible. She achieved this successfully by the 2nd day. Other tasks followed week by week. These can be seen in Table 21.2.

Of the first 10 tasks selected, Angela achieved success within a week on 8 of the tasks. The two failures were because the tasks were beyond her physical capabilities, i.e., the therapists and Angela were too ambitious in selecting the goals.

Meanwhile, Angela's mood improved, she no longer saw the psychiatrist, and appeared more cheerful and cooperative in sessions. She entered into the task selection and seemed to want to achieve success. She was discharged home in March 1982 with provisions made for her to attend a day center twice a week, and for home help to be provided.

FOLLOW-UP

I lost touch with Angela for several years, but in October 1994 I saw her again at a day center that she attends once a week. The first thing I noticed was how much Angela's speech had improved. We did not once use the Canon® communicator, all of her speech was quite intelligible. Angela was independent and mobile through use of an electric wheelchair. She welcomed me, arranged for one of the staff to make us some coffee, and we went into a quiet room for the interview and reassessment.

Table 21.2. Summary of Goals Achieved by Angela

DATE 1982	TASK SET	TASK ACHIEVED
Jan. 25	Drink half a cup of tea alone	Yes (just)
Jan. 25	Take off shoes	Yes
Feb. 1	Drink half a cup of tea alone	Yes
Feb. 1	Put on shoes	No: too hard
Feb. 1	Wash and dry hands	Yes
Feb. 8	Clean teeth	Yes
Feb. 15	Increase number of times wheelchair maneuvred around table	Yes
Feb. 22	Put tracksuit trousers on by self	Yes
Feb. 22	Further increase in number of times round table	Yes
March 1	Open door into and out of workshop	Yes out/No in

When asked what she saw as her main problems now, Angela listed four, in this order:

1. She said communicating was still a major problem (although communication difficulties were not apparent to me). Angela said the words sometimes came out in a jumble;
2. Problem number two was "emotional—I weep very easily";
3. The third problem was waterworks—"my bladder doesn't empty properly and certain foods cause a reaction"; and
4. The fourth problem Angela mentioned was balance. She said, "When I stand up its dreadful. I used to go to physio and it was like being 10 feet off the floor."

So, most of Angela's problems appeared to be physical—even the communication problem was probably due to dysarthria, caused by the brain stem damage and not to dysphasia, as she had no damage, as far as we knew, to the cortical areas.

I asked Angela to tell me what had happened since she left the rehabilitation center, some 12 yr earlier. She said she did very little except go to the day center once a week. Most of the time she stayed home and did a little bit of housework. She didn't go out much—the frequency and urgency of her need to go to the toilet made going out difficult. She lived in her own house and could get upstairs with help from her husband. He brought her to the day center and took her home again. She did a little cooking at the day center and socially found it useful as she saw no one else apart from her husband and two sons.

We repeated a number of the tests and these results can be seen in Table 21.1. On the Recognition Memory Test, Angela achieved an age scaled score of 13 for words (48/50) and 15 (48/50) for faces, very similar to the results obtained 12 yr before. She was also in the normal range on the Rivermead Behavioural Memory Test (standardized profile score = 20/24; screening score 10/12). She failed to recall one name and to remember to deliver the message. On the Raven's Standard Progressive Matrices Angela's raw score was 31 and her predicted IQ was 91. Previously she had achieved a raw score of 34. So, once again, there was very little change. It would appear that she did not have cognitive problems.

I asked if she was in touch with any friends from before her illness, "No," she said, "I used to cry so much at the beginning that I wouldn't have anything to do with them, and they drifted away." "What about new friends?" I asked. "Well, I have acquaintances with the staff and some of the patients here. I've always had acquaintances rather than friends." I then asked Angela if she ever got bored, she said, "Not really, I'm relieved I don't have to do things any more. I'm quite content to sit still and muse." "Do you ever get lonely?" I asked next. "Frequently," she said, "I feel alone because I'm not good with my husband. I don't like company, I'm a loner."

I then went on to ask about specific problems. First, I asked Angela if she thought she had any problems with attention and concentration these days. She thought she was just beginning to get better here, and volunteered, "I could never read a book since my illness, but now I can read a little." She thought her memory was bad and she couldn't trust it. Her performance on tests of memory, however, was in the normal range. "Do you have any problems with thinking, thinking things through, or working things out?" I asked. "No," said Angela, very emphatically, "I think too much." "What about finding the right word?" She replied, "Sometimes, if I don't think first, the wrong word comes out."

When asked whether she had reading problems, she said she did because she couldn't follow the words easily, she could not scan. She thought her writing was better than it was, although she had to use her left hand now (she was right-handed before becoming ill). "Do you have any difficulty understanding what you see, do things look strange or distorted, or as if part of the picture is missing?" I asked next. "Yes, I have terrible double vision and my eyes bounce up and down, so its difficult to read or write." She said she never had problems with her bowels, but her bladder was a big problem as she had said earlier. Sleeping had caused her problems for many years, but about 4 mo earlier she had been given antidepressants to "help her sleep" and since then things had gotten much better. Financially she was secure, the farm had been sold and she had a disability allowance. One of her sons was still at school, and the other working on a local farm. Her husband did most of the housework and Angela felt reasonably content with her life, although she was sometimes lonely. She appeared to have accepted her disabilities and most certainly did not want any more rehabilitation. She had not enjoyed her time at the rehabilitation center, and simply wanted to be left alone.

22

SARAH: LEARNING SOME SELF-CARE SKILLS AFTER AN ANESTHETIC ACCIDENT

BACKGROUND

In 1983, Sarah was 19 yr old and halfway through her 2nd yr at a multilingual secretarial college. She spoke French and German in addition to English and was an intelligent, kind young woman although a "bit of a loner" according to her aunt. Sarah lived with her aunt, uncle, and cousins as both her parents and sister had been killed in a train fire when Sarah was 16 yr old. Her aunt had promised her sister (Sarah's mother) that if anything ever happened to Sarah's parents, Sarah would live with her aunt and uncle. Her aunt felt Sarah was just beginning to get over the loss of her parents and sister when another tragedy occurred.

In February 1983, Sarah needed to have a wisdom tooth removed. She went into a private hospital for this minor operation and sustained a terrible anesthetic accident resulting in massive hypoxic brain damage. She was transferred to another hospital where she was on a ventilator for a month and in a coma for 6 wk. When she came around, she was unable to do anything for herself. She had severe sensory, motor, and cognitive deficits. Her aunt felt she was aware of certain things and could distinguish her aunt from other people.

In June 1983, Sarah was admitted to a rehabilitation center at the insistence of her aunt. The doctor who saw her first said in the admission summary "severely disabled with gross impairment of motor and sensory function and ataxia; coordination and power not possible to assess, able to stand unsteadily with myoclonic jerks. She cannot dress or feed herself. She is usually continent of urine and feces. Higher mental functions: dysarthria, dysphasia, cannot name simple objects, obeys only very simple commands."

Sarah was referred for a psychological assessment of her intellectual ability the week following her admission. She was always pleasant and cooperative although found almost every task extremely difficult.

INITIAL ASSESSMENT

During the first assessment in June 1983, we observed that Sarah seemed unable to coordinate her eye movements, so was unable to look voluntarily at objects or words. She was unable to point to or manipulate objects. She had a noticeable dysarthria making her speech slurred, although she was, on the whole, intelligible. She walked unaided but seemed rather clumsy and she appeared to have a marked problem with spatial awareness. Thus, if she had to walk round an object in the room she did not seem to know how far away from her it was or how to circumnavigate it. If she tried to sit in a chair she could not place herself in the correct position in relation to the chair. She could not read because she appeared to be unable to focus on the words. In other words she would look to the wrong point in space. If single letters were placed wherever her eyes were pointed she could read at least some of them, for example, the first letter of her name.

Although Sarah was unable to participate in the traditional neuropsychological tests we were able to establish baselines for a few basic cognitive functions. She had lost a considerable amount of general knowledge so appeared to have a semantic memory impairment. For example, she did not know her date of birth or how many legs birds have. Not only was she unable to count the number of objects or dots on a page, she made errors in counting aloud. She could not recite the alphabet. She managed A to G after which she could go no further. She could, however, tell us the name of the present Prime Minister. She was unable to read, write, or draw. Of seven objects shown to her she could name only one correctly (a toy car). When simple descriptions of these objects were provided Sarah managed to identify six out of seven objects. She correctly named car, clock, horse, cat, button, and dog. She failed on pencil. In retrospect it would have been better to have avoided the model animals as these appear to be particularly difficult for people with semantic memory difficulties, i.e., whose general knowledge about the world has been affected (see Jason, Chapter 9, Jenny, Chapter 15, and Kirsty, Chapter 17). She could not identify a single line drawing or photograph. She could not match faces or shapes. When asked about her vision Sarah usually said, "it all meets together." When words were spelled to her she correctly identified 9 out of 20 from the Schonell Graded Word Reading Test (tree, little, milk, egg, book, suit, playing, bin, road). The final test administered during this first assessment was the Vineland Social Maturity Scale (Doll, 1953) which assesses self-help skills, communication, socialization, locomotion, and occupation in people from birth to adulthood. Sarah's occupational therapist was the informant for completion of the Vineland. Sarah's overall mental age was at the $1-1\frac{1}{2}$-yr-old level. Her first failures were in the 0–1-yr-age group (grasping objects within reach; reaching for nearby objects, and grasping with thumb and finger). Her highest successes were at the 2–3-yr-old level (asks to go to the toilet; relates experiences).

What we did not appreciate at the time was that Sarah almost certainly had Balint's syndrome. We missed this because her problems were so widespread it was difficult to tease out one from another. Balint's syndrome (Balint, 1909) is comprised of three elements. First there is a psychic paralysis of gaze, i.e., an inability to look voluntarily into the peripheral field. Second, there is optic ataxia manifested by an inability to localize in space or manually point to visually presented objects. Third, there is a shrinking of the attentional field so that patients are typically only able to report one object or part of one object at a time. Rubens (1979) said, "It is as though they had bilateral visual neglect with macular sparing. Their problem is compounded by an inability to relate small portions of what they see to the remainder of the stimulus by scanning" (p. 239). De Renzi (1996) uses the term Balint-Holmes' syndrome in recognition of the contribution made by Gordon Holmes (1919) to the understanding of the disorder.

In retrospect Sarah certainly appeared to have this syndrome. She could not look voluntarily at stimuli or objects pointed out to her, she could not reach accurately and she could only perceive one letter at a time when trying to read. Balint's syndrome is associated with large bilateral parietal lesions (De Renzi, 1996; Rubens, 1979) and these lesions are known to occur following hypoxic brain damage.

SECOND ASSESSMENT

In October 1983, Sarah was reassessed by one of the clinical psychology trainees working under my supervision. She had improved in all areas tested 4 mo earlier as can be seen in Table 22.1. Her overall Vineland score was now at the 2–3-yr-old level with her first failure at the 1–2-yr-old level (pulls off socks, transfers objects, drinks from glass unassisted, and unwraps candy). Her highest success was at the 11–12-yr-old level (enjoys books, newspapers, magazines). Although Sarah still had problems reading, she would try to read and her reading had improved to some degree.

One of the questions we were trying to answer at this stage was whether or not Sarah had a visual object agnosia, like Jenny in Chapter 15. It will be remem-

Table 22.1. Results from Sarah's First Two Assessments

TASK	JUN. 1983	OCT. 1983
Orientation		
Own name	Succeeded	Succeeded
Year born	Failed	Succeeded
Own age	Failed	Succeeded
Present Prime Minister	Succeeded	Succeeded
Present US President	Failed	Succeeded
Writing	Failed	Succeeded
Drawing/copying	Failed	Failed
Reading	A few single letters	Most letters OK and four simple words
Reciting alphabet	A–G √	A–Z with 3 errors (K,U,V)
Naming from description (Coughlan & Warrington)	3/10 Correct	11/15 Correct
Naming actual objects	1/7 Correct (Toy car)	6/12 / 8/12 (Rotated)
Naming object when simple description provided	6/7 (Failed pencil)	7/7
Spelling (Words spelled aloud by tester)	9 Correct	10 Correct
Vineland Social Maturity Scale (Informant: occupational therapist)		
Raw score	21.5	42
Overall social age	1–1½ yr	2–3 yr
First failure	0–1 yr	1–2 yr
Highest success	2–3 yr	11–12 yr

bered that agnosia is a disorder of object recognition that is not due to poor eyesight, a naming or language disorder, or to general intellectual deterioration. Sarah certainly had some intellectual deterioration as a result of her anesthetic accident but was this sufficient to explain her difficulty with real objects and pictures of objects? No, we argued because Sarah was aware of her surroundings, she had some insight into the nature of her problems (for example, she said that she felt stupid when she could not do basic self-care activities); she was able to recall some of what had taken place in her therapy sessions and she was able to engage in a simple conversation in French. Was her object recognition difficulty due to poor eyesight? Again, although she had difficulty orienting her attention, she could name colors, read some words and letters, and could match colors. She was unable to count the number of dots on a page or match faces or shapes. However, this was probably due to her optic ataxia and problems with spatial localization. Could a naming or language problem explain Sarah's inability with objects and pictures? Many people with naming difficulties are able to say something about an object, to demonstrate they have recognized it, even if they cannot name it. For example, they might say, "It's a-a-thingummy—you eat it," or they might mime the use of the object. Sarah would not have been able to mime easily because she had difficulty organizing her movements but she could have described the object and its function, had she recognized it. She did not do this. On an unpublished test (devised by an earlier trainee Jacky Knibbs) in which she had to point to the correct picture from one of four (see Figure 22.1), Sarah was correct on only 27 out of 60.

In this task four kinds of responses can be made—the correct response (bucket), a random error (feather), a visually similar error (flowerpot), or a semantically similar error (spade). Sarah made 4 random errors, 15 visual errors, and 14 semantic errors. This pattern is not typical of someone with dysphasia and a naming disorder. Such a person would make more semantic errors than visual errors. Of course Sarah's performance was hampered by scanning, attentional, and localizational problems—but her object recognition difficulty was probably not due to a naming or language disorder.

Jenny in Chapter 15 had a particular type of agnosia, namely associative agnosia. One of the characteristics of associative agnosia is that people can match to sample. Another characteristic is that they can copy or draw the object they are unable to recognize. Jenny could do both these things but Sarah could not. If she had an agnosia, it was probably an even rarer kind of agnosia called apperceptive agnosia in which people cannot match to sample, or copy, or draw the unrecognized object. Such people may be considered blind. Sarah was not considered blind but she was considered to have very poor vision, which was not substantiated on our tests. She could read small print if she did not have to voluntarily direct her gaze to it. Furthermore it has been observed that Balint's syndrome (or elements of it) have been involved in cases of apperceptive agnosia (Rubens, 1979). It seems likely then that Sarah had an apperceptive agnosia as a result of Balint's syndrome.

Another question of interest was whether Sarah had a surface dyslexia, i.e., a difficulty reading and spelling irregular words. She was, at this time, unable to spell COUGH although she could read this word. We administered a lexical decision task whereby Sarah had to read a word and decide if it was a real word or not. From a list of 49 words, she correctly identified 34, made 4 false positives, and 11 false negatives. We felt the high error rate was due to her oculomotor difficulties. She made no errors when the words were read aloud to her. She also made many errors including homophone errors on a homophone list provided by Max Coltheart. This happened both when Sarah was reading the words herself and when we spelled them to her. She was asked to read (or we spelled to her)

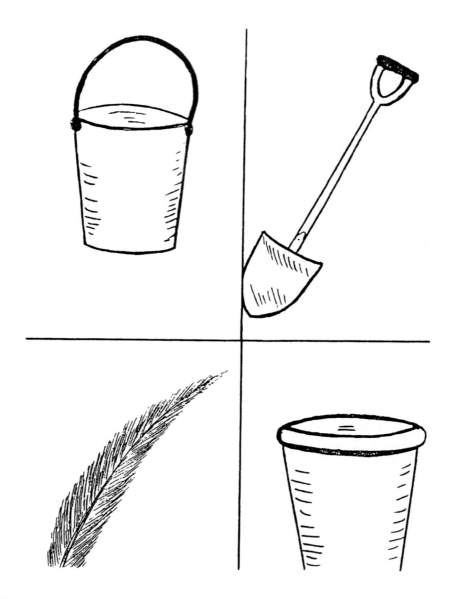

Figure 22.1. Example of a test to detect visual and semantic errors (Knibbs, unpublished).

two homophones, for example, break and brake, for Sarah to define. When asked to define P–O–R–E she said, "poor—penniless." Homophone confusions as we saw in Chapter 15 are characteristic of people with surface dyslexia. Sarah found the reading assessment very difficult and tiring. She was extremely slow because of the scanning problems and took a long time to see the word. She was unable to write so all words she was asked to spell to us had to be spelled aloud. Although she had a reasonable immediate memory, Sarah sometimes forgot where she was up to in spelling a word, so we did not pursue the reading and spelling as much as we might have. There were elements of surface dyslexia and surface dysgraphia but Sarah's problems were more widespread and compounded by the oculomotor and spatial localization difficulties.

The final question addressed in this second assessment was whether or not Sarah had apraxia. Apraxia can be defined as a movement disorder that cannot be explained by paralysis, weakness, poor comprehension, or refusal to cooperate. Sarah was unable to feed herself, drink unassisted, or dress herself yet she could walk and talk. She was never incontinent and always said when she needed to go to the toilet despite needing help when she was there. She could raise her arms above her head, she had a strong grip (not under voluntary control), and appeared to be well motivated to care for herself. Thus, she fulfilled the exclusion criteria for apraxia. She had a movement disorder (she could not initiate, sequence, or carry out motor activities) despite having the strength and range of movements required for the task. The disorder was not due to paralysis or weakness. She understood the task. Observing her attempts to sit on a chair, drink from a cup, or put on a coat left one in no doubt she understood what was required—she simply could not do it. However, the question remains to what extent did her poor scanning, reaching, and mislocalization cause the self-care and motor problems? I do not know how to tease these apart. Probably Sarah had Balint's syndrome *and* apraxia with the former exacerbating the latter. In any case the time had come to get on with some treatment despite the failure to fully explain all the basic underlying problems. In real life she could not do things for herself and this is where we started. We took things at face value and tried to tackle the problems head on.

REHABILITATION

The most distressing problem for Sarah was her almost total inability to do anything for herself. Improving her self-care skills therefore became a priority for treatment. She had by now been at the rehabilitation center for 4 mo and had been receiving occupational and physical therapy twice daily, 5 days a week, throughout this time. The therapists were experienced in working with brain injured people yet Sarah had learned no self-help skills during that time. A psychology student Anne Watson and I worked together with Sarah's occupational therapist to try to teach her some basic tasks. We used the results from the Vineland Social Maturity Scale to select our first treatment goal, namely Sarah's inability to drink from a cup unaided. The first stage involved direct observation. What actually happened when Sarah tried to drink from a cup? One common error was that she failed to reach the cup accurately. Her hand missed the cup and went too far to the left or to the right or in front of the cup. Another error occurred when Sarah managed to reach the cup. Typically she would hold the very top of the cup so that it was unstable. A third kind of error occurred when she found and touched the handle but was not able to grip it. The fourth kind of error occurred when she tried to release the cup after having drunk—she was unable to put it back on the table. The combination of Balint's syndrome and apraxia is consistent with these four types of error.

In the absence of guidance from published rehabilitation literature on how to treat someone with Sarah's pattern of deficits, we turned to the field of learning disability and decided to modify the chaining approach which is often used to teach self-care skills. Chaining involves breaking a task down into small steps and teaching one step in the chain first then a second step, then chaining the two together before teaching the third step in the chain, and so forth. We modified the procedure, however, by breaking the task into steps but teaching Sarah all the steps together.

The procedure was as follows: the task of drinking from a cup was broken down into nine steps selected partly through our observations or Sarah's behavior and partly through clinical intuition as to what would enable Sarah to succeed. The nine steps were:

1. Put your hand flat on the table,
2. Keep your hand low,
3. Put your thumb through the handle of the cup,
4. Grasp the handle,
5. Lift the cup to your mouth,
6. Drink,
7. Put the cup down on the table,
8. Open your fingers,
9. Release your fingers and take your thumb out of the handle.

After the seventh teaching session an additional step was added between steps 5 and 6. This step was 5a. Look for the red rim (a red strip was placed on the rim of the cup nearest to her mouth). This step was required because Sarah often held the further rim of the cup to her mouth, thus causing most of the liquid to pour down the front of her clothes.

Each step was scored as follows:

1. Step completed without help,
2. Verbal prompt required,
3. Slight physical prompt (a nudge in the right direction), and
4. Full physical guidance required, i.e. Sarah's hand was placed in the correct position.

Treatment took place each morning during Sarah's occupational therapy session. It began 8 mo following the anesthetic accident. She was seated at a table with a half-filled cup of coffee or fruit juice in front of her. First she was asked to drink the coffee or juice. If she then placed her hand flat on the table without help she would score 1 for this step. If she failed to carry out this step after 10 sec or if she made an incorrect response, she was given the verbal prompt: "put your hand flat on the table." If Sarah succeeded following a verbal prompt, the step was scored 2. If she failed to complete the step with a verbal prompt the therapist gently nudged her hand in the right direction. Success here would score 3. If Sarah still failed to complete the step, her hand was moved to the correct place and position and a score of 4 awarded. The same procedure was followed for each successive step. Thus it was possible to see for each step how much help Sarah required.

As can be seen from Figure 22.2, Sarah learned fairly quickly to drink from a cup unaided. The first time the program was implemented she was able to complete only one step alone (drink) and for 5 of the 9 steps she needed full physical guidance. However, by the third attempt (45 min later), she was completing all the steps unaided. In the following sessions during the 1st wk, Sarah's performance was variable, but by the following week she was doing all the steps unaided and was independent in drinking from a cup.

Since that time Sarah has always been able to drink from a cup although her movements are not smooth and fluent. She was able to generalize to other cups and to glasses. Given the rapidity and dramatic nature of the successful completion of this task, we wondered whether it was just a fluke and that Sarah was, perhaps, just at the right stage for learning to drink alone and our treatment was coincidental. We decided to follow the same procedure for a completely different task, namely pulling in her chair to the table. We also enrolled the help of a different therapist, Sarah's physiotherapist, to carry out the prompting.

Four mo earlier Sarah was unable to seat herself on a chair without help. Once again this appeared to be due partly to her apraxia and partly to the spatial localization problems. It was not due to weakness, paralysis, or failure to understand what was required of her. Sarah moved around the chair but would be unable to position herself correctly in relation to the seat of the chair. By October, Sarah was able to sit on the chair without help but was unable to pull the chair she was sitting on closer to the table. She could not position her hands correctly or move correctly in order to carry out the operation. Once again we broke the task down into steps and used the same procedure as before.

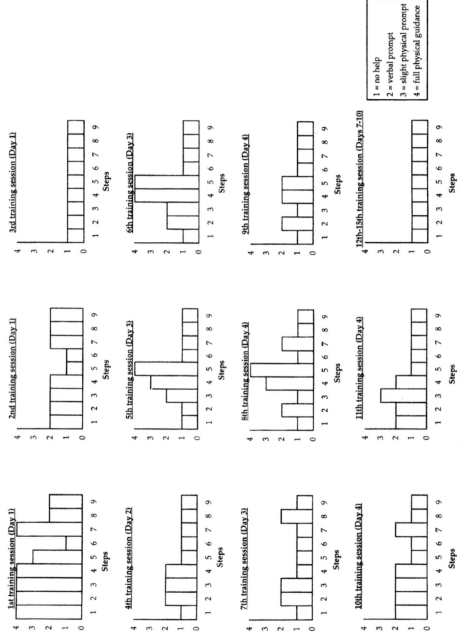

Figure 22.2. Amount of help required in drinking from a cup alone.

The steps were:

1. Stand up
2. Bend over slightly
3. Put one hand at the side of the chair
4. Grasp the chair
5. Put the other hand at the side of the chair
6. Grasp the chair
7. Put your head up and look where you are going
8. Walk forward with little steps while holding the chair
9. Put your head up and look where you are going
10. When your arms touch the table sit down.

This task was learned in a similar manner to the previous one. The results can be seen in Figure 22.3.

We felt that natural recovery could not account for the success as Sarah never learned to complete a self-help task without a similar structured program. She seemed unable to hold a plan of action in her mind in order to initiate and carry out an activity. Certain types of apraxia have indeed been considered as disorders of planning by some neuropsychologists. For example, one of the earlier writers on apraxia, Liepmann (1920) believed that ideational apraxia resulted from an impairment of the idea or plan of movement. Luria (1966, 1973) claimed that frontal apraxia was due to a disruption of both the plan or intention for action and of the ability to compare one's performance with the plan to see if the goal has been achieved. Heilman (1979) has a rather different explanation for ideational apraxia. He suggests it is due to a disorder of the verbally mediated motor sequence selector.

Both hypotheses may explain (or partially explain) Sarah's difficulties. If she is unable to plan her actions because of problems experienced in selecting the correct sequence, which is often verbally mediated, then providing a verbal prompt may overcome this deficit. Although Sarah did not overtly verbalize the action (nor did she covertly verbalize as far as we can tell), she was nevertheless able to perform the task once she had been taken through it several times. So the step-by-step approach may have provided an overall plan of the motor sequence and the verbal prompts may have been useful in unconsciously providing a mediator for the right action.

In retrospect, a third explanation may be invoked, namely errorless learning. Errorless learning as its name implies involves learning without errors. First described in the 1960s in work with pigeons (Terrace, 1963, 1966), errorless learning was soon used for people with developmental learning difficulties (Sidman and Stoddard, 1967; Walsh and Lamberts, 1979). In the 1990s the principle was used with brain injured memory impaired people (Wilson et al., 1994; Wilson

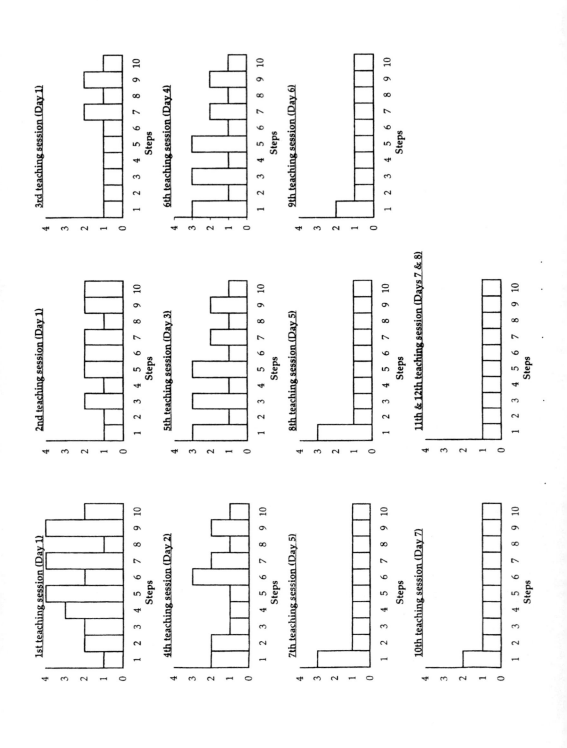

and Evans, 1996). This work followed on from a theoretically driven experiment in which Baddeley and Wilson (1994) posed the question, "Do amnesic subjects learn better if prevented from making mistakes during the learning process?" Three groups of subjects were given three trials in each of two tasks. In one task subjects were required to generate guesses, i.e., make mistakes, while in the other task the correct answer was provided before they could guess, i.e., mistakes were avoided. For the two control groups (one group of young and one group of elderly subjects) there was no significant difference between scores on nine test trials that followed the three learning trials. All 16 amnesic subjects, however, did better on the errorless learning trials, i.e., when mistakes were avoided.

Errorless learning may explain the success of other rehabilitation programs, even though the investigators were not aware they were using this method. Kime et al. (1996), for example, taught a young brain injured woman to use a personal organizer very effectively. During the learning process, she was not allowed to fail. Support and structure were provided at each step until she took over the steps herself. Errorless learning appears to work with memory impaired people because they cannot benefit from their mistakes. In order to learn from one's errors, one needs to remember such errors. In the absence of episodic memory, errors tend to be repeated and so should be avoided in the first place.

The errorless learning principle might explain Sarah's success. She was unable to remember how to carry out a motor task; the step-by-step procedure enabled her to successfully complete each step and this enhanced learning.

Sarah was discharged from the rehabilitation center soon after this in order to go to a center for people with physical handicaps where she spent 2 yr as a weekly boarder.

FOLLOW-UP

In April 1984, Sarah returned to the rehabilitation center for a reassessment. She cooperated well and her ability to manipulate objects seemed to have improved, so too had her reading. She now scored at a $14^{1}/_{2}$-yr-old level on the British Ability Scales word reading list. Although her counting, reciting the alphabet, naming objects, and naming to description were virtually unchanged, her Vineland overall score had now increased to a 4–5-yr-old level.

Six months later, i.e., 20 mo after the anesthetic accident, Sarah came back again for a further reassessment. This time we concentrated on her reading skills and object recognition. Sarah's behavior was described as cooperative and friendly, more alert, and oriented, and her speech easier to understand. Her ability to point accurately was better and she seemed to have fewer problems with her vision.

Discussing her reading skills I said these still appeared to be improving. The results suggested she had features of attentional dyslexia and approximate visual access (Coltheart, 1985). She could identify single letters but misidentified letters when these were embedded in words. Consequently she misread words, for example she read MASTERY as "MYSTERY." Although she tended to make more mistakes when reading irregular rather than regular words, this was not as strong an effect as say Jason in Chapter 9. Sarah's spelling of irregular words was not always typical of someone with surface dyslexia or dysgraphia. For example, she spelled BEACH as BEAH and BRICK as WRKK, which seemed to be attentional errors, although on other occasions her errors were phonetic, for example, RANE for RAIN. She also made homophone confusions such as BEET—defined as "a policeman's beat."

With regard to her agnosia, it was not possible to say for certain whether Sarah had a true visual object agnosia because we could not adequately assess her vision. She could define the names of objects she could not recognize directly; she was better at recognizing real objects than photographs and she had a very severe problem with the identification of model animals. All these characteristics were seen in Jenny in Chapter 15 and are consistent with agnosia. Sarah, however, could not recognize by touch possibly because of her apraxia and poor manipulation, she could not copy for the same reason and her naming to description was not perfect. Thus it was difficult to say whether she could recognize through another modality, which is required for a diagnosis of agnosia.

The following year in 1985, 30 mo after the anesthetic accident, Sarah was readmitted for a month to see if we could teach her some more basic self-care skills. Three tasks were selected:

1. Putting on her coat,
2. Putting on her track-suit pants, and
3. Making a cup of coffee.

Sarah was involved in the selection of these goals. She chose 2 and 3 with the rehabilitation team choosing the first goal. Once again each task was broken down into steps and an increasing amount of help given with each step as required. Scoring was the same as before. Making a cup of coffee for example was broken down into 18 steps. She always needed help pouring boiling water into the cup because her hand was not steady enough and we felt we could not take the risk. Sarah never learned the task without error but she was able to complete 14 of the 18 steps alone. She was, however, able to put her coat on independently and could sometimes manage her track-suit pants. We felt we had proved the efficacy of the approach and offered to teach the method to the staff at the center Sarah was attending. They did not take us up on this offer.

The next time I saw Sarah was in December 1988 when she agreed to take part in an Italian television program on brain injury. The Italian crew came to film her.

Her apraxia was still very marked and we did not have time for any neuropsychological tests. Sarah also seemed more aware of her problems and embarrassed at being asked to carry out tasks she could not do. For example, when asked to demonstrate how to wave good-by she said, "Don't ask me to do that—you know I can't do it and it makes me feel stupid." Thus her insight appeared to have increased and at the same time, her mood had worsened.

For 3 yr I lost touch with Sarah but contacted her again for a long-term follow-up study I was doing on 101 patients seen between 4–12 yr earlier (Wilson, 1995b). Sarah and her aunt agreed to take part. In 1990 Sarah received a large sum in compensation for the anesthetic accident. This will ensure adequate care for the rest of her life but the money cannot purchase treatment for Sarah's problems. When asked what they saw as Sarah's main problems in 1991, Sarah said, "[it was] steps—it's difficult getting up and down steps." This had been a problem since the early days as Sarah could not tell where, in space, objects were. Her aunt felt there were problems with bathing, dressing, and communication but the biggest problem was frustration at being helped. Sarah wanted to do everything independently and when she was helped she became frustrated, which brought on black moods.

Sarah had remained at the center for people with physical handicaps for about 3 yr before going to another center, which did not work out. She then started going to a day center and, at the time of my visit, was going 5 days a week. Transport was provided by social services. I repeated some of the tests from the earlier assessment. Sarah had continued to improve in some areas. For example, her naming to description was now 14 out of 15 and her NART score had increased from 13 out of 50 correct to 22 out of 50 correct. In other areas, things had not changed a great deal. Sarah was still unable to write or count the number of dots on a page. Her spelling was very phonetic and she had great difficulty recognizing objects.

Sarah herself was sad about her situation. She lives in a beautiful house with caring relatives and has obviously come a long way since the early days, but there is no doubt she remains very disabled and with increased insight has realized for herself the extent of her problems.

SARAH TODAY

I last saw Sarah in November 1996 to discuss this chapter with her aunt and uncle, and later with Sarah herself. "What does Sarah enjoy doing now?" I asked her aunt,

"She likes going to the local pub, she likes fashion magazines, and nice perfumes. Sometimes she goes to the shops. She can't do anything for herself and I am very reluctant to leave her in the house by herself. I don't even like to garden when she's in the house. If she wants me in the garden she will do a huge detour to avoid a step. Her self-preservation instincts are good!"

"What about friends?" I asked. "Her friends fizzled away apart from one friend from schooldays who is willing to have Sarah to stay. She last saw her about 2 yr ago."

Her aunt went on to explain that one of the main problems with Sarah was that she could not sort out fact from fiction. She sometimes imagined things and thought they had really happened. Sarah did not like to talk about the anesthetic accident but had become resigned to her situation. Her aunt and uncle both believed that Sarah was definitely aware of what she had lost.

Sarah joined us after her return from the day center. I asked her how she felt about her present situation. She replied,

"I can't do things for myself now. I'm jealous of other people. I can't do my maths now. I can't take a walk. I can't read easily. I also fall down the steps and have mishaps. I'm mentally and physically disabled. I'm very angry."

Sarah has obviously come a long way from the girl I first met in 1983 but there is little hope of further change and this young woman of 34 yr of age will remain extremely disabled.

23

CONCLUSIONS

In this book I have described 20 people who sustained an injury or insult to the brain, and I have explained in detail the subsequent rehabilitation that was carried out to make their daily living more manageable and less distressing. I have tried to describe as fully as possible the problems these people experienced both before and after rehabilitation, and I have given an account of their successes and failures over a period of several years. Wherever possible I have included written or tape recorded accounts from the brain injured people themselves, or their relatives, in the belief that their voices should be heard and their perspectives understood.

While the rehabilitation described in this book has centered in the main on cognitive problems, such as memory or reading difficulties, I hope I have been able to show that brain injured people are first and foremost people whose cognitive problems are only part of the whole context that makes up their daily lives and interaction with family and friends. They are not to be regarded simply as neuropsychological cases.

The book includes sections on the pure amnesic syndrome, memory with other cognitive disorders, language, acquired disorders of reading, perceptual, and visuospatial problems, and behavior and self-care skills. Because of the nature of brain injury there is, inevitably, overlap between these sections.

The major concern of rehabilitation is to reduce disability and handicap rather than initial impairment. Impairments are deficits caused by damage to physical and mental structures. Thus a patient with bilateral hippocampal damage will do poorly on tests of episodic memory. Improving performance on these tests, however, is not the point of rehabilitation. Instead we focus on the disability, i.e., how the memory problems manifest themselves in real life, e.g., forgetting to use a notebook, getting lost around the neighborhood, or having difficulty learning a new skill. Rehabilitation may well reduce the disability yet have no impact on the impairment. In addition to decreasing the disability, rehabilitation may also reduce the level of handicap, i.e., the extent to which memory problems prevent successful return to society. So a memory impaired person, such as Jay (Chapter 4), who compensates well and therefore has little handicap in real life, is able to live independently and earn his own living. Martin (Chapter 7) however, is handicapped by his problems and needs to live under close supervision.

I have chosen to focus on cognitive functions rather than diagnostic groups, such as head injury or stroke, as the behavioral manifestations of cognitive deficits cross diagnostic boundaries. Take, for example, Jack (Chapter 3) and Jay (Chapter 4). In many ways they are similar, particularly with regard to their neuropsychological test profiles, yet Jack sustained anoxic brain damage and Jay a posterior cerebral artery infarct. Sarah (Chapter 22) who also had anoxic brain damage experienced very different problems, needing particular help with self-care skills. People with traumatic head injury, not surprisingly, showed a wide variety of deficits. Although one needs to be aware of the diagnostic group and bear this in mind (because, for example, people with encephalitis are likely to achieve their optimum level of functioning much sooner than people with traumatic head injury), identification of rehabilitation goals is not determined by a diagnostic group but by assessment of need, deficit, patient and family desires, and so forth.

As I mentioned earlier, rehabilitation is a two-way process in which the brain injured person works together with health service staff and others to achieve optimum levels of physical, psychological, and social well-being (McLellan, 1991). Often in neurological or neuropsychological rehabilitation we cannot restore people back to their level of functioning before the insult. This is true of all 20 people described in this book. None achieved their former level of functioning. However, they all achieved something. Typically they were taught to compensate for or get around their difficulties, either through using residual skills more efficiently, or through finding an alternative way to achieve a goal, or through a combination of these.

The three people with a pure amnesic syndrome (Jack, Jay, and Alex) all compensated well. This is not surprising as memory impaired people without additional cognitive deficits are more likely to be independent and more likely to employ compensatory aids or strategies effectively (Wilson & Watson, 1996). In contrast, none of the four people with severe memory impairments together with additional cognitive difficulties (Clive, Martin, Lorna, and Jason) were able to compensate well. In the case of Clive, environmental restructuring together with modifications of staff behavior were the only ways found to help reduce Clive's emotional problems. He was also able to learn a few things through his relatively intact implicit memory. Martin and Jason were both able to learn some new information provided this was structured and taught through mnemonics or errorless learning. This was also true of Lorna although to a lesser extent. Lorna, it will be remembered had a slowly progressive cognitive decline so learned with increasing difficulty over time.

What about the compensatory abilities of the other patients whose main area of cognitive deficit was not memory? The Oxford English Dictionary definition of "compensate" is "to offset a disability by development in another direction." This can be said of Bill (Chapter 10) who was able to offset his inability to communicate by developing (with help from the speech therapist and myself) the means to communicate with a pictorial system. To put this another way, Bill was able to find an alternative method to reach the goal of communicating with others.

Laurence (Chapter 11) did not compensate through using alternative methods although he was, perhaps, using his residual skills more efficiently. He was always a good communicator despite his severe language problems, so it could be argued that he was using his residual communication skills to compensate for the word finding and comprehension deficits experienced. Ron (Chapter 12) would appear to be following a similar pattern. With a number of cognitive problems, he was still able, for the most part, to make people understand him by rewording or miming the concept he wanted to get across. Furthermore, Ron frequently resorted to his knowledge of the order of the alphabet, numbers, days of the week, and months of the year to help him compensate and retrieve the word or letter he wanted. So, for example, when asked, "What date is it today?," he would mutter under his breath "One, two, three, four, five, SIX . . . it's January, February, March, APRIL SIX."

Ted (Chapter 13) could have used to a much greater extent his ability to read initial letters if he traced them first with his finger to compensate for his inability to read initial letters through vision. Ted was very reluctant to use this method, however, wanting to read by the method he had always used in the past. His closest approach to compensation was through the use of text to help him understand the word. Thus if he saw the single word LOG he did not know whether the word was BOG, DOG, FOG, HOG, LOG, or whatever. Reading the same word in a prose passage, would in most cases enable him to read the word correctly because of the context.

Derek (Chapter 14) originally used the tracing method to help him after his successful attempt at learning to read. He needed this only for a short time though and soon managed with vision alone. Derek and Jenny (Chapter 15) may come closest, of all those in this book, to achieving restoration of function, progressing from being completely alexic after sustaining severe head injuries through to reading at the level of a $13^1/_2$- and a $12^1/_2$-yr-old respectively. However, even these dramatic improvements only partially restored the function of reading as both Derek and Jenny always read letter-by-letter and were always better at regularly spelled than irregularly spelled words.

Because Paula (Chapter 16) was discharged from rehabilitation early at the request of her father, who would not allow any follow-up, it is difficult to say much about her ability to compensate over the years. What we do know is that her attempts to use her relatively intact verbal skills to compensate for her poor object recognition did not work. When she saw a picture of a thimble she tried to verbally describe it by saying, "It's white and bumpy." Unfortunately her interpretation of a white and bumpy object was "a cauliflower." Similarly on another occasion I showed her a picture of a sofa with two round cushions on it. Paula looked carefully at the picture and said, "There's a round thing like a wheel" (this was one of the cushions). When asked what else she could see she said, "There's another one" (this was the second cushion). "So what do you think it is?" I asked. "A bicycle," said Paula. There is no doubt that Paula's physiotherapist and I reduced her fear of exercises through shaping, i.e., gradually working towards the final goal. It would be difficult I think to argue this was compensatory behavior rather than simply an anxiety management or fear reduction process.

With Kirsty (Chapter 17), compensation was perhaps responsible for some of her progress at least initially. She improved her ability to name objects if she was able to touch them rather like Ted (Chapter 13) and his tactile letter reading. As she showed greater recovery, however, Kirsty no longer needed to depend on the tactile route.

Richard (Chapter 18) benefited from several methods to compensate for his difficulties. One of the most fruitful was environmental adaptation. With his poor scanning, Richard was helped greatly if his coffee mug was on a different shelf from other mugs and his socks were kept separate from his pajamas. Richard was also able to use external memory aids, particularly later on in his rehabilitation when the aids took into account his visuospatial problems. Dolly (Chapter 19) had a number of problems similar to Richard's and she was taught to scan more efficiently to enable her to compensate for her unilateral neglect.

The last three people, Jim, Angela, and Sarah (Chapters 20, 21, and 22, respectively), showed varying degrees of compensatory behavior. Jim was able, to some extent, to use his better verbal skills to help compensate for his poor visuospatial skills. Changing the environmental demands also reduced his behavior problems. Both Angela and Sarah were helped to achieve some self-care skills through breaking functions or tasks down into smaller steps. With Angela this was achieved at a more global level, i.e., her ability to be independent was broken down into smaller steps such as learning to drink a cup of tea alone or open the door by herself. With Sarah the individual tasks themselves required breakdown so that in order to drink alone from a cup we had to start by teaching her to find the table and place her hand on it. Is this compensation? I would argue that it is as both Angela and Sarah achieved their final goals through an alternative route and, as I suggested above, this is one of the ways to achieve compensation.

I have tried to show the importance of assessment, both for building up a picture of an individual's strengths and weaknesses (typically achieved through standardized tests), and for identifying the disabilities or everyday problems typically achieved by functional or behavioral measures that help determine the rehabilitation goals. Jim (Chapter 20) is a good example of how standardized and functional measures can go hand in hand to help plan treatment. Sarah (Chapter 22) is a good example of how behavioral assessment and behavioral treatment are often inextricably linked. The assessment of how Sarah performed each step of the self-care tasks taught her was also the treatment strategy itself and it would be impossible to say when the assessment ended and the treatment began.

With many of the other people in this book the link between assessment and treatment may be less explicitly stated but it is always there. Once again I stress the need to treat , reduce, or ameliorate functional consequences, which are the problems faced by individuals and their families in their daily lives, rather than impairments identified by standardized tests. We do not and we should not engage in rehabilitation simply in order to enable people to improve their scores on neuropsychological tests. Nor should we use results from these tests to evaluate the success of our rehabilitation programs. Memory impaired people can improve the way they function by using a personal organizer or pager to remind them to keep appointments while still failing to improve on standardized tests of memory. The purpose of memory rehabilitation is to enable people to be more independent and not to simply pass a standardized test. People can improve their scores on neuropsychological tests yet remain functionally disabled in their daily lives. Although conventional tests can help us plan rehabilitation through building up a picture of cognitive functioning, and ecologically valid tests can predict which people are likely to experience everyday problems, we need greater precision than they can offer in order to identify treatment goals. The relationship between cognitive impairments as measured on tests and cognitive failures in everyday life is too weak to base our rehabilitation programs on the results obtained from the former. Until we can show that treating *impairments* reduces *disability* we should avoid using the results from standardized tests to evaluate responses to rehabilitation.

In conclusion, I would like to look ahead to the year 2000 and beyond and consider future developments in the field. We must above all ensure ethical and effective neuropsychological rehabilitation. We should address the cognitive, emotional, motivational, social, and other sequelae resulting from neurological impairment. Cognition should not be divorced from noncognitive functions because feelings, social situations, self-esteem, and so forth affect how we think and how we behave. As I said before, we must focus on disability rather than impairment, that is we should address problems faced by the individual and not address a deficit identified by a test or series of tests.

Despite the fact that at present neuropsychologists have different concepts and terminology than occupational therapists, speech and language therapists, and other disciplines, we need to develop a greater dialogue between the various professions engaged in rehabilitation. The challenge is to develop a common language and a broader as well as deeper theoretical understanding. For this we shall need a wider theoretical spectrum on which to base our rehabilitation programs, and we should not be confined by our own conceptual frameworks.

It is probably true to say that the main theoretical influences on neuropsychology and neuropsychological rehabilitation have come from (1) the study of neuropsychology itself, which provides us with an understanding of how the brain is organized; (2) cognitive (neuro)psychology, which provides us with theoretical models to help explain phenomena and predict patterns of behavior; and (3) behavioral psychology, which has provided us with a number of intervention strategies that can be modified or adapted for use with brain injured people. Behavioral psychology has also provided strategies to help us assess everyday manifestations of neuropsychological impairments, analyze problems, and evaluate the efficacy of treatments. One branch of behavioral psychology in particular, learning theory, has been important in helping neuropsychologists improve learning in people with brain injury.

There are of course numerous other perhaps less powerful sources of influence on the development of neuropsychology and neuropsychological rehabilitation, including neurology, psychiatry, gerontology, occupational therapy, linguistics, ergonomics, information technology, and others; all of them serving to emphasize the fact that neuropsychology and neuropsychological rehabilitation are areas requiring a broad theoretical base, or perhaps one should say, several theoretical bases (Wilson, 1997). It is apt, I think, to point out here that it is simply not sufficient for cognitive psychologists to suggest that neuropsychological rehabilitation should be driven by theories solely from their own discipline. The danger of following one model or theoretical approach too closely, without considering other possible influential sources, is that we might become too narrow and constrained.

The interaction between theory and clinical practice needs to be strengthened. Theory can sometimes predict which methods to use but we often require clinical experience and observation to tell us how to implement theoretical findings. We also need to ensure proper evaluation of neuropsychological rehabilitation programs at a number of levels, from the general (Are these programs effective?) to the specific (Is this patient changing as a result of our intervention?).

How do research findings change our clinical behavior? Often this is in subtle ways of which we may not be aware. No psychologist working with memory impaired clients today would assume that someone with a good digit span and poor delayed memory was hysterical or faking, or malingering. Yet 20 yr ago a psychiatrist claimed this about a woman who became amnesic following coal–gas poisoning. This woman had the classic combination of normal immediate memory together with a grossly impaired ability to learn new information. For some time she was classified as a hysterical amnesic because her pattern of symptoms "was inconsistent with her psychiatrist's totally incorrect concept of the structure and breakdown of human memory" (Baddeley, 1984, p. 6). Since the development of cognitive models of memory, I doubt that this particular misdiagnosis would happen today.

In other areas, the change in our clinical behavior as a result of research is perhaps more deliberate. In the early 1990's Alan Baddeley and I began some research into the usefulness of errorless learning in the rehabilitation of memory impaired people. Errorless learning is a technique whereby errors are avoided, as far as possible, during the learning process. Our work had been influenced by two different fields within psychology. The first being errorless discrimination learning from behavioral psychology, and the second being research into implicit memory and learning from cognitive neuropsychology. Our work, then, was certainly theoretically driven. In the first of our studies most participants and *all* of the densely amnesic people learned more when prevented from guessing (Baddeley and Wilson, 1994). Once I saw that 100% of amnesic people did better when prevented from guessing, I changed my clinical behavior overnight. I used to say to severely memory impaired people, "Can you remember my name? No? Well have a guess," or words to that effect. Now, unless test requirements demand otherwise, I say, "I don't want you to guess, only tell me if you are sure." In the absence of episodic memory it would appear to be best to avoid trial-and-error learning. We went on to establish that errorless learning principles could be used to teach amnesic patients relevant everyday information (Wilson et al., 1994; Wilson and Evans, 1996).

In contrast to the above examples, where research has initially informed practice, we can consider the evaluation of a new memory aid, (Wilson et al., 1997). This small pager, and the software that drives it, have been of real benefit to a number of brain injured people, enabling some to get back to work, some to return to college, and others to lead a more independent life. While research backs up these findings, the development of the pager and the subsequent research to confirm its benefits were entirely patient driven. It would be hard to make a case that the study was theoretically driven unless one used an ergonomic type of theoretical explanation, that in order to achieve maximum benefit the compensatory device should be active, immediate, specific, and timely.

In the above examples I have tried to show that theory and practice are complementary in the sense that both can, and indeed must, inform each other. Professionals themselves can go one further by accepting that the very work in which they are engaged may not only inform their future attitudes and practices but may also contribute in some small way to the development of future theory. As a student I was told, "Every patient you see should be capable of being written up for a journal," and, even if this is a little ambitious, it is a good general rule to follow. Most clinicians plan treatments, take notes, and monitor progress. The information gathered in this way can form the basis for action or self-directed research. Research provides feedback on clinical effectiveness and productivity; it can show us how to use time more efficiently; it allows us to confirm or disconfirm theoretical predictions; and it can extend the boundaries of neuropsychological knowledge.

Our rapidly expanding knowledge of the brain and how it works is likely to continue in the early years of the next century and beyond, and as a result of this we can expect many new treatments for brain injury. These are likely to include medicines, drugs, new technology, transplants, and even genetic manipulation. However, one thing is certain, and that is that these new treatments will have to be measured by their effectiveness in alleviating the problems of brain injured people in their everyday lives. This can only be done by observing and assessing brain injured people in the kinds of rehabilitation programs I have been describing in this book. There is a great chance for theorists, researchers, and clinicians to use our increasing knowledge of the brain, together with more sophisticated and theoretically informed methods of rehabilitation, to work more effectively on issues relating to brain injury, medication, treatment, and rehabilitation.

Finally, we need to ensure that rehabilitation is available to all who need it. As a British politician said in 1973, "An improvement in rehabilitation can mean more to millions of people than almost any other medical advance" (Sir Keith Joseph).

References

Albert, M. L. (1979). Alexia. In K. M. Heilman & E. Valenstein (Eds.), *Clinical neuropsy-chology.* New York: Oxford University Press.

Alderman, N. & Burgess, P. (1994). A comparison of treatment methods for behaviour dis-order following herpes simplex encephalitis. *Neuropsychological Rehabilitation, 4,* 31–48.

Alderman, N. & Ward, A. (1991). Behavioural treatment of the dysexecutive syndrome: Reduction of repetitive speech using response cost and cognitive overlearning. *Neu-ropsychological Rehabilitation, 1,* 65–80.

Alderman, N., Fry, R. K. & Youngson, H. A. (1995). Improvement of self-monitoring skills, reduction of behaviour disturbance and the dysexecutive syndrome: Compari-son of response cost and a new programme of self-monitoring training. *Neuropsycho-logical Rehabilitation, 5,* 193–221.

Anastasi, A. (1982). *Psychological Testing, 5th edition.* New York: Collier/Macmillan.

Baddeley, A. D. (1984). Memory theory and memory therapy in B. A. Wilson, N. Moffat (eds.), *Clinical Management of Memory Problems* (pp. 5–27). London: Croom Helm Ltd.

Baddeley, A. D. (1992). Memory theory and memory therapy. In B. A. Wilson & N. Mof-fat (Eds.), *Clinical management of memory problems, 2nd edition* (pp. 1–31). London: Chapman & Hall.

Baddeley, A. D. (1993). A theory of rehabilitation without a model of learning is a vehicle without an engine: A comment on Caramazza and Hillis. *Neuropsychological Reha-bilitation, 3,* 235–244.

Baddeley, A. D. Emslie, H. & Nimmo-Smith, I. (1992). *The Speed and Capacity of Lan-guage Processing (SCOLP) Test.* Bury St. Edmunds, Suffolk: Thames Valley Test Com-pany.

Baddeley, A. D. & Hitch, G. (1974) Working memory. In G. H. Bower (Ed.), *The psychology of learning and motivation, vol. 8* (pp. 47–89). New York: Academic Press.

Baddeley, A. D. & Wilson, B. A. (1986). Amnesia, autobiographical memory and confabulation. In D. Rubin (Ed.) *Autobiographical memory* (pp. 225–252). New York: Cambridge University Press.

Baddeley, A. D. & Wilson, B. A. (1994). When implicit learning fails: Amnesia and the problem of error elimination. *Neuropsychologia, 32,* 53–68.

Balint, R. (1909). Seelenhamung des 'Schauens', optische ataxie, raumlische storung des aufmersamkeit. *Monatsschrift für Psychiatrische Neurologie, 25,* 51–81.

Bauer, R. M. & Rubens, A. L. (1985). Agnosia. In K. M. Heilman & E. Valenstein (Eds.), *Clinical neuropsychology, 2nd edition* (pp. 187–241). New York: Oxford University Press.

Ben-Yishay, Y. (1978). Working approaches to remediation of cognitive deficits in brain damaged persons. *Rehabilitation Monograph No. 59.* New York: New York University Medical Center.

Bennett-Levy, J. (1984). Determinants of performance on the Rey-Osterreith Complex Figure Test: An analysis and a new technique for single-case assessment. *British Journal of Clinical Psychology, 23,* 109–119.

Benson, D. F. & Geschwind, N. (1969). The alexias. In P. J. Vinken & G. W. Bruyn (Eds.), *Handbook of clinical neurology, vol. 4* (pp. 112–140). Amsterdam: North Holland Publishing Co.

Benton, A. L., Van Allen, M. W., Hamsher, K. de S. & Levin, H. S. (1975) *Test of Facial Recognition.* Iowa City: Department of Neurology, University of Iowa Hospitals.

Best, W., Howard, D., Bruce, C. & Gatehouse, C. (1997). Cueing the words: A single case study of treatments for anomia. *Neuropsychological Rehabilitation, 7,* 105–141.

Bickerstaff, E. R. (1957). Brain stem encephalitis—further observations on a grave syndrome with benign prognosis. *British Medical Journal, 1,* 1384–1387.

Bird, T. D., Follett, C. and Griep, E. (1983). Cognitive and personality function in myotonic muscular dystrophy. *Journal of Neurology, Neurosurgery, and Psychiatry, 46,* 971–48.

Bishop, D. V. M. (1982). *Test for Reception of Grammar.* Abingdon: Thomas Leach Ltd.

Bishop, D. & Byng, S. (1984). Assessing semantic comprehension: Methodological considerations and a new clinical test. *Cognitive Neuropsychology, 1,* 233–243.

Black, J. E., Sirevaag, A. M. & Greenough, W. T. (1987). Complex experience promotes capillary formation in young rat visual cortex. *Neuroscience Letters, 83,* 351–355.

Bluma, S., Shearer, M., Frohman, A. & Hilliard, J. (1976) *Portage guide to early education.* Wisconsin, USA: Co-operative Educational Service Agency.

Bogousslavsky, J. & Caplan, L. (1995). *Stroke syndromes.* Cambridge: Cambridge University Press.

Booraem, C. D. & Seacat, G. F. (1972). Effects of increased incentive in corrective therapy. *Perceptual and Motor Skills, 34,* 125–126.

Bower, G. H. (1972). A selective review of organizational factors in memory. In E. Tulving & W. Donaldson (Eds.), *Organization of memory.* New York: Academic Press.

British Psychological Society Report (1989). *Services for young adult patients with acquired brain damage.* Leicester: BPS.

Brooks, D. N. (Ed.) (1984). *Closed head injury: Social, psychological and family consequences.* Oxford: Oxford University Press.

Brooks, D. N. (1991). The effectiveness of post-acute rehabilitation. *Brain Injury, 5,* 102–149.

Brooks, D. N. & Baddeley, A. (1976). What can amnesic patients learn? *Neuropsychologia, 14,* 111–122.

Byng, S. & Coltheart, M. (1986). Aphasia therapy research: methodological requirements and illustrative results. In E. Hjelmquist & L. N. Nilsson (Eds.), *Communication and handicap* (pp. 383–398). Hillsdale, N.J.: Erlbaum.

Cameron, R. J. & White, M. (1987). *The Portage Early Education Programme.* Windsor: NFER-Nelson UK.

Camp, C. J. (1989) Facilitation of new learning in Alzheimer's Disease. In G. Gilmore, P. Whitehouse & M. Wykle (Eds.), *Memory and aging: Theory, research and practice.* New York: Springer.

Camp, C. J. & Schaller, J. R. (1989). Epilogue: Spaced retrieval memory training in an adult day-care center. *Educational Gerontology, 15,* 641–648.

Camp, C. J. & Stevens, A. B. (1990). Spaced retrieval: A memory intervention for dementia of Alzheimer type (DAT). *Clinical Gerontologist, 10,* 58–61.

Caramazza, A. (1989). Cognitive neuropsychology and rehabilitation: an unfulfilled promise? In X. Seron, & G. Deloche (Eds.), *Cognitive approaches in neuropsychological rehabilitation* (pp. 383–398). Hillsdale, N.J.: Erlbaum.

Censori, B., Provinciali, L., Danni, M., Chiaramoni, L., Maricotti, M., Foschi, N., Del-Pesce, M. & Salvolini, U. (1994). Brain involvement in myotonic dystrophy: MRI features and their relation to clinical and cognitive condition. *Acta Neurologica Scandinavica, 90,* 211–217.

Cermak, L. S. (1980). Comments on imagery as a therapeutic mnemonic. In L. W. Poon, J. L. Fozzard, L. S. Cermak, D. Arenberg, & L. W. Thompson (Eds.), *New directions in memory and aging.* Hillsdale, N.J.: Lawrence Erlbaum Associates.

Chang, L., Anderson, T., Migneco, O. A., Boone, K., Mehringer, C. M., Villanueva-Meyer, J., Berman, N., & Mena, I. (1993). Cerebral abnormalities in myotonic dystrophy: Cerebral blood flow, magnetic resonance imaging, and neuropsychological tests. *Archives of Neurology, 50,* 917–923.

Chomsky, N. (1972). *Language and mind.* New York: Harcourt, Brace & World.

Christensen, A-L. & Teasdale, T. W. (1995). A clinical and neuropsychological led post-acute rehabilitation programme. In M. A. Chamberlain, V. C. Newman, and A. Tennant (Eds.), *Traumatic brain injury rehabilitation: Initiatives in service delivery, treatment and measuring outcome* (pp. 88–98). New York: Chapman & Hall.

Ciminero, A. R., Calhoun, K. S. & Adams, H. E. (Eds.), (1977). *Handbook of behavioral assessment.* New York: Wiley.

Clare, L. & Wilson, B. A. (1997). *Coping with memory problems: A practical guide for people with memory impairments, relatives, friends and carers.* Bury St. Edmunds: Thames Valley Test Company.

Collins, F. L., Ricci, J. A. & Burkett, P. A. (1981). Behavioural training for myopia: Long term maintenance of improved acuity. *Behavioural Research and Therapy, 19,* 265–268.

Coltheart, M. (1985). Cognitive neuropsychology and reading. In M. Posner & O. S. M. Marin (Eds.), *Attention and performance XI* (pp. 3–37). Hillsdale, N.J.: Erlbaum.

Coltheart, M. (1991). Cognitive psychology applied to the treatment of acquired language disorders. In P. Martin (Ed.), *Handbook of behavior therapy and psychological science: An integrative approach* (pp. 216–226). New York: Pergamon Press.

Coltheart, M., Bates, A. & Castles, A. (1994). Cognitive neuropsychology and rehabilitation. In M. J. Riddoch & G. W. Humphreys (Eds.), *Cognitive neuropsychology and cognitive rehabilitation* (pp. 17–37). Hove: Lawrence Erlbaum Associates.

Cope, D. N., Cole, J. R., Hall, K. M. & Barkan, H. (1991). Brain injury: Analysis of outcome in a post-acute rehabilitation system. *Brain Injury, 5,* 111–139.

Cope, N. (1994). Traumatic brain injury rehabilitation outcome studies in the United States. In A.-L. Christensen & B. P. Uzzell (Eds.), *Brain injury and neuropsychological rehabilitation: International perspectives* (pp. 201–220). Hillsdale, NJ: Lawrence Erlbaum Associates.

Cot, F., Degiovani, R., & Hirsbrunner, T. (1993). In D. Lafond, R. Degiovani, Y. Joanette, J. Ponzio & M. T. Sarno (Eds.), *Living with aphasia.* San Diego: Singular Publishing Group.

Coughlan, A. K. & Warrington, E. K. (1978) Word comprehension and word-retrieval in patients with localized cerebral lesions. *Brain, 101,* 163–185.

Craik, F. I. M. & Lockhart, R. S. (1972). Levels of processing: A framework for memory research. *Journal of Verbal Learning and Verbal Behavior, 11,* 671–684.

Crovitz, H. (1979). Memory retraining in brain damaged patients: The airplane list. *Cortex, 15,* 131–134.

Cullen, C. N. (1976). Errorless learning with the retarded. *Nursing Times,* 25th March 1976.

Cummings, J. L. & Benson, D. F. (1992). *Dementia: A clinical approach, Second edition.* Boston: Butterworth-Heinemann.

Davidoff, J. & Wilson, B. A. (1985). A case of associative visual agnosia showing a disorder of pre-semantic visual classification. *Cortex, 21,* 121–134.

de Partz, M. P. (1986). Re-education of a deep dyslexic patient: Rationale of the method and results. *Cognitive Neuropsychology, 3,* 149–177.

De Renzi, E. (1996). Balint-Holmes' syndrome. In C. Code, C-W. Wallesch, Y. Joanette, A. R. Lecours (Eds.), *Classic cases in neuropsychology* (pp. 123–143). Hove: Psychology Press.

Denes, F. G., Semenza, C., Stoppa, E., & Lis, A. (1982). Unilateral spatial neglect and recovery from hemiplegia: A follow up study. *Brain, 105,* 543–552.

Dennis, M. & Kohn, B. (1975). Comprehension of syntax in infantile hemiplegics after cerebral hemidecortication: Left hemisphere superiority. *Brain and Language, 2,* 472–482.

Diller, L. (1976). A model for cognitive retraining in rehabilitation. *The Clinical Psychologist, 29,* 13–15.

Diller, L. (1994). Changes in rehabilitation over the past 5 years. In A.-L. Christensen & B. P. Uzzell (Eds.), *Brain injury and neuropsychological rehabilitation: International perspectives* (pp. 1–15). Hillsdale, NJ: Lawrence Erlbaum Associates.

Diller, L. & Gordon, W. A. (1981). Rehabilitation and clinical neuropsychology. In S. B. Filskov & T. J. Boll (Eds.), *Handbook of clinical neuropsychology* (pp. 702–733). New York: Wiley.

Diller, L., & Weinberg, J. (1977). Hemi-inattention in rehabilitation: The evolution of a rational remediation program. In E. A. Weinstein & R. P. Friedland (Eds.), *Advances in neurology, vol. 18* (pp. 63–82). New York: Raven Press.

Doll, E.A. (1953). *The measurement of social competence.* Minneapolis: Educational Publishers.

Dunn, L. M. & Dunn, L. M. (1982). *British Picture Vocabulary Scale.* Windsor: NFER-Nelson Publishing Company Ltd.

Eames, P. (1989). Head injury rehabilitation: towards a 'model' service. In R. Ll. Wood & P. Eames (Eds.), *Models of brain injury rehabilitation* (pp. 48–58). London: Chapman.

Elliot, C. D., Murray, D. J. & Pearson, L.S. (1977). *British Ability Scales.* Windsor: NFER-Nelson.

Ellis, A. W. & Young, A. W. (1997). *Human cognitive neuropsychology: A textbook with readings*. Hove: Psychology Press.

Eson, M. E., Yen, J. K. & Bourke, R. S. (1978). Assessment of recovery from serious head injury. *Journal of Neurology, Neurosurgery and Psychiatry, 41*, 1036–1042.

Evans, J. J. & Wilson, B. A. (1992). A memory group for individuals with brain injury. *Clinical Rehabilitation, 6*, 75–81.

Evans, J. J., Wilson, B. A., Schuri, U., Baddeley, A. D., Canavan, T., Laaksonen, R., Bruna, O., Lorenzi, L., Della Sala, S., Andrade, J., Green, R. & Taussik, I. A comparison of 'errorless' and 'trial and error' learning methods for teaching individuals with acquired memory deficits. [Manuscript submitted to *Neuropsychological Rehabilitation*].

Farah, M. J. (1990). *Visual agnosia*. Cambridge, MA: The MIT Press.

Freund, D. C. (1889). Ueber optische aphasie und seelenbllindheit. *Arch. J. Psychiat. u Nervenkr., 20*, 276–297.

Frith, C. D. (1992). *The cognitive neuropsychology of schizophrenia*. Hove: Lawrence Erlbaum Associates.

Gainotti, G. (1993). Emotional and psychosocial problems after brain injury. *Neuropsychological Rehabilitation, 3*, 259–277.

Gardner, H., Zurif, E. B., Berry, T. & Baker, E. (1976). Visual communication in aphasia. *Neuropsychologia, 14*, 275–292.

Gentile, A. M., Green, S., Neiburgs, A., Schmelzer, W. & Stein, D. G. (1978). Disruption and recovery of locomotor and manipulative behaviour following cortical lesions in rats. *Behavioral Biology, 22*, 417–455.

Geschwind, N. (1965). Disconnexion syndromes in animals and man. *Brain, 88*, 237–294.

Gianutsos, R. (1992). The computer in cognitive rehabilitation: It's not just a tool any more. *Journal of Head Trauma Rehabilitation, 7*, 26–35.

Gianutsos, R. & Gianutsos, J. (1987) Single case experimental approaches to the assessment of interventions in rehabilitation psychology. In B. Caplan (Ed.) *Rehabilitation psychology* (pp. 453–470). Rockville, MD: Aspen Corp.

Glisky, E. L. (1995). Computers in memory rehabilitation. In A. D. Baddeley, B. A. Wilson, & F. N. Watts (Eds.), *Handbook of memory disorders* (pp. 557–575). Chichester: John Wiley.

Glisky, E. L., Schacter, D. L., & Tulving, E. (1986). Computer learning by memory impaired patients: Acquisition and retention of complex knowledge. *Neuropsychologica, 24*, 313–328.

Godden, D., & Baddeley, A. D. (1975). Context-dependent memory in two natural environments: on land and under water. *British Journal of Psychology, 66*, 325–331.

Goodglass, H. & Kaplan, E. (1983). *The assessment of aphasia and related disorders, 2nd edition*. Philadelphia: Lea & Febiger.

Gray, J. M., Robertson, I. H., Pentland, B. & Anderson, S. (1992). Microcomputer-based attentional training after brain damage: A randomised group controlled trial. *Neuropsychological Rehabilitation, 2*, 97–115.

Greenwood, R. J. & McMillan, T. M. (1993). Models of rehabilitation programmes for the brain-injured adult—I: Current provision, efficacy and good practice. *Clinical Rehabilitation, 7*, 248–255.

Gruneberg, M. M. (1973). The role of memorization techniques in finals examination preparation: A study of psychology students. *Educational Research, 15*, 134–139.

Gunzburg, H. C. (1973). *Social competence and mental handicap, 2nd edition*. London: Bailliere Tindall.

Hageman, A. T. M., Gabreels, F. J. M., Liem, K. D., Renkawek, K. & Boon, J. M. (1993).

Congenital myotonic dystrophy: A report on thirteen cases and a review of the literature. *Journal of the Neurological Sciences, 115,* 95–101.

Halligan, P. W. & Marshall, J. C. (Eds.) (1994). *Neuropsychological Rehabilitation: A Special Issue: Spatial neglect: Position papers on theory and practice.* Hove: Lawrence Erlbaum Associates Limited.

Halstead, W. C. (1947). *Brain and intelligence.* Chicago: University of Chicago Press.

Hanlon, R., Clontz, B. & Thomas, M. (1993). Management of severe behavioural dyscontrol following subarachnoid haemorrhage. *Neuropsychological Rehabilitation, 3* 63–76.

Harper, P. S. (1989). Myotonic dystrophy, second edition. London: Saunders.

Hecaen, H. & Albert, M. L. (1978). *Human neuropsychology.* New York: Wiley.

Heilman, K. M. (1979). Apraxia. In K. M. Heilman and E. Valenstein (Eds.), *Clinical neuropsychology* (pp. 159–185). New York: Oxford University Press.

Heilman, K. M. & Valenstein, E. (Eds.) (1985). *Clinical Neuropsychology, 2nd edition.* New York: Oxford University Press.

Hendrickson, J., Roberts, M. & Shores, R. E. (1978). Antecedent and contingent modeling to teach basic sight vocabulary to learning disabled children. *Journal of Learning Disabilities, 11,* 524–528.

Hersh, N. & Treadgold, L. (1994). NeuroPage: The rehabilitation of memory dysfunction by prosthetic memory and cueing. *NeuroRehabilitation, 4,* 187–197.

Higbee, K. L. (1978). Some pseudo-limitations of mnemonics. In M. M. Gruneberg, P. E. Morris & R. N. Sykes (Eds.), *Practical aspects of memory* (pp. 147–154). London: Academic Press.

Hodges, J., Patterson, K., Oxbury, S. & Funnell, E. (1992a). Semantic dementia: Progressive fluent aphasia with temporal lobe atrophy. *Brain, 115,* 1783–1806.

Hodges, J., Salmon, D. P. & Butters, N. (1992b). Semantic memory impairment in Alzheimer's disease: Failure of access or degraded knowledge? *Neuropsychologia, 30,* 301–314.

Holmes, G. (1919). Disturbances of visual space recognition. *British Medical Journal, 2,* 230–233.

Hopkins, R. O., Kesner, R. P. & Goldstein, M. (1995). Memory for novel and familiar spatial and linguistic temporal distance information in hypoxic subjects. *Journal of the International Neuropsychological Society, 1,* 454–468.

Howard, D. & Patterson, K. (1992). *Pyramids and Palm Trees.* Bury St Edmunds: Thames Valley Test Company.

Humphreys, G. W. and Riddoch, J. (1987). *To see but not to see: A case study of visual agnosia.* London: Lawrence Erlbaum Associates.

Huppert, F. A., Brayne, C. & O'Connor, D. W. (Eds.) (1994). *Dementia and normal ageing.* Cambridge: Cambridge University Press.

Ince, L. P. (1969). A behavioural approach to motivation in rehabilitation. *Psychological Record, 19,* 105–111.

Ince, L. P. (1976). *Behavior modification in rehabilitation medicine.* Baltimore: Williams & Wilkins.

Jackson, W. T. & Gouvier, W. D. (1992). Group psychotherapy with brain-damaged adults and their families. In C. J. Long & L. K. Ross (Eds.), *Handbook of head trauma: Acute care to recovery* (pp. 309–327). New York: Plenum Press.

Jastak, J. R. & Jastak, S. R. (1965). *The Wide Range Achievement Test.* Arlington, DE: Guidance Associates of Delaware.

Jennett, B. & Teasdale, G. (1981). *Management of head injuries.* Philadelphia: F. A. Davis.

Jones, R. S. P. & Eayrs, C. B. (1992). The use of errorless learning procedures in teaching people with a learning disability. *Mental Handicap Research, 5,* 304–312.

Jones, R. S. P. & Eayrs, C. B. (1994). Errorless learning revisited: Towards an effective teaching strategy. *Mental Handicap Research, 7*, 160–161.

Kanfer, F. H. & Saslow, G. (1969). Behavioural diagnosis. In C. Franks (Ed.), *Behaviour therapy: Appraisal and status* (pp. 417–444). New York: McGraw-Hill.

Kapur, N. (1988). *Memory disorders in clinical practice.* London: Butterworths.

Kapur, N. (1997). *Injured brains of medical minds.* Oxford: Oxford University Press.

Kapur, N., Barker, S., Burrows, E. H., Ellison, D., Brice, J., Illis, L. S., Scholey, K., Colbourn, C., Wilson, B. A. & Loates, M. (1994). Herpes simplex encephalitis: Long term magnetic resonance imaging and neuropsychological profile. *Journal of Neurology, Neurosurgery, and Psychiatry, 57*, 1334–1342.

Kapur, N. & Pearson, D. (1983). Memory symptoms and memory performance of neurological patients. *British Journal of Psychology, 74*, 409–415.

Kapur, N., Young, A., Bateman, D. & Kennedy, P. (1989). Focal retrograde amnesia: A long term clinical and neuropsychological follow-up. *Cortex, 25*, 387–402.

Katz, R. B. & Sevush, S. (1989). Positional dyslexia. *Brain and Language, 37*, 266–289.

Kerkoff, G., Münßinger, U., Eberle-Strauss, G., & Stögerer, E. (1992). Rehabilitation of hemianopic alexia in patients with postgeniculate visual field disorders. *Neuropsychological Rehabilitation, 2*, 21–42.

Kertesz, A. (1979). *Aphasia and associated disorders.* New York: Grune and Stratton.

Kime, S. K., Lamb, D. G. & Wilson, B.A. (1996). Use of a comprehensive program of external cuing to enhance procedural memory in a patient with dense amnesia. *Brain Injury, 10*, 17–25.

Kinsella, G. & Ford, B. (1980). Acute recovery patterns in stroke patients. *Medical Journal of Australia, 2*, 663–666.

Kløve, H. & Cleeland, C. S. (1972). The relationship of neuropsychological impairment to other indices of head injury. *Scandinavian Journal of Rehabilitation Medicine, 4*, 55–60.

Kohn, B. & Dennis, M. (1978). Selective impairments of visuospatial abilities in infantile hemiplegics after right cerebral hemidecortication. *Neuropsychologia, 12*, 505–512.

Kolb, B. (1992). Mechanisms underlying recovery from cortical injury: reflections on progress and directions for the future. In F. D. Rose & D. A. Johnson (Eds.), *Recovery from brain damage: Reflections and directions* (pp. 169–186). New York: Plenum.

Kopelman, M. D. (1995). The assessment of psychogenic amnesia. In A. D. Baddeley, B. A. Wilson & F. N. Watts (Eds.), *Handbook of memory disorders* (pp. 427–448). Chichester: John Wiley.

Kopelman, M., Wilson, B. A. & Baddeley, A. D. (1989). The autobiographical memory interview: A new assessment of autobiographical and personal semantic memory in amnesic patients. *Journal of Clinical and Experimental Neuropsychology, 11*, 724–744.

Kopelman, M., Wilson, B. A. & Baddeley, A. D. (1990). *The Autobiographical Memory Interviews.* Bury St Edmunds: Thames Valley Test Company.

Landauer, T. K. & Bjork, R. A. (1978). Optimum rehearsal patterns and name learning. In M. M. Gruneberg, P. E. Morris & R. N. Sykes (Eds.), *Practical aspects of memory* (pp. 625–632). London: Academic Press.

Lezak, M. D. (1995). *Neuropsychological assessment, 3rd edition.* New York: Oxford University Press.

Lhermitte, F. and Beauvois, M-F. (1973). A visual-speech disconnexion syndrome: Report of a case with optic aphasia, agnosic alexia and colour agnosia. *Brain, 96*, 695–714.

Liepmann, H. (1920). Apraxia. *Ergebnisse der gesammten Medizin, 1*, 516–543.

Lincoln, N. B. (1978). Behaviour modification in physiotherapy. *Physiotherapy, 64*, 265–267.

Lindgren, M., Hagstadius, S., Abjornsson, G., Ørbaek, P. (1997). Neuropsychological rehabilitation of patients with organic solvent-induced chronic toxic encephalopathy: A
pilot study. *Neuropsychological Rehabilitation, 7,* 1–22.

Lishman, A. W. (1987). *Organic psychiatry, 2nd edition.* Oxford: Blackwell Scientific
Publications.

Livingston, M. A., Brooks, D. N. & Bond, M. (1985). Three months after severe head injury: Psychological and social impact on relatives. *Journal of Neurology, Neurosurgery, and Psychiatry, 48,* 870–875.

Luria, A. R. (1966). *Higher cortical functions in man.* London: Tavistock.

Luria, A. R. (1973). *The working brain.* New York: Basic Books.

Luria, A. R., Naydin, V. L., Tsvetkova, L. S. & Vinarskaya, E. N. (1969). Restoration of
higher cortical functions following local brain damage. In P. J. Vinken & G. W. Bruyn
(Eds.), *Handbook of clinical neurology, volume 3* (pp. 368–433). New York: Elsevier.

Malamud, N. & Skillicorn, S. A. (1956). Relationship between the Wernicke and the Korsakoff Syndrome. *Archives of Neurology and Psychiatry, 76,* 585–596.

Malloy, P., Mishra, S. K. & Adler, S. H. (1990). Neuropsychological deficits in myotonic
muscular dystrophy. *Journal of Neurology, Neurosurgery, and Psychiatry, 53,* 1011–
1013.

Marr, D. (1982). *Vision.* San Francisco: Freeman.

Marshall, J. C., & Newcombe, F. (1966). Syntactic and semantic errors in paralexia. *Neuropsychologia, 4,* 169–176.

Marshall, J. C. & Newcombe, F. (1973). Patterns of Paralexia: a psycholinguistic approach. *Journal of Psycholinguistic Research, 2,* 175–199.

Mayer, E., Brown, V. J., Dunnett, S. B. & Robbins, T. W. (1992). Striatal graft-associated
recovery of a lesion-induced performance deficit in the rat requires learning to use the
transplant. *European Journal of Neuroscience, 4,* 119–126.

McKenna, P. & Warrington, E. K. (1983). *The Graded Naming Test.* Windsor: NFER-
Nelson.

McKinlay, W. W., Brooks, D. N., Bond, M. R., Martinage, D. P. & Marshall, M. M.
(1981). The short-term outcome of severe blunt head injury as reported by relatives
of the injured persons. *Journal of Neurology, Neurosurgery, and Psychiatry, 44,* 527–
533.

McLellan, D. L. (1991). Functional recovery and the principles of disability medicine.
In M. Swash & J. Oxbury (Eds.), *Clinical neurology* (pp. 768–790). Edinburgh:
Churchill Livingstone.

McMillan, T. M., & Greenwood, R. J. (1993). Model of rehabilitation programmes for the
brain-injured adult—II: Model services and suggestions for change in the UK. *Clinical
Rehabilitation, 7,* 346–355.

Mehlbye, J. & Larsen, A. (1994). Social and economic consequences of brain damage
in Denmark. In A.-L. Christensen & B. P. Uzzell (Eds.), *Brain injury and neuropsychological rehabilitation: International perspectives* (pp. 257–267). Hillsdale, NJ:
Lawrence Erlbaum Associates.

Meichenbaum, D. (1977). *Cognitive-behaviour modification: An integrative approach.*
New York: Plenum Press.

Mendelow, A. D. (1991). Management of open/basal injuries. In M. Swash & J. Oxbury
(Eds.), *Clinical neurology* (pp. 689–692). Edinburgh: Churchill Livingstone.

Mielke, R., Herholz, K., Fink, G., Ritter, D. & Heiss, W. D. (1993). Positron emission tomography in myotonic dystrophy. *Psychiatry Research—Neuroimaging, 50,* 93–99.

Miller, E. (1984). *Recovery and management of neuropsychological impairments.* Chichester: Wiley.

Mitchum, C. C. & Berndt, R. S. (1995). The cognitive neuropsychological approach to treatment of language disorders. *Neuropsychological Rehabilitation, 5,* 1–16.

Moffat, N. (1989). Home based cognitive rehabilitation with the elderly. In L. W. Poon, D. C. Rubin, & B. A. Wilson (Eds.), *Everyday cognition in adulthood and late life* (pp. 659–680). Cambridge: Cambridge University Press.

Moody, S. (1988). The Moyer reading technique re-evaluated. *Cortex, 24,* 473–476.

Moore, B. E. & Ruesch, J. (1944). Prolonged disturbances of consciousness following head injury. *New England Journal of Medicine, 230,* 445–452.

Moyer, S. B. (1979). Rehabilitation of alexia: A case study. *Cortex, 15,* 139–144.

Nelson, H. E. (1976). A modified card sorting test sensitive to frontal lobe defects. *Cortex, 12,* 313–324.

Nelson, H. E. (1982). *The National Adult Reading Test (NART).* Windsor: NFER-Nelson.

Newcombe, F. (1996). Very late outcome after focal wartime brain wounds. *Journal of Clinical and Experimental Neuropsychology, 18,* 1–23.

Nickels, L. A. (1992) The autocue? Self-generated phonemic cues in the treatment of a disorder of reading and naming. *Cognitive Neuropsychology, 9,* 155–182.

Oldfield, R. C. & Wingfield, A. (1965). Response latencies in naming objects. *Quarterly Journal of Experimental Psychology, 17,* 273–281.

Osterreith, P. A. (1944). Le test de copie d'une figure complexe. *Archives de Psychologie, 30,* 206–256.

Oxbury, J. & Swash, M. (1991). Viral diseases. In M. Swash and J. Oxbury (Eds.), *Clinical neurology* (pp. 792–800). Edinburgh: Churchill Livingstone.

Palmer, B. W., Boone, K. B., Chang, L., Lee, A. & Black, S. (1994). Deficits and personality patterns in maternally versus peternally inherited myotonic dystrophy. *Journal of Clinical and Experimental Neuropsychology, 16,* 784–795.

Parenté, R., Anderson-Parenté, J. K. & Shaw, B. (1989). Retraining the mind's eye. *Journal of Head Trauma Rehabilitation, 4,* 53–62.

Parkin, A. (1984). Amnesic syndrome: A lesion specific disorder? *Cortex, 20,* 479–508.

Parkin, A. J., Miller, J. & Vincent, R. (1987). Multiple neuropsychological deficits due to anoxic encephalopathy: A case study. *Cortex, 23,* 655–665.

Patterson, K. E. (1994). Reading, writing and rehabilitation: A reckoning. In M. J. Riddoch & G. W. Humphreys (Eds.), *Cognitive neuropsychology and cognitive rehabilitation* (pp. 425–447). Hove: Lawrence Erlbaum Associates.

Patterson, K. & Hodges, J. R. (1995). Disorders of semantic memory. In A. D. Baddeley, B. A. Wilson & F. N. Watts (Eds.), *Handbook of memory disorders* (pp. 167–186). Chichester, Sussex: John Wiley & Sons.

Patterson, K. E. and Kay, J. (1982). Letter-by-letter reading: Psychological descriptions of a neurological syndrome. *Quarterly Journal of Experimental Psychology, 34A,* 411–41.

Patterson, K. E. & Wilson, B. A. (1990). A ROSE is a ROSE or a NOSE: A deficit in initial letter identification. *Cognitive Neuropsychology, 7,* 447–477.

Phillips, W. A. (1983). Short-term visual memory. *Philosophical Transactions of the Royal Society, B302,* 295–309.

Pommerenke, K. & Markowitsch, H. J. (1989). Rehabilitation training of homonymous visual field defects in patients with postgeniculate damage of the visual system. *Restorative Neurology and Neuroscience, 1,* 47–63.

Ponsford, J. (1995). Mechanisms, recovery and sequelae of traumatic brain injury: A foundation for the REAL approach. In J. Ponsford, S. Sloan & P. Snow (Eds.), *Traumatic brain injury: Rehabilitation for everyday adaptive living* (pp. 1–31). Hove: Lawrence Erlbaum Associates.

Ponsford, J. & Kinsella, G. (1992). The use of a rating scale of attentional behaviour. *Neuropsychological Rehabilitation, 1,* 241–257.

Ponsford, J., Sloan, S. & Snow, P. (1995). *Traumatic brain injury: Rehabilitation for everyday adaptive living.* Hove: Lawrence Erlbaum Associates.

Prigatano, G. P. (1986). Personality and psychosocial consequences of brain injury. In G. P. Prigatano & Others (Eds.), *Neuropsychological rehabilitation after brain injury* (pp. 29–50). Baltimore and London: The Johns Hopkins University Press.

Prigatano, G. P. (1994). Individuality, lesion location, and psychotherapy after brain injury. In A.-L. Christensen & B. P. Uzzell (Eds.), *Brain injury and neuropsychological rehabilitation* (pp. 173–186). Hillsdale, N.J.: Lawrence Erlbaum Associates.

Prigatano, G. P. (1995). Personality and social aspects of memory rehabilitation. In A. D. Baddeley, B. A. Wilson & F. N. Watts (Eds.), *Handbook of memory disorders* (pp. 603–614). Chichester: John Wiley.

Ratcliff, G. (1970). *Aspects of disordered space perception.* Unpublished DPhil thesis, University of Oxford.

Ratcliff, G. (1979). Spatial thought, mental rotation and the right cerebral hemisphere. *Neuropsychologia, 17,* 49–54.

Ratcliff, G. & Newcombe, F. (1982). Object recognition: Some deductions from the clinical evidence. In A. W. Ellis (Ed.), *Normality and pathology in cognitive functions.* New York: Academic Press.

Raven, J. C. (1960). *Guide to the Standard Progressive Matrices.* London: Lewis.

Rawles, R. E. (1978). The past and present of mnemotechny. In M. M. Gruneberg, P. E. Morris & R. N. Sykes (Eds.), *Practical aspects of memory* (pp. 164–171). London: Academic Press.

Reitan, R. M. & Davison, L. A. (1974). *Clinical neuropsychology: Current status and applications.* New York: Hemisphere.

Renfrew, E. (1975). *Word finding, 3rd edition.* Oxford: Renfrew Language Test Publishers.

Riddoch, M. J. & Humphreys, G. W. (Eds.) (1994), *Cognitive neuropsychology and cognitive rehabilitation.* Hove: Lawrence Erlbaum Associates.

Robertson, I. (1990). Does computerised cognitive rehabilitation work? A review. *Aphasiology, 4,* 381–405.

Robertson, I. H. & Cashman, E. (1991). Auditory feedback for walking difficulties in a case of unilateral neglect: A pilot study. *Neuropsychological Rehabilitation, 1,* 175–184.

Robertson, I. H., Hogg, K. & McMillan, T. M. (1998). Rehabilitation of unilateral neglect: Reducing inhibitory competition by contralesional limb activation. *Neuropsychological Rehabilitation, 8,* 19–30.

Robertson, I. H. & North, N. (1993). Active and passive activation of left limbs: Influence on visual and sensory neglect. *Neuropsychologia, 31,* 293–300.

Robertson, I. H., Tegnér, R., Tham, K., Lo, A. & Nimmo-Smith, I. (1995). Sustained attention training for unilateral neglect: Theoretical and rehabilitation implications. *Journal of Clinical and Experimental Neuropsychology, 17,* 416–430.

Robertson, I. H., Ward, T., Ridgeway, V. & Nimmo-Smith, I. (1996). The structure of normal human attention: The Test of Everyday Attention. *Journal of the International Neuropsychological Society, 2,* 525–534.

Robertson, I. H. & Wilson, B. A. (in press). Neuropsychological rehabilitation. J. W. Fawcett, A. E. Rosses, & S. B. Dunnett (Eds.), *Brain damage, brain repair,* Oxford: Oxford University Press.

Robinson, F. P. (1970). *Effective study.* New York: Harper and Row.

Ross, E. D. (1983). Right-hemisphere lesions in disorders of affective language. In A. Kertesz (Ed.), *Localization in neuropsychology* (pp. 493–508). New York: Academic Press.

Rowntree, D. (1983). *Learn how to study.* New York: Harper & Row.

Rubens, A. B. (1979). Agnosia. In K. M. Heilman & E. Valenstein (Eds), *Clinical neuropsychology.* New York: Oxford University Press.

Schacter, D. & Crovitz, H. (1977). Memory function after closed head injury: A review of the quantitative research. *Cortex, 13,* 105–176.

Schonell, F. J. & Schonell, F. E. (1963). *Diagnostic attainment testing.* Edinburgh: Oliver & Boyd.

Seron, X. & Deloche, G. (Eds.) (1989). *Cognitive approaches in neuropsychological rehabilitation.* Hillsdale, N.J.: Lawrence Erlbaum Associates.

Shallice, T. & Evans, M. E. (1978). The involvement of the frontal lobes in cognitive estimation. *Cortex, 14,* 294–303.

Shallice, T. & Warrington, E. K. (1977). Auditory-verbal short-term memory impairment and conduction aphasia. *Brain and Language, 4,* 479–491.

Shiel, A., McLellan, D. L., Wilson, B. A., Evans, J. J. & Pickard, J. (submitted). The effect of rehabilitation on violent behaviour after severe head injury. Manuscript submitted to *Brain Injury.*

Sidman, M. & Stoddard, L. T. (1967). The effectiveness of fading in programming simultaneous form discrimination for retarded children. *Journal of Experimental Analysis of Behavior, 10,* 3–15.

Sisler, G. & Penner, H. (1975). Amnesia following severe head injury. *Canadian Psychiatric Association Journal, 20,* 333–336.

Skelly, M. (1979). *Ameri-Ind gestural code based on universal American Indian hand talk.* New York: Elsevier.

Skinner, C. (1996). Assessment of impaired language. In L. Harding and J. R. Beech (Eds.), *Assessment in neuropsychology* (pp. 111–124). London: Routledge.

Slaven, G. (1996) *"Smart" houses.* Personal communication.

Snow, P. & Ponsford, J. (1995). Assessing and managing impairment of consciusness following traumatic brain injury. In J. Ponsford, S. Sloan & P. Snow (Eds.), *Traumatic brain injury: Rehabilitation for everyday adaptive living* (pp. 33–64). Hove: Lawrence Erlbaum Associates.

Sohlberg, M. M. & Mateer, C. (1989). Training use of compensatory memory books: A three-stage behavioural approach. *Journal of Clinical and Experimental Neuropsychology, 11,* 871–891.

Sturm, W. & Willmes, K. (1991). Efficacy of a reaction training on various attentional and cognitive functions in stroke patients. *Neuropsychological Rehabilitation, 1,* 259–280.

Stuss, D. T., Kates, M. H. & Poirier, C. A. et al. (1987). Evaluation of information-processing speed and neuropsychological functioning in patients with myotonic dystrophy. *Journal of Clinical and Experimental Neuropsychology, 9,* 131–146.

Talbott, R. (1989). The brain injured person and the family. In R. Ll. Wood & P. Eames (Eds.), *Models of brain injury rehabilitation* (pp. 3–16). London: Chapman and Hall.

Taub, E., Miller, N. E., Novack, T. A., Cook, E. W., Fleming, W. C., Nepomuceno, C. S., Connell, J. S. & Crago, J. E. (1993). Technique to improve chronic motor deficit after stroke. *Archives of Physical Medicine and Rehabilitation, 74,* 347–354.

Taylor, G. P. & Parsons, R. W. (1970). Behaviour modification techniques in a physical medicine and rehabilitation center. *Journal of Psychology, 74,* 117–124.

Teasdale, G. (1991). Epidemiology. In M. Swash and J. Oxbury (Eds.), *Clinical neurology* (pp. 670–671). Edinburgh: Churchill Livingstone.

Teasdale, G. & Jennett, B. (1974) Assessment of coma and impaired consciousness: a practical scale. *Lancet, 2,* 81–84.

Teddy, P. (1991). Haemorrhagic disorders. In M. Swash and J. Oxbury (Eds.), *Clinical neurology* (pp. 985–1020). Edinburgh: Churchill Livingstone.

Terrace, H. S. (1963). Discrimination learning with and without "errors". *Journal of Experimental Analysis of Behavior, 6,* 1–27.

Terrace, H. S. (1966). Stimulus control. In W. K. Honig (Ed.), *Operant behaviour: Areas of research and application* (pp. 271–344). New York: Appleton-Century-Crofts.

Thomas, D., Barnard, R. O., Darling, J. L., Godlee, J. N., Kendall, B. E. & McKeran, R. O. (1991). *Cerebral tumours.* In M. Swash and J. Oxbury (Eds.), Clinical neurology (pp. 1022–1095). Edinburgh: Churchill Livingstone.

Thurstone, L. L. & Jeffrey, T. E. (1956). *Flags: A test of spatial thinking.* Illinois: Industrial Relations Center.

Tompkins, K. (1978). *The alphabet kids.* Waitsfield, Vermont: Essex Publishing Company.

Trexler, L. E. (Ed.) (1982). *Cognitive rehabilitation: Conceptualization and intervention.* New York: Plenum Press.

Tulving, E. (1983). *Elements of episodic memory.* Oxford: Oxford University Press.

Tulving, E. & Schacter, D. L. (1990). Priming and human memory systems. *Science, 247,* 301–306.

Uzzell, B. P. & Gross, Y. (1986). *Clinical neuropsychology of intervention.* Boston: Martinus Nijhoff.

Victor, M., Adams, R. D. & Collins, G. H. (1971). *The Wernicke-Korsakoff syndrome.* Oxford: Blackwell Scientific Publications.

von Cramon, D. & Matthes-von Cramon, G. (1992). Reflections on the treatment of brain injured patients suffering from problem-solving disorders. *Neuropsychological Rehabilitation, 2,* 207–230.

Wade, D., Langton Hewer, R., Skilbeck, C. & David, R. (1985). *Stroke: A critical approach to diagnosis, treatment and management.* London: Chapman & Hall.

Walsh, B. F. & Lamberts, F. (1979). Errorless discrimination and fading as techniques for teaching sight words to TMR students. *American Journal of Mental Deficiency, 83,* 473–479.

Warrington, E. K. (1984). *The Recognition Memory Test.* Windsor: NFER-Nelson.

Warrington, E. K. & James, M. (1967). An experimental investigation of facial recognition in patients with unilateral cerebral lesions. *Cortex, 3,* 317–326.

Warrington, E. K. & James, M. (1991). *The Visual Object and Space Perception Battery.* Bury St Edmunds: Thames Valley Test Company.

Warrington, E. K. & Shallice, T. (1984) Category specific semantic impairments. *Brain, 107,* 829–854.

Warrington, E. K. and Taylor, A. M. (1978). Two categorical stages of object recognition. *Perception, 7,* 695–705.

Wearing, D. (1992). Self help groups. In B. A. Wilson & N. Moffat (Eds.) *Clinical management of memory problems, second edition* (pp. 271–301). London: Chapman and Hall.

Wechsler, D. (1945). A standardized memory scale for clinical use. *Journal of Psychology, 19,* 87–95.

Wechsler, D. (1955) *Wechsler Adult Intelligence Scale Manual.* New York: The Psychological Corporation.

Wechsler, D. (1981a) *Manual for the Wechsler Adult Intelligence Scale-Revised.* New York: The Psychological Corporation.

Wechsler, D. (1981b) *Wechsler Adult Intelligence Scale.* New York: The Psychological Corporation.

Wechsler, D. (1987). *The Wechsler Memory Scale-Revised.* San Antonio: The Psychological Corporation.

Weinberg, J., Diller, D., Gordon, W. A., Gerstman, L. J., Lieberman, A., Hodges, G. & Ezrachi, O. (1979). Training sensory awareness and spatial organisation in people with right brain damage. *Archives of Physical Medicine and Rehabilitation, 60,* 491–496.

Weinstein, E. A. (1991). Anosognosia and denial of illness. In G. P. Prigatano & D. L. Schacter (Eds.), *Awareness of deficit after brain injury* (pp. 240–257). New York: Oxford University Press.

Wilson, B. A. (1981). A survey of behavioural treatments carried out at a rehabilitation centre for stroke and head injuries. In G. Powell (Ed.), *Brain function therapy.* Aldershot: Gower.

Wilson, B. A. (1982). Success and failure in memory training following a cerebral vascular accident. *Cortex, 18,* 581–594.

Wilson, B. A. (1984) Memory therapy in practice. In B. A. Wilson & N. Moffat (Eds.), *Clinical management of memory problems* (pp. 89–111). London: Croom Helm.

Wilson, B. A. (1985). Adapting 'Portage' for neurological patients. *International Rehabilitation Medicine, 7,* 6–8.

Wilson, B. A. (1987a). Identification and remediation of everyday problems in memory impaired adults. In O. A. Parsons, N. Butters & P. E. Nathan (Eds.), *Neuropsychology of alcoholism: Implications for diagnosis and treatment* (pp. 322–337). New York: Guilford Press.

Wilson, B. A. (1987b). Neuropsychological rehabilitation in Britain. In M. J. Meier, A. L. Benton, & L. Diller (Eds.), *Neuropsychological rehabilitation* (pp. 430–436). London: Churchill Livingstone.

Wilson, B. A. (1987c). Single case experimental designs in neuropsychological rehabilitation. *Journal of Clinical and Experimental Neuropsychology, 9,* 527–544.

Wilson, B. A. (1987d). *Rehabilitation of memory.* New York: Guilford Press.

Wilson, B. A. (1987e). The measurement of perceptual impairment. *Clinical Rehabilitation, 1,* 169–173.

Wilson, B. A. (1989a). Coping strategies for memory dysfunction. In E. Perecman (Ed.), *Integrating theory and practice in neuropsychology* (pp. 155–172). Hillsdale, N.J.: Lawrence Erlbaum Associates.

Wilson, B.A. (1989b). Designing memory-therapy programs. In L. Poon, D. Rubin & B. Wilson (Eds.), *Everyday cognition in adulthood and late life* (pp. 615–638). Cambridge: Cambridge University Press.

Wilson, B. A. (1989c). Improving recall of health service information. *Clinical Rehabilitation, 3,* 275–279.

Wilson, B. A. (1989d). Management of problems resulting from damage to the Central Nervous System. In S. Pearce & J. Wardle (Eds.), *The practice of behavioural medicine* (pp. 51–81). Oxford: Oxford University Press.

Wilson, B. A. (1989e). *Memory problems after head injury.* Nottingham: National Head Injuries Association.

Wilson, B. A. (1989f). Models of cognitive rehabilitation. In R. Ll. Wood & P. Eames (Eds.), *Models of brain injury rehabilitation* (pp. 117–141). London: Chapman & Hall.

Wilson, B. A. (1989g). Remediation and management of disorders of memory. In M. van der Linden & R. Bruyer (Eds.), *Neuropsychologie de la memoire humaine* (pp. 160–176). Societe Neuropsychologie de Langue Francais.

Wilson, B. A. (1991a). Behaviour therapy in the treatment of neurologically impaired adults. In P. R. Martin (Ed.), *Handbook of behavior therapy and psychological science: An integrative approach* (pp. 227–252). New York: Pergamon Press.

Wilson, B. A. (1991b). Long term prognosis of patients with severe memory disorders. *Neuropsychological Rehabilitation, 1,* 117–134.

Wilson, B. A. (1991c). Psychological tests—What does the therapist want? *Therapy Weekly,* April 4th 1991.

Wilson, B. A. (1991d). Theory, assessment and treatment in neuropsychological rehabilitation. *Neuropsychology, 5,* 281–291.

Wilson, B. A. (1992). Memory therapy in practice. In B. A. Wilson & N. Moffat (Eds.), *Clinical management of memory problems, Second edition* (pp. 120–153). London: Chapman & Hall.

Wilson, B. A. (1994). Remediation of acquired dyslexia: A 6–10 year follow-up study of seven brain injured people. *Journal of Clinical and Experimental Neuropsychology,* 16, 354–371.

Wilson, B. A. (1995a). Dealing with memory problems. *Reviews in Clinical Gerontology, 5,* 457–463.

Wilson, B. A. (1995b). Life after brain injury: Long-term outcome of 101 people seen for rehabilitation 5–12 years earlier. In J Fourez and N Page (Eds.), *Treatment issues and long-term outcomes: Proceedings of the 18th Annual Brain Impairment Conference* (Hobart, Australia, 1994) (pp. 1–6). Bowen Hills, Queensland: Australian Academic Press.

Wilson, B. A. (1995c). Management and remediation of memory problems in brain-injured adults. In A. D. Baddeley, B. A. Wilson, & F. N. Watts (Eds.), *Handbook of memory disorders* (pp. 451–479). Chichester: John Wiley.

Wilson, B. A. (1995d). Memory rehabilitation: Compensating for memory problems. In R. A. Dixon and L. Bäckman (Eds.), *Compensating for psychological deficits and declines: Managing losses and promoting gains* (pp. 171–190). Mahwah, N.J.: Lawrence Erlbaum Associates.

Wilson, B. A. (1995e). Recent developments in neuropsychological rehabilitation. *Clinical Psychology Forum, 85,* 11–13.

Wilson, B. A. (1996). Cognitive functioning of adult survivors of cerebral hypoxia. *Brain Injury, 10,* 863–874.

Wilson, B. A. (1997a). Cognitive rehabilitation: How it is and how it might be. *Journal of the International Neuropsychological Society, 3,* 487–496.

Wilson, B. A. (1997b). Management of acquired cognitive disorders. In B. A. Wilson and D. L. McLellan (Eds.), *Rehabilitation studies handbook* (pp. 243–261). Cambridge: Cambridge University Press.

Wilson, B. A. (1997c). Research and evaluation in rehabilitation. In B. A. Wilson and D. L. McLellan (Eds.), *Rehabilitation studies handbook* (pp. 161–187). Cambridge: Cambridge University Press.

Wilson, B. A. (1997d). Semantic memory impairments following non-progressive brain damage: A study of four cases. *Brain Injury, 11,* 259–269.

Wilson, B. A., Baddeley, A. D., Evans, J. J. & Shiel, A. (1994). Errorless learning in the rehabilitation of memory impaired people. *Neuropsychological Rehabilitation, 4,* 307–326.

Wilson, B. A., Baddeley, A. D. & Kapur, N. (1995). Dense amnesia in a professional musician following herpes simplex virus encephalitis. *Journal of Clinical and Experimental Psychology, 17,* 668–681.

Wilson, B. A., Baddeley, A. D., Shiel, A. & Patton, G. (1992). How does post traumatic amnesia differ from the amnesic syndrome and from chronic memory impairment? *Neuropsychological Rehabilitation, 2,* 231–243.

Wilson, B. A., Clare, L., Young, A. & Hodges, J. (1997). Knowing where and knowing what: A double dissociation. *Cortex, 33,* 529–541.

Wilson, B. A. & Cockburn, J. (1988). The Prices Test: A simple test of retrograde amnesia. In M. Gruneberg, R. Morris & R. Sykes (Eds.), *Practical aspects of memory: Current research and issues, vol. 2* (pp. 46–51). Chichester: John Wiley & Sons.

Wilson, B. A. & Cockburn, J. (1997). A seven- to fourteen-year follow-up study of adults with very severe intellectual impairment following a neurological insult. *Journal of Rehabilitation Outcomes Measurement, 1,* 60–66.

Wilson, B. A., Cockburn, J. & Baddeley, A. D. (1985). *The Rivermead Behavioural Memory Test.* Bury St. Edmunds: Thames Valley Test Company.

Wilson, B. A., Cockburn, J. & Halligan, P. (1987). The development of a behavioural test of visuospatial neglect. *Archives of Physical Medicine and Rehabilitation, 68,* 98–102.

Wilson, B. A., Cockburn, J. & Halligan, P. W. (1988). *The Behavioural Inattention Test.* Bury St Edmunds: Thames Valley Test Company.

Wilson, B. A. & Davidoff, J. (1993). Partial recovery from visual object agnosia: A 10 year follow-up study. *Cortex, 29,* 529–542.

Wilson, B. A. & Evans, J. J. (1996). Error free learning in the rehabilitation of individuals with memory impairments. *Journal of Head Trauma Rehabilitation, 11,* 54–64.

Wilson, B. A., Evans, J. J., Bremner, S., Brentnall, S., Keohane, C. & Williams, H. (in press). The Oliver Zangwill Centre for Neuropsychological Rehabilitation: A partnership between healthcare and rehabilitation research. To appear in A-L. Christensen & B. Uzzell (Eds.). *Neuropsychological rehabilitation.* New York: Plenum Publishing Company.

Wilson, B. A., Evans, J. J., Emslie, H. & Malinek, V. (1997). Evaluation of NeuroPage: A new memory aid. *Journal of Neurology, Neurosurgery, and Psychiatry, 63,* 113–115.

Wilson, B. A. & Moffat, N. (1984). Running a memory group. In B. A. Wilson & N. Moffat (Eds.), *Clinical management of memory problems.* London: Croom Helm.

Wilson, B. A. & Moffat, N. (Eds.) (1984). *Clinical management of memory problems.* London: Croom Helm.

Wilson, B. A. & Patterson, K. E. (1990). Rehabilitation and cognitive neuropsychology: Does cognitive psychology apply? *Journal of Applied Cognitive Psychology, 4,* 247–260.

Wilson, B. A. & Powell, G. E. (1994). Neurological problems: treatment and rehabilitation. In S. J. E. Lindsay & G. E. Powell (Eds.), *The handbook of clinical adult psychology, Second edition* (pp. 688–701). London: Routledge.

Wilson, B. A., Shiel, A., Watson, M., Horn, S. & McLellan, D. L. (1994). Monitoring behaviour during coma and post traumatic amnesia. In A.-L. Christensen & B. Uzzell (Eds.), *Progress in the rehabilitation of brain-injured people* (pp. 85–98). Hillsdale: Lawrence Erlbaum Associates.

Wilson, B. A. & Watson, P. C. (1996). A practical framework for understanding compensatory behaviour in people with organic memory impairment. *Memory, 4,* 465–486.

Wilson, B. A. & Wearing, D. (1995). Prisoner of consciousness: A state of just awakening following Herpes Simplex Encephalitis. In R. Campbell & M. Conway (Eds.), *Broken memories* (pp. 14–30). Oxford: Blackwell.

Wilson, J. T. L. (1993). Visual short-term memory. In F. J. Stachowiak, R. De Bleser, G. Deloche, R. Kaschel, H. Kremin, P. North, L. Pizzamiglio, I. Robertson, & B. A.

Wilson, (Eds.), *Developments in the assessment and rehabilitation of brain-damaged patients: Perspectives from a European Concerted Action* (pp. 107–110). Tübingen: Gunter Narr Verlag.

Wolpert, I. (1924). Die simultanagnosie: Storung der Gesamtauffassung. *Zeitschrift fur die gesante Neurologie and Psychiatrie, 93,* 397–415.

Wood, R. Ll. (1984). Behaviour disorders following severe brain injury: Their presentation and psychological management. In D. N. Brooks (Ed.) *Closed head injury: Social, psychological and family consequences.* Oxford: Oxford University Press.

Wood, R. Ll. (1988). Management of behaviour disorders in a day treatment setting. *Journal of Head Trauma Rehabilitation, 3,* 53–62.

Woodward, J. B. III, Heaton, R. K., Simon, D. B. & Ringel, S. P. (1982). Neuropsychological findings in myotonic dystrophy. *Journal of Clinical Neuropsychology, 4,* 335–342.

Yates, F. A. (1966). *The art of memory.* London: Routledge & Kegan Paul.

Yule, W. & Carr, J. (Eds.) (1987). *Behaviour modification for people with mental handicaps.* London: Croom Helm.

Zangwill, O. L. (1947). Psychological aspects of rehabilitation in cases of brain injury. *British Journal of Psychology, 37,* 60–69.

Zangwill, O. L. (1977). The amnesic syndrome. In C. W. M. Whitty and O. L. Zangwill (Eds.), *Amnesia* (pp. 104–117). London: Butterworths.

Zigmond, A. S. & Snaith, R. P. (1983). The Hospital Anxiety and Depression Scale. *Acta Psychiatrica Scandinavica, 67,* 361–370.

Zihl, J. (1995). Visual scanning behaviour in patients with homonymous hemianopia. *Neuropsychologia, 33,* 287–303.

INDEX